Atlas of the
HUMAN BRAIN

Atlas of the

HUMAN BRAIN

JÜRGEN K. MAI

Department of Neuroanatomy
Heinrich–Heine University of Düsseldorf
4001 Düsseldorf, Germany

JOSEPH ASSHEUER

Institute for Magnetic Resonance Imaging
Cologne, Germany

GEORGE PAXINOS

School of Psychology
The University of New South Wales
Sydney 2052, Australia

ACADEMIC PRESS

Harcourt Brace & Company

San Diego   London   Boston   New York   Sydney   Tokyo   Toronto

This book is printed on acid-free paper.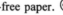

Copyright © 1997 by ACADEMIC PRESS

Academic Press
a division of Harcourt Brace & Company
525 B Street, Suite 1900, San Diego, California 92101-4495, USA
http://www.apnet.com

Academic Press Limited
24-28 Oval Road, London NW1 7DX, UK
http://www.hbuk.co.uk/ap/

Library of Congress Cataloging-in-Publication Data

Mai, Jürgen K.
    Atlas of the human brain / by Jürgen K. Mai, Joseph Assheuer,
  George Paxinos.
          p.   cm.
    Includes bibliographical references and index.
    ISBN 0-12-465360-X (case : alk. paper). -- ISBN 0-12-465361-8
  (pbk. : alk. paper)
    1. Brain--Anatomy--Atlases.   2. Neuroanatomy--Atlases.
  I. Assheuer, Joseph   II. Paxinos, George, date.   III. Title.
    [DNLM: 1. Brain--atlases.   WL 17 M217a 1997]
  QM455.M347   1997
  611'.81--dc21
  DNLM/DLC
  for Library of Congress   97-10171
                                                   CIP

PRINTED IN THE UNITED STATES OF AMERICA
97   98   99   00   01   02   NE   9   8   7   6   5   4   3   2

Contents

Preface

The great neuroanatomists of the first part of this century determined the structural plan of the brain by investigating post mortem tissue with classic staining methods. Recent imaging techniques (especially magnetic resonance imaging, MRI) make it possible to view the structure of the living brain. The ability to anneal the structural plan with imaging data would enhance our understanding of the relationship between structure and function. The primary aim of this book is to transfer the information from the classical studies to the cross-sectional brain *in situ* and juxtapose this information with MR images obtained from the same brain, thus taking advantage of this wealth of detailed information to increase the resolution of imaging modalities. An additional aim is to provide a myeloarchitectonic atlas of coronal sections with detail sufficient to satisfy the needs of those using sensitive immunohistochemical and autoradiographic methods.

The present book consists of a series of maps, each featuring (different aspects of) brain morphology and topography. The surface anatomy of each brain is presented in the Talairach (coordinate) space together with the exact location of the sections. This correlation with the Talairach atlas is important because this atlas is becoming the standard with regard to stereotaxic space. The reader can advance from the surface view of the gyri and sulci to the section level.

PART 1
TOPOGRAPHIC AND
TOPOMETRIC ATLAS

Part 1 consists of serial macroscopic sections of MRI-scanned human heads. First the surface anatomy of the brain is presented together with a topometric grid; in addition, the locations of the sections are indicated thereon. Second, *in situ* sections of the entire head, with delineations not in excessive detail but with emphasis on the brain, are shown. The *in situ* sections guarantee that no significant deformation of the brain occurred and allow correlation to bony landmarks and blood vessels. They are placed over a stereotaxic grid that gives a real image of the same brain and the user sees not only the gross morphology but also the identifying labels of the structure.

Therefore, on all these plates, only relevant features are labeled extensively. This presentation of macroscopic sections forms a unique set of a numerous sections combining the following features:

1. The sections are cut at regular intervals in all planes of section. The regularity and comprehensiveness of the sets of sections place our book above those from other publications.

2. Because the sections are thick (1 cm), both sides of every section are shown. The reverse sides present additional information and the viewer can thus follow any structure through the sequence of sections.

3. Every section includes radiologic images (X-ray from the same head and MR images with different weighting from a healthy volunteer) showing the same plane of section. Structures seen in the skull/brain sections can be correlated with those clearly visible in MR tomography. The MR images are of low magnification and therefore cannot compete with the images in modern dedicated MR tomography books. However, it is rare that detailed gyral and nuclear anatomy and histology of sections accompany these images. The "typical" MR images obtained *in vivo* can also be compared with the *in vitro* images. For those who are interested, correlations between *in vivo* and *in vitro* parameters are included. To our knowledge the combination of the above features is unique in the literature and renders this part of our book attractive to all those interested in the relationship between human brain structure and its surroundings.

A. Horizontal sections of the brain in the head: Full presentations of 11 sections depict those parts of the head having direct relationships with the brain. The continuing sections (levels below the base of the skull/axis) are not of significance in an understanding of brain topography, yet these sections will be of interest to students of anatomy and radiology; therefore these levels through the skull (showing the topography of the blood vessels, nerves, and ganglia related to the brain) are presented only as diagrams and are not accompanied by photographs through the biological tissue. Delineation of the brain, and especially the cortex, is depicted *in situ* (once as seen within the section, and once in addition on its own, so that the surface anatomy can be seen and compared with the surface drawings of the brain).

B. Coronal sections (−20° angulation): This head was sectioned such that the plane of section is parallel to the brainstem axis; thus, this plane corresponds to the major ascending and descending fiber tracts. For this reason radiological analysis often is based on this plane.

C. Sagittal sections: This plane of sectioning shows most clearly the external landmarks of the brain. It is, however, rarely used in human neuroanatomy and therefore only sections representing one hemisphere are depicted.

PART 2
MYELOARCHITECTONIC ATLAS

Part 2 consists of 69 photographs of myelin-stained coronal sections placed opposite to the corresponding schematic diagrams. The brain in these photographs was cut perpendicular to the intercommissural line (the line connecting the anterior and the posterior commissure). The plates depict mainly subcortical structures; the inclusion of the entire hemisphere in the photographs would have reduced the resolution of the depicted elements to an unacceptable level. The accompanying diagrams are of the same size and define the position, extent, and relationship of nuclei and pathways of the forebrain and mesencephalon.

This atlas is unique for the following reasons:

1. It provides the most comprehensive delineations available. It was derived by the authors after consideration not only of the material presented but also of the serial sections between the represented levels (which will be made available on electronic media).

2. It is based on many experimental studies using comparably prepared, serially sectioned brains and thus features major, recent conceptual advances in the organization of the brain. Preliminary versions of these line drawings have already been used in several published articles dealing with the structural and histochemical organization of the brain. Their suitability for the mapping of neurotransmitters, neuropeptides, receptors, and functional data has thus been tested.

3. The tissue sections have been meticulously studied over the past years; this brain served as a reference brain and was evaluated by preeminent neuroanatomists such as the Vogts, Brockhaus, Hassler, Wahren, Hopf, and Sanides. Indeed, multiple architectonic and morphometric studies published in the past contain data from this particular brain. A list of references (related to publications referring to this brain) is included so that dedicated neuroscientists can gain an in-depth understanding of the basis of our delineation.

Although a person outside this field may consider it a handicap to use old tissue stained by the Vogts, any scientist in the field will agree that this is a significant asset.

4. A set of 36 figures (4 pages of figures) of reduced cortical gyrification and subcortical detail is included for use as templates by researchers who prefer a more probabilistic approach to cerebral localization.

Reproduction of Figures by Users of the Atlas

Reproduction of any part of this book is subject to the usual restrictions of copyright. However, we can assure researchers that the publisher will attend promptly to any written request to reproduce the figures in the atlas. Please identify the figures you wish to use and allow approximately 4 weeks for your request to be processed. Please contact the publisher at the following address:

ACADEMIC PRESS
Permissions Department
6277 Sea Harbor Drive
Orlando, Florida 32887
Telephone: 407-345-3994
Fax: 407-345-4058

The authors request that users of the atlas send them reprints of publications (to the address of J.K. Mai) in which the atlas was used and which can shed light on the organization of regions.

Acknowledgments

The authors were fortunate to receive assistance from a number of collegues. We are particularly grateful to L. Lanta, who assisted in the description of the macroscopic sections, prepared the corresponding line drawings, and delineated the vasculatory territories of brain arteries; to H. Lange, who made invaluable contributions to the macroscopic and microscopic delineation of cortical areas; and to T. Longerich and T. Sievert for making available their studies on the *in vivo/ in vitro* correlation in magnetic resonance imaging. Significant improvements in this atlas were due to the expert help of C. Hartz-Schütt, A. Walter, S. Morres, and F. Forutan, especially in the delineation of forebrain structures. The brilliant work of T. Voß and J. Bongartz in converting the atlas data into electronic files is highly appreciated.

Our special thanks go to those persons who by their last will provided their bodies for educational and research purposes (in anatomy). We are grateful to H. Goslar and H. Hartwig for supporting the goals of this study and for allowing the use of such cadavers. We are indebted to R. Wedemeier for preparation and fixation and for his assistance during sectioning of the cadaver heads. E. Tödter donated the macrotome and designed and constructed the cryosectioning and photographing devices. This and his endless help, together with the invaluable assistance of E. Baseler and P. Sillmann, were crucial to mastering technical problems during the preparation of the first part of the atlas. All photographs of frozen sections and all histological and histochemical procedures were performed with superb skill by S. Lensing-Höhn and V. Holler. Photographs of the archival section material used in this atlas were prepared with masterful excellence by A. Fahnenstich and Hong-Qin Wang.

This long endeavor was made possible not only by the initiative, continued interest, and help of many persons but also by their patience during our preoccupation with this work. We thank H.-J. Freund in Düsseldorf, P. Mattmann in Zürich, and J. Reed and S. Krajewski in La Jolla, among many others. We especially thank J. Huston, who helped navigate the project through the critical phases.

We owe special thanks to A. Hopf, former head of the C. and O. Vogt Institute and Department of Neuroanatomy and manager of the C. and O. Vogt Gesellschaft für Hirnforschung. He continuously supported this project and together with K. Zilles made possible the use of the archival material. We greatly appreciate the financial support for this project, which was provided by the C. and O. Vogt Society for Brain Research.

Finally we are indebted to Academic Press for allowing us to use expected royalties to develop this atlas.

1 INTRODUCTION

1.1 Cerebral (Functional) Localization

The term "cerebral localization" refers to the concept that different parts of the brain contribute differently to bodily functions and behavior and mental processes and its corollary, that dysfunction of localized brain areas is correlated with typical forms of diseases. The concept of cerebral localization (which does not exclude dynamic or plastic interactions) is based on a long history of philosophical projection, clinical observation, and experimental examination. Scientific evaluation of the significance of brain areas (in question) started around the end of the last century. It was founded on comparative studies, microscopic evaluation of architectonics of the brain, and physiological and psychological experiments and neurological observation. Histologists, physiologists, and clinicians worked together to resolve the problem of central representation of perception, emotionality, planning, thinking, and consciousness. By defining criteria for such functions, it became possible to ascribe even subtle aspects of functional deviations to proposed areas of cerebral lesioning. Determining the degree of disturbance of a function became a prerequisite for surgical intervention and rehabilitation procedures.

Imaging techniques, studies of gene expression, and improvements in clinical and psychological methods have extended our knowledge of physiological and psychological processes and accordingly provided excellent tools for clinical diagnostics and for therapeutic and preventional procedures.

1.2 The Problem of Interindividual Variability

Modern imaging techniques provide excellent macroscopic resolution in a short time. When the image data are present in metric 3-D coordinates, they can be integrated into a computerized reference brain atlas. However, it is an absolute requirement that interindividual differences be constrained.

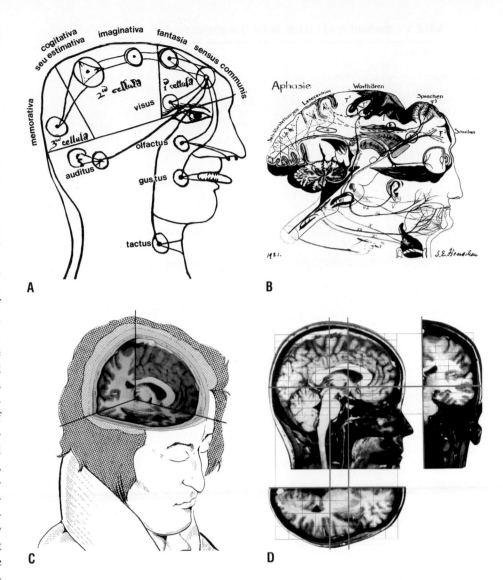

FIGURE 1 (**A**) In antiquity and middle ages, the soul, as well as the perception and motoric performances, were speculatively localized in the ventricles of the brain. Percepts produced by sense organs (sensus communis: tactus, gustus, olfactus, auditus, visus) were transferred to the lateral ventricles of the brain (first cellule) where they were thought to be integrated with imagination (imaginary power, "fantasia"). The resulting images were projected (translocated) to the second cellule where they were impacted on motivation and rational thinking. This integration resulted in the planning and execution of action. Items not passed over to planning and actions were relegated to memory. (Modified from Avicenna.) (**B**) Until the 19th century the most conspicuous and (in terms of function and according to current appreciation) most important part of the human brain, the pallium, remained neglected (unregarded). Its importance and relation to higher cognitive function was at least speculatively recognized by F. J. Gall. He thought of the brain as a complex mosaic of mental organs, each of which comprising (containing) mental faculties which were anatomically localized within the cortex. Influenced by his teachings and the clinical findings of P. Broca, the search for brain structures as "carriers" for brain function was intensified. Those examinations were in most instances based on observations of changes in neural structure within the autopsy brain after focal brain injury. With the advent of those examinations, the inclusion of subcortical structures and the peripheral fiber tracts became more and more important (Henschen, 1922). (**C**) Following a period of nonempirical thinking and of scientifically oriented examinations of autopsied brains, modern imaging techniques enabled a nondestructive view into the (living) brain. In order to successfully navigate within the brain space and its highly complex structure, applicable rules for orientation were required. Cartographic reference points were provided by external and internal landmarks. During this time, the anterior and posterior commissures (AC, PC) were most commonly used as internal landmarks. They provided the basis for 2-dimensional coordinate nets superimposed on tomographic images which could then be extended to achieve segmentation of 3-D imaging values. In this figure an orthogonal reference is centered (X, Y, Z: 0) on the AC. The axes are defined as follows: Z, by the line through the centers of both commissures (intercommissural line, ICL); Y, by the vertical line through the AC and oriented in the symmetrical axis; X, by the horizontal line through the AC. (**D**) Three-dimensional grid system obtained by such manipulation, represents a series of static (metric or proportional nets) overlaid onto a dynamic and individual brain structure. The accuracy of date integration (adjusting individual and model brains) is therefore inherently limited. This restriction is taken into account by new approaches in which the large interindividual variability of the brain is appreciated.

TABLE 1   Variability of Linear Brain Dimensions

(A) MRI Brains

	F-AC	AC-PC	PC-O	L	CR-IC	IC-CA	H	W
MEAN	75.3	25.8	75.3	75.5	41.6	117.2	66.4	
n	26	13	26	26	26	26	26	
SD	3.3	2.2	3.6	6.8	4.2	2.4	4.7	2.3
MAX	73	29	86	185	81	45	123	70
MIN	62	21	70	160	58	37	108	62
Range	11	8	16	25	13	8	15	8

(B) Autopsy Brains

	F-AC	AC-PC	PC-O	L	CR-IC	IC-CA	H	W
MEAN	65.4	24.8	76.1	166.6	63.7	34.9	98.6	65.8
n	25	17	25	25	25	25	25	25
SD	4.0	1.9	4.5	7.9	5.3	3.8	5.8	3.8
MAX	74	28	82	179	72	43	106	76
MIN	59	22	67	149	55	28	85	59
Range	15	6	15	30	17	15	21	17

(C) Talairach et al.

	F-AC	AC-PC	PC-O	L	CR-IC	IC-CA	H	W
MEAN	70	25	76	171	78	43	121	68

(**A**) MR images were made from 26 hemispheres of healthy volunteers (Mai *et al.*, 1992). (**B**) Determination in autopsy brains were made on 1:1 photographs of brains from the Vogt Collection in Düsseldorf (modified from Sievert, 1992). (**C**) List of the corresponding measures derived from a group of several hundred patients reported by Talairach *et al.* (1967) and Talairach and Tourmoux (1988). The differences in the mean dimensions between the autopsy brains and the patient brains apparently corresponds to the volume deficit induced during fixation and post mortem morphological alterations. (Abbreviations: AC-PC, anterior to posterior commissure; CR-IC, crown to intercommissural plane; F-AC, frontal pole to anterior commissure; H, brain height; IC-CA, intercommissural plane to base of brain; LE, brain length; PC-O, posterior commissure to occipital pole; W, width of one hemisphere.)

1.2.1 The Degree of Variation of Brain Structures and Dimensions

It is well known that both the surface morphology of the brain and the linear dimensions show great variation. In Table 1 we show values derived from our studies compared with results from Talairach and co-workers (1967, 1988).

These values underline the high degree of interindividual variability and the influence of the conditions (*in vivo* brains, postmortem brains *in situ* and fixed autopsy brains) under which such determinations are made. The variation among the brains becomes even more impressive when surface contours around brain nuclei are plotted with respect to comparable planes of sectioning. Under these conditions, correspondingly small areas of overlap are observed (Delmas and Pertuiset, 1959; Paul, 1965; van Buren and Borke, 1972; Schaltenbrand and Wahren, 1977; Sievert, 1992). This situation holds true regardless of whether such comparisons are based on MR images or on histological sections (Sievert, 1991; Mai *et al.*, 1992). Sections (obtained from either MRI or anatomy) from different brains cannot therefore be compared directly but must be manipulated by transformation algorithms.

1.2.2 Compensation of Interindividual Variability by Standardization/Transformation Procedures

The degree of intersubject variability in

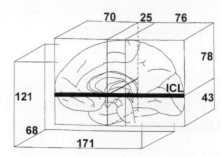

FIGURE 3 Graphic presentation of the Talairach standard proportional grid system. The cerebral space is defined by orthogonal horizontal, sagittal, and verticofrontal reference planes. The distances between the reference planes are defined as follows: Horizontal planes, intercommissural plane (ICL) through the upper limit of the anterior (AC) and lower limit of the posterior commissures (PC), parallel planes through the highest and lowest points of the hemisphere. Sagittal planes, median-sagittal plane and parallel planes through the lateralmost points of the hemispheres. Verticofrontal planes, through the center of the AC (VAC), through the center of the PC (VPC), through the frontal and occipital poles. The fronto-occipital extent between the VAP and the VCP is defined in all hemispheres as 2.5 cm.

brain structure demands that interindividual differences must be compensated for by application of a transformation mode. When searching for a suitable transformation system (Assheuer *et al.*, 1990) one must consider that when a linear transformation is chosen, the stretching factors for the three dimensions in a brain must be different (van Buren *et al.*, 1972; Sievert, 1992). Further, the transformation not only must be based on the outline dimensions of a brain (the pial-CSF interface) but also must include reference points inside the brain.

These reference points must be clearly visualized in clinical imaging (MRI) and must have a constant position in relation to the rest of the brain structures *in vivo* as well as *in vitro* (i.e., histologic sections). After construction of the model brain, this reference and transformation system must meet the need to be dynamically fitted to the individual patient's images. This means that the reference and transformation model must be universally valid intraindividually for the course of histological preparation, intraindividually for sequential patient imaging, and interindividually for a collective of autopsy brains and the corresponding histological material. Last but not least, the system and its contents (histological data) must be stored in a computer for use in computer-aided imaging with

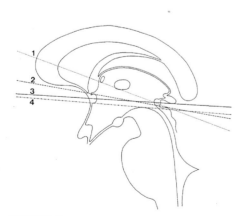

FIGURE 2 Some orientation points and reference lines proposed for application in stereotaxic surgery. 1, Hassler and Riechert (1954); 2, Talairach *et al.* (1952); 3, Schaltenbrand and Bailey (1954); 4, Delmas and Pertuiset (1959). From Assheuer *et al.* (1990).

TABLE 2 Dimensions of the Thalamus as Determined *In Vivo* (MRI) and *In Vitro* (Fixed Brain)

A. MRI without Transformation

	frontal	occipital	cranial	caudal	medial	lateral
MEAN	+35	+35.4	+19.7	-29	0	21.0
n	26	26	26	26	26	26
SD	1.7	3.9	1.5	1.3	0	2.5
MAX	+6	+43	+22	-5	0	26
MIN	0	+31	+17	-1	0	17
Range	6	12	5	4	0	9

B. MRI with Transformation

	frontal	occipital	cranial	caudal	medial	lateral
MEAN	+3.4	+34.7	+20.3	-3.0	0	21.5
n	26	26	26	26	26	26
SD	1.7	4.5	1.3	1.3	0	2.3
MAX	+6	+42.7	+22.3	-5.2	0	26.4
MIN	0	+28	+18.3	-1.1	0	18.5
Range	6	14.7	4	4.2	0	7.9

C. Sectioned Material without Transformation

	frontal	occipital	cranial	caudal	medial	lateral
MEAN	+4.4	+33.8	+16.7	-3.5	1.1	26.9
n	25	25	25	25	25	25
SD	1.7	3.0	2.3	1.8	0.8	2.5
MAX	+8	+41	+20	-6	3	31
MIN	+2	+29	+13	0	0	23
Range	6	12	7	6	3	8

D. Sectioned Material without Transformation

	frontal	occipital	cranial	caudal	medial	lateral
MEAN	+4.3	+33.7	+20.5	-4.4	1.2	28.1
n	25	25	25	25	25	25
SD	1.6	1.7	2.8	2.3	0.9	2.0
MAX	+7	+37	+25	-8	3	32
MIN	+2	+31	+15	0	0	24
Range	5	6	10	8	3	8

Values indicate the maximal extensions of the thalamus in the three dimensions. (**A, B**) Estimates of thalamic dimensions in MRT brains. (**A**) Statistics of thalamus outlines without transformation (coordinates [mm] in gridmodel). (**B**) Statistics of thalamus outlines with transformation (coordinates [mm] in gridmodel). (**C, D**) Estimates of thalamic dimensions in serially sectioned material. (**C**) Thalamus outlines calculated without transformation (coordinates [mm] in gridmodel). (**D**) Statistics of thalamus outlines with transformation (coordinates [mm] in gridmodel).

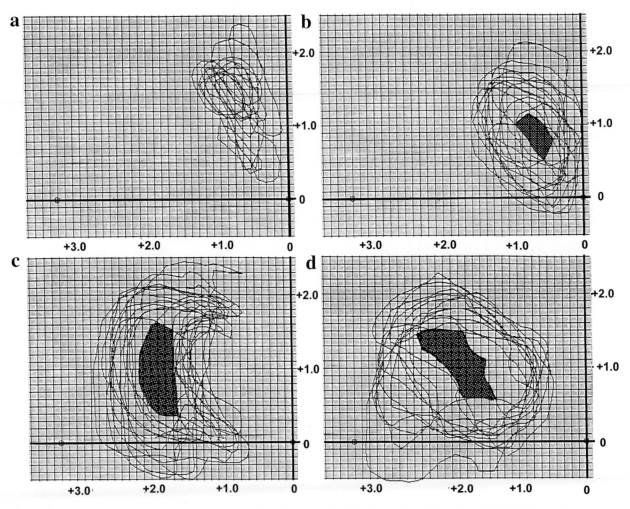

FIGURE 4 Interindividual comparison based on the outlines of individual and normalized thalamic nuclei. Interindividual curve groups were created separately for the anterior (**a**), mediodorsal (**b**), ventral thalamic nuclei (**c**) and pulvinar (**d**) in each plane. The curves of a group show the outlines of a subnucleus in the same standard plane of all evaluated individuals. These curve groups demonstrate the extent of the interindividual variability of the cross-sectional area in the standard grid. (Modified from Sievert, 1992, and Sievert *et al.*, 1989.)

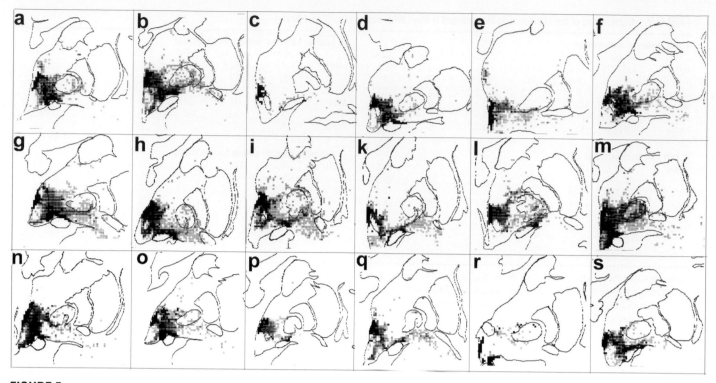

FIGURE 5 Distribution of ratings of neurophysin-positive cells and processes at the level of the anterior commissure. Note the variation of brain morphology as evidenced in myelin-stained paraffin sections (from which the delineations derived) as well as the variation of the immunohistochemical profiles (shaded squares). (Modified from Mai *et al.,* 1993.)

quick access to the data.

In the past, numerous models for localization have been developed, mostly as aids in stereotaxic surgery, X-ray evaluations, and tomographic imaging (see Assheuer *et al.,* 1990; Maziotta *et al.,* 1995; Toga *et al.,* 1996). Most commonly, equaling positions were used as landmarks and proportional linear transformations were performed (Talairach *et al.,* 1967, 1988). At present, the most

common reference systems are founded on the intercommissural line (ICL), connecting the anterior and posterior commissures (Figs. 2 and 3). This reference line, together with the symmetric plane, serves as a basis for orthogonal planes that define the space of any individual brain.

In a modification of the Talairach grid system, the center of the anterior commissure in the median plane is used

as zero point, and all dimensions are given as metric coordinates (Schaltenbrand and Wahren, 1977; Mai *et al.,* 1992; Fig. 3).

This modification appears helpful if interindividual comparisons of the discriminated (and outlined) structures (including size and position) are made, if additional reference points or trajectories are implemented in the analysis program, and if nonlinear transformation is applied.

During the preparation of this atlas we applied linear transformation in the Talairach space (see Section 2.2.8) because of its versatility and general applicability. With regard to precision, however, it is trivial that the adaptation of the coordinates of brain structures from the individual into a standardized grid system by application of linear transformation routines does not override the problem of individual variation. This fact, well known in the literature, is also stressed in our own studies, where we have evaluated the positional (topometric) accuracy of the individual versus the standardized grid system by comparing the degree of overlap of thalamic substructures (Table 2; Fig. 4). Two data sets, one from fixed (*in vitro*) brains, the other from MR images (*in vivo* brains), were tested. In these studies the outlines of the anterior, me-

TABLE 3 Methodologic Approaches toward a Human Reference Brain

Approaches	Disadvantages	Advantages
IN-VIVO BRAIN		
MRI	limited resolution, limited tissue characterization, comparatively large section thickness	large numbers of brains can be studied, non-invasive, biological and dynamic criteria, short acquisition time, high tissue contrast, 3D reconstruction routines available
IN-VITRO (AUTOPSY) BRAIN		
NON-EMBEDDED BRAIN Gross morphology MRT Serial (Frozen) sections	pre-end postmortem changes, freezing artifacts, expenses, immediate processing necessary	MRT, extraction of detailed morphological and histochemical parameters, tissue shrinkage negligible
EMBEDDED BRAIN Serial (Paraffin) sections	pre-end postmortem changes, preparatory (embedding and sectioning) artifacts	MRT of the autopsy brain possible before embedding, high number of serial sections, processing time is not limited
VIRTUAL (CALCULATED) BRAIN		
PROBABILISTIC ATLAS ATLAS BASED ON HOMOLOGY DEVELOPMENTAL ATLAS	?	?

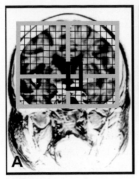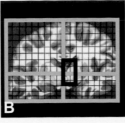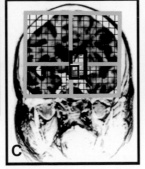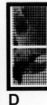

FIGURE 6 Concept for combining diagnostic imaging (**A**) and histoanatomical data (**B**) into a common data set (**C, D**). The MR image (**A**) is superimposed onto a corresponding histological image (**B**). The hypothalamic region of the merged image is shown in (**D**) within the diencephalon (black boxed area).

diodorsal, ventral thalamic nuclei, and pulvinar of the thalamus were determined on paraffin sections of 25 formalin-fixed hemispheres (Sievert, 1992) and also on MR images of 26 hemispheres of healthy individuals. As shown, the data from both of these studies resulted in very poor fitting of the contours of individual thalamic nuclei. Similar discouraging results became evident when the location and distribution of immunohistochemically labeled cells and profiles or areas of equidense substance P concentration were compared (Mai *et al.*, 1993; Proll, 1990; Fig. 5).

1.3 The Human Brain Reference Atlas

A reference atlas must take into account the interindividual variability and thus allow compensation by transformation routines. At this time, the most common procedure is that proportional or metric nets derived from a "reference" data set are fitted to the tomograms of the individual brain. The establishment of such a reference brain can be derived from different approaches (Table 3).

As noted in Table 3, tissue specificity and resolution obtained by current imaging techniques are not high enough to provide detailed information about tissue composition and organization. Therefore, it is necessary to supplement such image data with those from the microscopic examination of brain sections. Correlation of diagnostic imaging and histoanatomical findings then allows identification and circumscription of those functional areas, which either lie below the resolution of the imaging techniques (MRI, CT) or cannot be differentiated on the basis of contrast levels.

This correlation can be performed by overlaying the imagery with representative histochemical information of a reference brain, transformed to the individual dimensions of the patient brain (Fig. 6).

1.3.1 Histological Approach toward a Standardized Human Brain Atlas

Light microscopic analysis of histological and (immuno-) histochemical human brain sections provides detailed and specific information of normal and disease-affected structures. Correlation of the *in vitro* data with *in vivo* imaging would thus provide a much more detailed understanding of brain function. To use such data in clinical applications, histological and biochemical characteristics of a given tissue compartment should be made available during clinical routine imaging. This would allow maximum correlation between structure and function, especially in interpretation of lesions. The amount of correlation could be tested by physiological means.

1.3.2 Frozen vs. Paraffin Sections

Given that the high resolution provided by histological examination of sections is desired, two approaches to data collection are generally favored: Collection from frozen tissue or from autopsy brains embedded in wax, most commonly paraffin. The frozen sectioning technique, particularly of whole cadaver heads, avoids multiple disadvantages and artifacts that are inevitable when the brain is taken out of the skull and embedded (Talairach *et al.*, 1988). The embedding technique provides consistent series of thin, durable histological sec-

tions with excellent morphology.

Moreover, most histochemical techniques can be performed even after long storage times.

In both methodologies the correlation between data extracted from histological sections and those obtained from gross anatomy *in vivo* is limited by two groups of parameters: First, the events influencing brain morphology prior to fixation (by chemicals or by freezing) of the brain; second, all preparatory (procedural) steps from the initiation of fixation to inspection of the stained sections.

Post mortem (autolytic) changes in brain morphology and alterations during preparation of the autopsy brain. Even when still inside the skull (post mortem delay), the (unfixed) autopsy brain is altered (van Buren and Borke, 1972; Schaltenbrand and Wahren, 1977), leading to inconstant changes. Even the use of *in situ* fixation does not overcome this problem, as this method leads to initial swelling of the brain with a flattening of the surface of the hemispheres (Andrew and Watkins, 1969; Van Buren and Borke, 1972; Schaltenbrand and Wahren, 1977). Considering the findings of Mark and Yakovlev (1955), Brierley and Beck (1959) concluded that the inconstant post mortem artifacts, for example, due to the collapse of vessels and ventricles, cannot be eliminated by *in situ* fixation. Additional morphological alterations are inevitable following the mechanical forces when the brain is taken out of the skull.

A. Morphological Changes Due to Fixation: The next step leading to structural deviation is the fixation itself. Freezing induces initial swelling, with the degree dependent on the technique used. If the brain is frozen *in situ*, this often results in severe displacement of brain substance.

Additionally, the preservation of (particularly cortical) brain matter is inferior to that obtained after embedding in paraffin. Formalin fixation, on the other hand, causes a gradual, slight decrease in volume (shrinkage) after a short phase of initial swelling (see Longerich, 1989). Differences in the extent of shrinkage are related to formalin concentration, salt additives, and duration and temperature of fixation (Vogt 1940; Spiegel *et al.*, 1952; Brierley and Beck, 1959; Delmas and Pertuiset, 1959; van Buren and Maccubin, 1962;

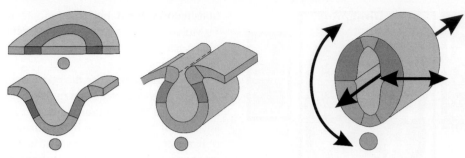

FIGURE 7 (**A**) Dorsal view of the trilaminar embryonic disc showing differentaition of the ectodermal layer into somatic and neural components (neural plate) and fate map of the presumptive location of various parts of the nervous system. (**B**) A fluid-filled neural tube separates from the neural plate that can be described to have a longitudinal, a circumferential (tangential), and a radial dimension (Nowakowski, 1987). In the longitudinal dimension, three major swellings (from which the forebrain, midbrain, and hindbrain arise) can be identified in the rostral half of the tube. In the circumferential (or tangential) dimension, four identified zones, or "plates," form in each side of the plane symmetry: the floor, the paired lateral, and the roof plates. These are related to the functional organization in sensory and motor subdivisions. The radial dimension is related to the proliferaition and translocation of cells. Along this dimension, the wall of the neural tube develops nuclei and laminae that are distinct for each subdivision.

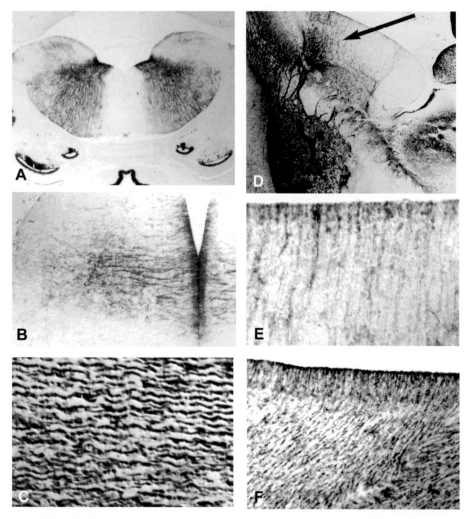

FIGURE 8 Photographs of immunohistochemically stained (CD15) sections from a mouse embryo (embryonal day 14, **A–C**) and from a human fetus (23 weeks of gestation, **D–F**). (**A**) Mouse hindbrain demonstrating the direct relationship between segments of the ventricular and pial surface. (**B**) Segment of radial glial fibers in a cross section through the prosencephalon. (**C**) Precise alignment of radial glial fibers in the tegmentum. (**D**) Location of radial glial cells in the human lateral ganglionic eminence with positive processes (arrow) extending towards the striatum. At the time of nuclear differentiation, the relationship between ventricular surface on the one hand, and nuclei and cortex on the other hand, is registered by the trajectories of radial glial fibers. (**E, F**) Higher magnification of radial glial cells and processes in the ganglionic eminence and subventricular zone, stressing the precise alignment of the processes (from Mai *et al.,* 1995; Mai and Lensing-Höhn, 1995).

Talairach and Szikla, 1967; Andrew and Watkins, 1969; Seligson and Nashold, 1969; van Buren and Borke, 1972; Schaltenbrand and Wahren, 1977; Hitchcock *et al.,* 1984). Estimates of the degree of shrinkage of the human brain are around 5% linear shrinkage or a maximum of 14% volume shrinkage (van Buren and Maccubin, 1962; van Buren and Borke, 1972; Andrew and Watkins, 1969; Fox *et al.* 1985).

B. Morphological Changes Due to Paraffin Embedding of Macrotomic Blocks and Sectioning and Staining of the Histological Sections: When the brain is taken out of the skull, morphological alterations occur, as during autopsy, separation of the hemispheres, and the macrotome-sectioning of the hemispheres to blocks. Pressure is exerted along the sectioning direction, which leads to a flattening in this direction, especially of structures exposed on the surface.

When the linear dimensions of the fixed brain and of mounted sections are compared, the freezing technique causes only negligible artificial shrinkage of less than 5% (Schaltenbrand and Wahren, 1977; Willis and Grossman, 1977).

Using paraffin results (together with the deparaffination) in a linear shrinkage of 30% in each direction, 20% celloidin and 5% wax. The amount of shrinkage during dehydration of the macrotome blocks and their embedding depends on the embedding technique (Schaltenbrand and Wahren, 1977). Andrew and Watkins (1969) found a linear shrinkage of 7% (20% volume shrinkage) for paraffin embedding. Some authors have additionally calculated the effect of microtomic sectioning. Van Buren and Borke (1972) used celloidin embedding and found linear shrinkage of 20% along the direction of sectioning, 16% and 21% respectively for the other directions, equaling 47% volume shrinkage. Fox *et al.* (1985) found 20% linear shrinkage for paraffin-embedded material (volume reduction nearly 50%). Finally, the sections are mechanically distorted by the process of fitting them to a glass surface (for example, by smoothing and brushing). The classical staining techniques available for frozen and paraffin-embedded material are both roughly the same; the mounting and staining procedures, however, affect the frozen sections much more than the paraffin sections.

This is because the adherence of some brain parts is poor and parts of the frozen section can therefore float away; additionally, the sections may be tracted, distorted, or sheered.

In summary, despite swelling during freezing, the processed sections show almost *in vivo* dimensions (Schaltenbrand and Wahren, 1977). This advantage is outweighed by the multiple artifacts, mostly related to distortions of brain substance.

Quantification of the corresponding influences seems to be nearly impossible, and using this technique for the development of a reference brain is therefore limited. The use of formalin-fixed, paraffin-embedded autopsy brains results in a (nonlinear) shrinkage of approximately 50% and thus adds severe inevitable artifacts caused during fixation, embedding, sectioning, and mounting of the brain sections. Nevertheless, although paraffin sections do not represent the exact stereological position of a structure in the brain (*in situ*), the relative positions of brain structures are always preserved, so that a direct correlation between histomorphology in the section examined and the *in situ* situation can in principle be calculated. In addition, information about human brain structure has been gained in the past mainly by examination of microscopic sections of formalin-fixed and paraffin-embedded autopsy brains. Therefore, a huge number of studies are based on this technique.

For this atlas we have applied frozen sectioning as well as the paraffin-embedding technique (see Section 2, Material and Methods). The disadvantages of the former technique, including difficulties in consistently fitting consecutive hemispheric sections on one hand, and anticipation that application of available computer technology will enable reformatting of histological sections to *in vivo* conditions, on the other hand, have led us to favor the histological approach based on embedded material. At present, this technology offers the best preconditions for combining a detailed stereological description of the structural and histochemical architecture (topistics) with a standardized spatial reference system (topometry). The particular brain that we have selected (Section 4) offers the additional advantage that detailed and valuable information (qualitative and morphometric studies) already exists.

1.4 Future Directions

1.4.1 Application of the Transformation Mode to Brain Structures

It is desirable that the atlas plates do not serve only as templates for comparison of structures identified either by their structural properties (here the myeloarchitecture) or by their relationship to identifiable landmarks in two dimensions. Therefore, the 3-D organization of the major structures presented in this atlas has been evaluated. These reconstructions help in the interpretation of material available in different planes of sectioning. Transformation of image data presented in this way to the material under study will be accomplished by interactive routines. As this material is not yet available, we have included in this atlas a series of sections that are transformed to the dimensions of the Talairach space (Talairach and Tournoux, 1988). It might be possible to combine the data of our myeloarchitectonic histological atlas with those of a probabilistic MRI atlas comprising data sets from homogeneous populations of individuals (Mazziotta *et al.,* 1995).

1.4.2 Nonlinear Transformation Based on Structural Homology and Developmental Parameters

Going further, whether comparison of adult brains is the appropriate approach to interpreting the evidently complex and individually different structures of the human brain might, in principle, be questioned. This complexity of brain structure poses an almost impenetrable obstacle to the analysis of brain organization and to understanding its function. The cortex in particular poses great difficulties, because the gyri are often tortuous and concealed within cortical sulci. The disclosure of similarities of cortical organization in different species has opened the possibility of defining cerebral structures in experimental species and describing homologous structures in the human brain (Carman *et al.,* 1995). It is anticipated that new modalities that will make it unnecessary to analyze the convolution in much detail will emerge.

Moreover, the fields of developmental and molecular biology are describing rules that are principally similar in all higher species. Basic design principles (perhaps even the "fundamental plan") of the vertebrate system may eventually emerge by considering the major components before they undergo their own, more or less, elaborate pattern of differentiation. This may in turn yield more effective ways to represent the components of the adult nervous system.

Because the brain acquires its complex configuration out of a very simple basic structure by way of consecutive morphogenetic events, analysis of the early stages of development makes the interpretation much more lucid. At the beginning of development, the prospective nervous system takes the shape of an essentially flat, elliptical sheet of ectodermal cells. Development then progresses through the formation of a (neural) tube and the eventual differentiation into brain and spinal cord (see Swanson, 1992). It is possible to relate the major subdivisions, including nuclear structures, of the developed brain and spinal cord to the presumptive location of the primordial cell groups in the neural plate and tube by tracing the trajectories of migrating neurons toward their location at later stages of development. These trajectories can help in establishing a virtual atlas. This involves the construction of a ventricular map and the establishment of (radial) trajectories to only single landmarks, which are more easily defined than the complex structures.

1.5 References

Andrew, J., and Watkins, E. S. *A Stereotaxic Atlas of the Human Thalamus and Adjacent Structures.* The Williams & Wilkins Co., Baltimore (1969).

Assheuer, J., Lanta, L., Longerich, U. J. J., Sievert, T., and Mai, J.K. Standardisierung der cerebralen Bilddarstellung in der Magnetresonanztomographie (MRT). *RöFo,* **153,** 296-302 (1990).

Assheuer, J., Longerich, U., and Mai, J. K. Correlations of relaxation curves under in vivo and in vitro conditions. *2nd European Congress of NMR in Medicine and Biology,* Berlin (1988).

Brierley, J. B., and Beck, E. The significance in human stereotactic brain surgery of individual variation in the diencephalon and globus pallidus. *J. Neurol. Neurosurg. Psychiat.* **22,** 287-298 (1959).

Carman, G. J., Drury, H. A., and Van Essen, D. C. Computational methods for reconstructing and unfolding the cerebral cortex. *Cereb. Cortex.* **5,** 506-517 (1995).

Delmas, A., and Pertuiset, B. *La Topometrie Cranio-Encephalique chez l'Homme.* Masson & Cie, Paris; C.L. Thomas, Springfield, Ill. (1959).

Fox, C. H., Johnson, F. B., Whiting, J., and Roller, P. P. Formaldehyde fixation. *J. Histochem. Cytochem.* **33,** 845-853 (1985).

Henschen, S. E. Klinische und anatomische Beitrige zur Pathologie des Gehirns. Teil VII: In *Über motorische Aphasie und Agraphie,* (pp. 1-319). Selbstverlag, Stockholm (1922).

Hitchcock, E., and Cadavid, J. Third ventricular width and thalamo-capsular laterality. *Acta Neurochir., Suppl. 33,* 547-551 (1984).

Lanta, L. *Topometrie cerebraler Läsionen: Anwendung des Proportionalitätsgrids nach Talairach" zur Präzisierung der Struktur-Funktionszuordnung.* Thesis, Medical Faculty, Düsseldorf (1989).

Longerich, U. *MRI-Untersuchungen an in vivo und in vitro Gehirngewebe: Einfluß von Fixierung und Temperatur auf das Relaxationsverhalten, die Protonendichte und das Kontrast-verhalten.* Thesis, Medical Faculty, Düsseldorf (1989).

Longerich, U., Sievert, T., and Mai, J. K. *Topometric and topistic analysis of the human brain. I. Development of a model brain using MRI-Imaging.* Neurobiologisches Colloquium, Nancy (1989).

Longerich, U., Mai, J. K., and Assheuer, J. Einfluß der Formalinfixierung auf die Kontrastierung der Magnetresonanztomographie Sequenzen. *Verh. Anat. Ges.* Ulm (1989).

Mai, J. K., Voß, T. A., Assheuer, J., Lanta, L., Sievert, T., Teckhaus, L. A histological approach towards a human brain reference atlas for computer assisted imaging techniques. *Abstr. Soc. Neurosci.* **22,** 408-417 (1992).

Mai, J. K., Berger, K., and Sofroniew, M. V. Morphometric evaluation of neurophysin-immunoreactivity in the human brain: Pronounced interindividual variability and evidence for altered staining patterns in schizophrenia. *J. Hirnforsch.,* **34,** 133-154 (1993).

Mai, J. K., Andressen, C., Lensing-Höhn, S., Kazimierek, M., Voß, T., and Müller, G. CD15 positive radial glial fibers define prosomeric boundaries the mouse developing forebrain. *Eur. J. Neurosc.,* **90** (1995).

Mai, J. K., and Lensing-Höhn, S. Compartmental expression patterns of the CD15 epitope and of the epidermal growth factor receptor (EGFr) within the ganglionic eminence. *Soc. Neurosci.,* Abstr. 21, Vol.1. p. 800 (320.9), 1995.

Mark, V. H., and Yakovlev, P. I. A note on problems and methods in preparation of a human stereotaxic atlas. Including a report of measurements of the posteromedial portion of the ventral nucleus of the thalamus. *Anat. Rec.* 745-752 (1955).

Mazziotta, J. C., Toga, A. W., Evans, A., Fox, P., and Lancaster, J. A probabilistic atlas of the human brain: Theory and rationale for its development. *Neuroimage* **2,** 89-101 (1995).

Nowakowski, R. S. Basic concepts of CNS development. *Child Dev.* **58,** 568-595 (1987).

Paul, W. *Der thalamische Ventrooralkern im Kommissurensystem.* Thesis, Würzburg, 1965.

Proll, E. *Semiquantitative Untersuchung zur Verteilung der Substanz P-Immunreaktivät im Vorderhirn des Menschen: Ein Vergleich zwischen Gehirnen schizophren Erkrankter und einer Kontrollgruppe.* Thesis, Medical Faculty, Düsseldorf (1990).

Schaltenbrand, G., and Wahren, W. *Guide to the Atlas for Stereotaxy of the Human Brain.* Thieme Publ., Stuttgart (1977).

Seligson, D., and Nashold, B. S. Changes in the size and shape of the lateral ventricles with formalin fixation. *Confin. Neurol.* **31,** 209-218 (1969).

Sievert, T. *Topometrie des menschlichen Gehirns: Evaluation eines Verfahrens zur Integration morphologisch-funktioneller Daten aus histologischen Schnitten in die klinische Diagnostik.* Thesis, Medical Faculty, Düsseldorf (1992).

Sievert, T., Longerich, U. J. J., and Mai, J. K. Topometric and topistic analysis of the human brain. 2. Topometric evaluation of histologic brain sections. *Neurobiologisches Colloquium,* Nancy, (1989).

Spiegel, E. A., Wycis, H. T., and Baird, H. W.: Studies in stereoencephalotomy -I. Topical relationship of subcortical structures to the posterior commissure. *Confin. Neurol., 12,* 121-134 (1952).

Swanson, L. W. *Structure of the Rat Brain.* Elsevier, Amsterdam, London, New York, Tokyo (1992).

Talairach, J., and Szikla, G. *Atlas d'Anatomie stereotaxique du Telencephale.* Masson & Cie, Paris (1967).

Talairach, J., and Tournoux, P. *Co-planar stereotaxic atlas of the Human Brain.* G. Thieme, Stuttgart/New York (1988).

Toga, A. W., Thompson, P., and Payne, B. A. Modeling morphometric changes of the brain during development. In: *Developmental Neuroimaging. Mapping the Development of Brain and Behavior.* (Thatcher, R. W., Lyon, G. R., Rumsey, L. J., and Krasnegor, N., eds.) Academic Press, San Diego, 1996.

van Buren, J. M., and Maccubin, D. A. An outline atlas of human basal ganglia. *J. Neurosurg., 19,* 811-839 (1962).

van Buren, J. M., and Borke, R. C. *Variations and Connections of the Human Thalamus.* Springer Verlag, Berlin, Heidelberg, New York (1972).

Vogt, O. Über nationale Hirnforschungsinstitute. *J. Psychol. Neurol.* **50,** 1-10 (1940).

2 MATERIALS AND METHODS

2.1 Topographic and Topometric Atlas

2.1.1 Anatomical Preparations

The 17 heads used for this study were from bodies donated to the Department of Anatomy, H.-Heine University of Düsseldorf. The studies were performed in accordance with established ethical and human standards. The cadavers were perfused via the radial veins first with physiological saline and then with fixative. The composition of the fixative changed as the study progressed. The three heads presented in this atlas were perfused with a fixative containing 10% formalin, glycerol, and Incidin (Henkel, Düsseldorf). The heads were removed from the perfused cadavers within 36 hours after death and were placed in a wooden box with ear bars and head holders to allow exact positioning and fixing for subsequent sectioning; in this way the coordinates of the position box and the desired plane of anatomic sectioning were exactly aligned. The heads were covered with linen and fixative to prevent the preparation from drying out between performance of the MR imaging and the freezing process.

2.1.2 Magnetic Resonance Imaging (MRI)

Pilot MRI Scans: Pilot MRI scans were performed with the heads in the wooden position boxes to determine the effect of fixation and to detect pathological or artifactual changes. Of the 17 heads used for this part of the study, 4 showed severe neuropathological alterations, such as hemorrhage, focal lesions, or tumor, which were not known before the MRI was performed (see Assheuer *et al.,* 1987). Five heads were excluded for technical reasons: artifacts due to incomplete fixation, brain swelling, or insufficient image resolution (MR imaging started in 1984). Additionally, 2 heads were later discarded from this study because of problems with the sawing machine.

MR Scan Orientations: All heads were scanned in the horizontal, coronal, sagittal, and oblique coronal planes according to a standardizing protocol (Assheuer *et al.,* 1990). The corresponding section planes were defined (a) by the intercommissural line and their verticals, and (b) by the vertical to the brain stem axis (Meynert's plane). For defining additional planes, we used the cantho-meatal line and the orbital axis.

MR System and Scan Modes: For *in vitro* imaging and *in vivo/in vitro* correlation, scans and measurements were performed on a 0.15-Tesla superconductive magnet (Vista 2035, Picker International). For *in vitro* imaging we used a multislice double-echo sequence (spin-echo sequence (SE) 5000/40/160) with four excitations to render proton (N(H))- and T_2-weighted images. The slice thickness was 5 mm with a matrix of 256×256 and a field of view of 250 mm, resulting in a pixel size of 0.96 mm^2 and a voxel size of 4.8 mm^3. These scans are presented in the pages preceding the atlas figures of the horizontal, coronal, and sagittal sections (Sections 3.1, 3.2 and 3.3, respectively).

For *in vivo/in vitro* correlation, we used a single-slice technique with SE and inversion recovery (IR) sequences with the following parameters: SE (TR: 200, 800, 1600, 3200, 6400 ms combined with TE 30, 40, 60, 80, 120, 160 ms) and IR (TR 620, 1240, 2480 ms combined with TI 32, 100, 150, 200, 300, 400, 500, 600, 700 ms). The slice thickness was 5 mm with a matrix of 256×256 and a field of view of 250 mm.

For *in vivo* imaging we used a 1.0-Tesla superconductive magnet (Vista 2055 HPQ, Picker International) using (a) multislice, double-echo sequence, SE 3000/20/100, resulting in proton- and T_2-weighted images; (b) multislice sequence, IR 5000/600, resulting in T_1-weighted images; and (c) multislice partial saturation (PS) sequence, PS 500/10, resulting in T_1-weighted images with partial fat suppression. The slice thickness was 5 mm with a matrix of 256×256 and a field of view of 250 mm. These images are presented in Sections 3.1 to 3.3 facing each macroscopic anatomical section.

2.1.3 MR Images: *In Vivo/In Vitro* Correlation

In autopsy brains, relaxation times, signal-to-noise ratio, and contrast are altered due to the absence of flow effect, cessation of metabolism, and fixation procedures. To perform comparison analysis between living and postmortem tissue, parameters that influence signal intensity were measured under both *in vivo* and *in vitro* conditions.

For such a correlation, the heads of two volunteers and of two cadaver heads were scanned. The parameters of the IR and SE sequences and corresponding images of one image plane are shown in Fig. 1.

Examples of regression curves of *in vivo/in vitro* measurements of signal intensities are shown in Figs. 2 and 3. T_1 (spin-lattice) relaxation, T_2 (spin-spin) relaxation, and N(H) (proton density) of the *in vivo/in vitro* tissues are represented in Fig. 4.

Compared with the *in vivo* results, the *in vitro* tissues show large, nonlinear reduction in T_1 relaxation times and N(H) values, small (negligible) changes in T_2 relaxation times, and increased contrast (in IR images highly dependent on extrinsic parameters, TI, TR). A stable correlation between the variations seen under *in vitro* conditions and the *in vivo* relaxation curves exists.

The different gray-scale values determined from the same *in vivo* and *in vitro* structures can be explained by biophysical alterations in the different fractions of water ("three-fraction model," Grösch and Noack, 1976) by temperature, formalin fixation, additives to the fixative solution, and duration of tissue fixation (see Longerich, 1989).

These results show that the MR images of formalin-fixed cadaver heads not only are helpful in correlating *in vitro* tissues to the *in vivo* situation by means of structural gradients and contrast, but also can be used for image interpretation on a quantitative basis. Estimation of the signal changes after formalin fixation may thereby aid characterization of human brain tissue by MRI before it is laminated and neuropathologically evaluated. Moreover, the addition of paramagnetic substances or shift reagents to the perfu-

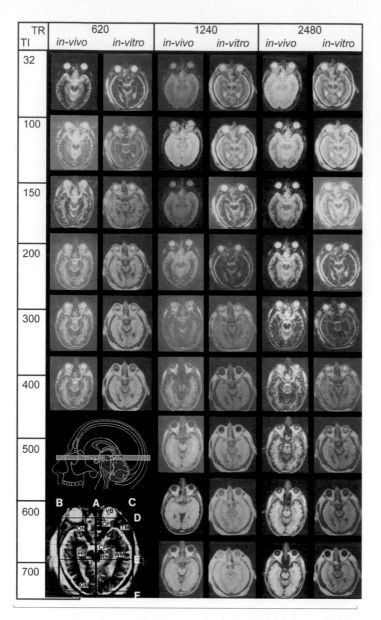

FIGURE 1 Sequence parameters used for in vivo/in vitro correlation. Measurements shown were taken from a 25-year-old volunteer (*in vivo*) and from a cadaver (*in vitro*). (**A**) TR (repetition time) and TI (spin-lattice relaxation) times for IR sequences. (**B**) TR and TE (spin-spin relaxation) times for SE-sequences. MR images obtained under *in vivo* and *in vitro* conditions exhibit striking differences. Upper inset shows the plane of sectioning. The lower inset shows every scan overlaid with a grid (**A–F**) to secure precise location of the same regions of interest throughout the series. (Abbreviations: CP, cerebral peduncle; GM, gray substance; Hi, hippocampus; Li, cerebrospinal fluid; OF, orbital fat; ON, optic nerve; RN, red nucleus; TM, temporalis muscle; VB, vitreous body; WM, white matter.)

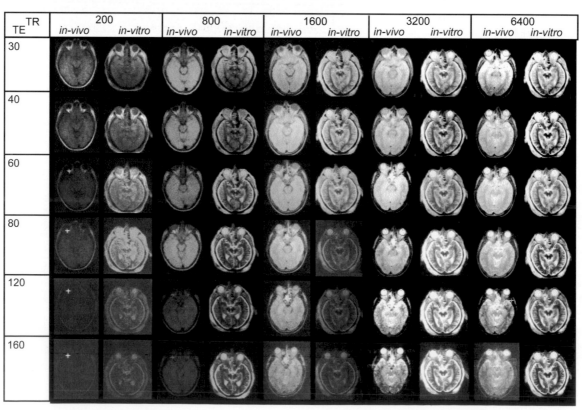

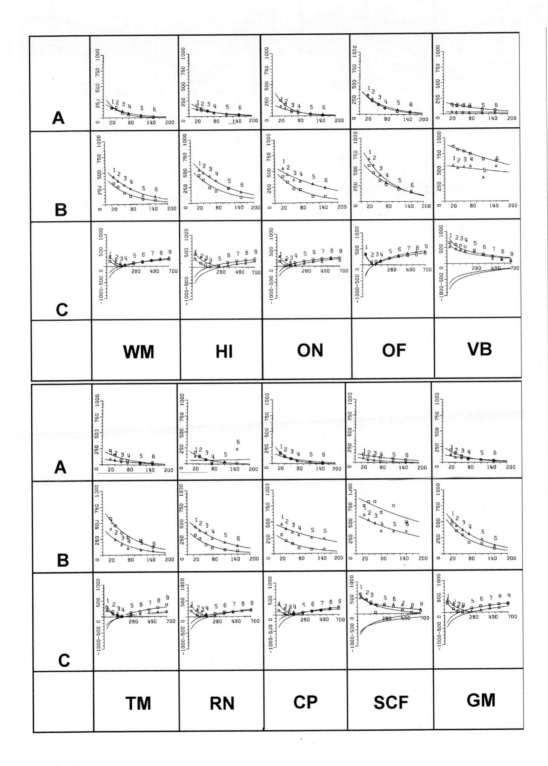

FIGURE 2 Regression curves of *in vivo* (open triangles) and *in vitro* (open squares) signal intensity measurements from 10 different tissues that show dependency of signal intensity (as gray values, *Y* axis) from TE (spinecho sequences, **A, B**) and TI (inversion recovery sequences, **C**) at constant TR (**A**: 200 ms; **B**: 5000 ms; **C**: 2500 ms). T_1 and T_2 relaxation times are calculated from these curves. Regions of interest: 1, white matter; 2, hippocampus; 3, optic nerve; 4, orbital fat; 5, vitreous body; 6, temporalis muscle; 7, red nucleus; 8, cerebral peduncle; 9, cerebrospinal fluid; 10, gray matter.

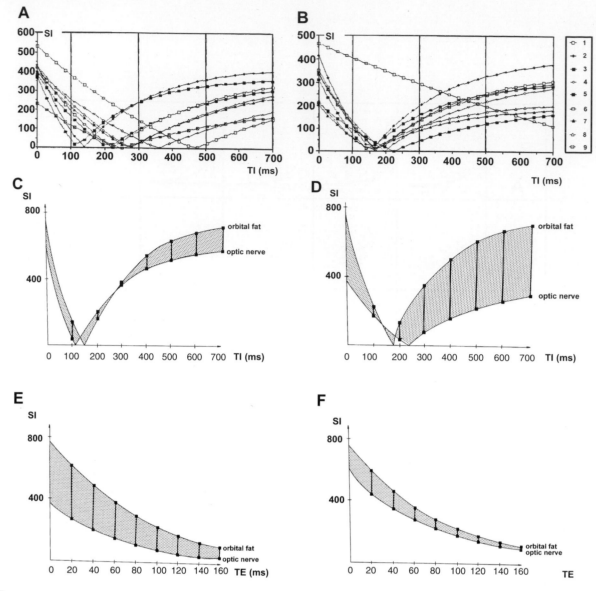

FIGURE 3 (**A, B**) Comparison between *in vivo* (**A**) and *in vitro* (**B**) signal intensity (SI) measurements using IR sequences with different TI (50–700 ms) at constant TR (500 ms) for the following tissues: 1, vitreous body; 2, orbital fat; 3, optic nerve; 4, hippocampus; 5, white matter; 6, gray substance; 7, cerebral peduncle; 8, red nucleus; 9, temporalis muscle. (**C–F**) Registration similar to (**A**) and (**B**) showing the ranges of signal intensities for tissues with short and long T_1 (**C, D**) and T_2 (**E, F**) relaxation under *in vivo* (**C, E**) and *in vitro* (**D, F**) conditions.

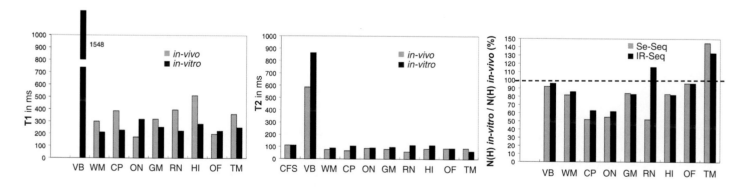

FIGURE 4 Comparison between *in vivo* and *in vitro* tissues (**A, B**) T_1 (spin-lattice relaxation, **A**) and T_2 (spin-spin relaxation, **B**) values (in ms) determined for the following regions of interest: VB, vitreous body; OF, orbital fat; ON, optic nerve; HI, hippocampus; WM, white matter; GM, gray matter; CP, cerebral peduncle; RN, red nucleus; TM, temporalis muscle; CSF, cerebrospinal fluid. (**C**) Relation between *in vitro* N(H) relative to *in vivo* N(H) (in %) for the regions of interest. (Abbreviations: IR-Seq., T_1 (spin-lattice relaxation); SE-Seq., T_2 (spin-spin relaxation).) Data from Longerich, 1989.

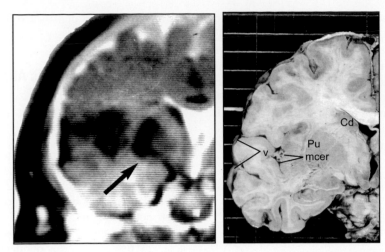

FIGURE 5 (**A**) Increase in signal intensity after addition of prussian blue into the perfusion medium. An increase in signal intensity is recognized in some blood vessels, but is particularly prominent in the stratium (arrow, unpublished results). (**B**) Corresponding anatomical section. (Abbreviations: Cd, caudate nucleus; mcer, middle cerebral artery; Pu, putamen; v, superficial vessels.)

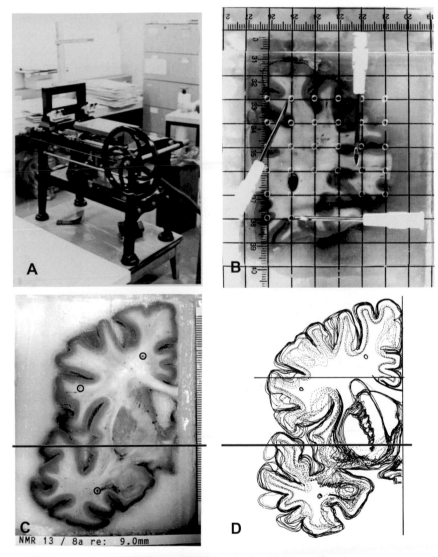

FIGURE 6 (**A**) Cyrosectioning device consisting of the Tetrander ("Pantomikrotom," see Vogt, 1905), freezing table, photograph stand, and tube holder for dry ice. (**B**) Frozen tissue block with matrix for perpendicluar orientation of canulas used for punch marking. (**C**) Fixed slice of the hemisphere (shown in Section 3.2) embedded in mythylcellulose and showing section surface with scales and punchmarks (fiducial marks used later for topographic adjustment of sections). (**D**) Drawings made from serial sections of one slice.

sion fluid can increase the regional contrast and demarcate areal boundaries that are not evident in regularly performed scans. Prussian blue, for example, has been found to increase the signal in basal ganglia structures, as shown in Fig. 5.

2.1.4 Macroscopic Anatomy and Correlations between Skull and Brain

Preparation and photography of 1-cm-thick anatomical sections: Immediately after the MR scans, the position box with the head fixed by plastic ear bars was filled with Styropore and water and then cooled to −45°C. Both the position box and the fixed head were sectioned at the desired plane at 1-cm thickness (cryomacrotomy). The head sections were then freed from the surrounding material, cleaned, and photographed together with rulers to indicate size. The thawed sections were preserved in modified Kaiserling's solution (Kaiserling, 1900).

Radiographs and visualization of blood vessels by radiopaque material: From the head slices, radiographs were prepared either from single sections or from stacks of multiple sections. Afterward, contrast media were injected into cut ends of larger blood vessels and the radiographs were repeated.

Staining: After photography and radiologic examination, the sections were block-stained in either sudan red or sudan black B. Sections were incubated in 1% stain solution in 70% alcohol and differentiated an average of 3 months (Romeis, 1968).

Dissection of anatomical slices and interpretation of cortical gyri: Before dissection of the head and neck structures, the brain slices were removed from the skull. The single brain sections were mounted according to their *in vivo* situation and photographs were then made to document the gyrification pattern. After the individual gyri and sulci were named, the brain was represented diagramatically, taking into account the loss of tissue due to the sawing process.

Documentation of gross morphological features: Drawings were based on enlarged photographs of the anatomical slices. Additional information revealed by the radiographs and during the process of dissection was later incorporated.

2.1.5 Preparation of 100-μm-Thick Frozen Histological Brain Sections

After removal from the skull case and photography of the assembled brain slices, the slices were immersed for 48 hours in a fixative containing 4% formalin and 30% sucrose. Each slice was then brought in a mold to a freezing table, 30 × 20 cm in size (Dipl. Ing. Tödter, Sandhausen, FRG). The mold, containing one single brain slice, was then filled with methylcellulose (dissolved in water and stained with various chromogens) and cooled to −20°C. Before sectioning, calibrated punch marks were made. Every section was photographed with a scale bar (Fig. 6).

The sections were then transferred into individual containers filled with phosphate-buffered saline (plus 30% sucrose). Mounting of the sections was aided by photographs taken from each section during the sectioning. For some brains all sections were mounted. Cells were stained with either toluidine blue or cresyl violet; myelinated fibers were demonstrated with hematoxylin (procedures of Weigert or of Spielmeyer) or with sudan black B (see Romeis, 1968).

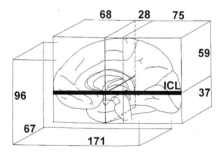

FIGURE 7 Diagram showing the midsagittal view of the right hemisphere (A58) in the Talairach space. The measurements shown were taken from 1 : 1 photographs of the formalin-fixed brain (compare with Fig. 3 in the Introduction).

Within each section the outlines of the area encompassing the basal ganglia together with the contours demarcating major nuclei were drawn onto a transparent sheet using a projection device with a magnification of ×6.5. By means of the punch marks, the singular sections were brought into register in a sequence from rostral to caudal.

2.1.6 Presentation of the Images

All anatomical head and brain slices (Sections 3.1 to 3.3) are mounted in the same way. Each series of sections begins with in vitro MR images of the head taken prior to sectioning. To provide a comprehensive view of the head, MR images are shown in all three orthogonal planes. This allows a better orientation in the three-dimensional space and aids in recognition of the topography of selected structures. Furthermore, comparisons between these *in vitro* images and the *in vivo* images presented next to the anatomical head and brain slices can be made. The following page presents two surface views of the brain, sectioned with the placement of sections indicated. The next page provides surface views of the brains showing their gross morphology together with the delineation of the most important gyri. Coloring on this page serves as a distinction between surface areas and differs from that applied in the sections. On drawings of the midsagittal views, the orthogonal reference planes, corresponding to the Talairach proportional grid system and defining the brain space, are included. Every brain structure can thus be adjusted to the defined spatial coordinate system. The main part of each topographic and topometric atlas presents anatomical head and brain slices. These are mounted to show every section from both sides. This allows the pursuit of any structure of interest throughout the series of sections. These representations are accompanied by four MR images of the corresponding plane and (normally) two images showing the real section, the radiograph of the real section, and/or the vasculatory territory within the brain section. MR images are performed from a healthy, 25-year-old volunteer. The MR images differ with respect to T_1, T_2, and proton density (N(H)) contrast.

2.2 Myeloarchitectonic Atlas (Histological Atlas)

2.2.1 Material

The histological reference brain (A58/right hemisphere) is based on the brain of a 24-year-old male (* 25.5.1905; + 7.11.1929). This brain belongs to the Vogt collection in Düsseldorf (brain weight at autopsy: 1383 g; fresh volume, 1316.3 cm³; cause of death, hypovolemic shock; death to fixation interval, 3 hours). The external morphology of the formalin-fixed brain was well documented (photographs of the convexity of the brain were published by Schulze, 1960). This brain was selected for presentation in this atlas because numerous researchers have analyzed and reported on its structures in the intervening decades (see Section 4.4).

2.2.2 Methods

Histological procedures: The brain was cut into blocks oriented vertically to the intercommissural plane and embedded in paraffin. The positions where these cuts were made in the right hemisphere are indicated in Fig. 1, page 268. The values of some linear measurements are given in Fig. 7.

Serial frontal sections of 20 μm were

TABLE 1
Reference of the Sections Used (R1 to R5 Refer to the Numbers of the Paraffin-Embedded Tissue Blocks)

1.	R1-902	19.	1476	37.	651	55.	501
2.	705	20.	1450	38.	599	56.	602
3.	501	21.	1425	39.	551	57.	700
4.	301	22.	1400	40.	504	58.	798
5.	102	23.	1352	41.	449	59.	901
6.	R2-1005	24.	1303	42.	406	60.	996
7.	901	25.	1251	43.	348	61.	1100
8.	800	26.	1204	44.	301	62.	1200
9.	700	27.	1151	45.	251	63.	1301
10.	601	28.	1102	46.	200	64.	1398
11.	499	29.	1050	47.	153	65.	R5-98
12.	407	30.	1006	48.	101	66.	298
13.	308	31.	949	49.	53	67.	499
14.	204	32.	902	50.	R4-103	68.	699
15.	103	33.	850	51.	151	69.	898
16.	49	34.	802	52.	200		
17.	R3-1555	35.	749	53.	301		
18.	1499	36.	701	54.	401		

prepared. Most were stained with either cresyl violet or hematoxylin. Some additional sections were stained according to the technique of Holzer or remained unstained. Some of these unstained sections were used for immunohistochemistry (e.g., substance P; see Mai *et al.*, 1986).

Estimates of volume changes: As outlined in the Introduction, volume changes in paraffin sections provide major obstacles in comparing these sections with the *in vivo* condition. Therefore, some efforts have been made to estimate tissue shrinkage and to transform the dimensions of this brain either to the approximate *in vivo* conditions or to the standard dimensions proposed by Talairach.

The volume changes due to formalin fixation could not be determined because the fresh volume was not known. Many researchers agree that the brain volume at an approximate fixation time of 3 to 4 weeks, the time when this brain was embedded, corresponds to the values determined at autopsy (see Longerich, 1989). It is therefore reasonable that the dimensions of the formalin-fixed brain (Fig. 7) represent the *in vivo* situation.

The volume deficit due to the histological preparation could be calculated. At the time this brain was processed, no effort was made to control the morphometric situation of the material during the procedure. A separate determination of the degree of shrinkage that occurred during dehydration, paraffin embedding, cutting and mounting of the sections (discussed in the Introduction) could thus not be made. The overall volumetric changes, however, could be calculated from differences in linear dimensions between the fixed, unembedded hemisphere (scaled photographs) and the serially sectioned hemisphere. Such calculations were made available by Lange and Thörner (1974) and by Sievert (1992) (see page 269).

2.2.3 Past Histological, Morphometric, and Immunohistochemical Studies

Numerous descriptive and quantitative studies were performed on sections from the brain presented in the myeloarchitectonic atlas. The relevant morphometric data (fresh volume, volume of serial sections, numeric cell density, volumetric cell density, absolute cell numbers) have been compiled and are listed together with the references in Section 4.4. Added to these data and the references is a set of drawings on which the most relevant of the original, published delineations were integrated (see Section 4.5). Delineations on these drawings are therefore not identical with those of the present atlas.

2.2.4 Nomenclature

It is difficult to incorporate the current spoken terminology into a logical hierarchical system. In the nomenclature now most commonly used (Paxinos and Watson, 1982; Paxinos and Huang, 1995), abbreviations often start with attributes (anterior, superficial, magnocellular, etc.) that are already specific or that might designate parcellations not in common use. To alleviate the problem, we have added a hierarchical tree on which the most important structures are diagrammatically, and sometimes arbitrarily, grouped. In some instances, synonyms have been added. In the Abbreviations sections, the latinized nomenclature is also provided.

2.2.5 Presentation of Images of the Paraffin-Embedded Brain (Myeloarchitectonic Atlas)

Photographs of hematoxylin stained sections and accompanying diagrams: The photographs and diagrams show the whole hemisphere at section levels where no relevant subcortical structures are recognized (magnification ×4.63). The main body of the photographs depicts subcortical structures (magnification ×7.9). The placement of each photograph and the relative position with respect to the Talairach space (see below) can be located on accompanying diagrams. The intersection of the midline with the approximate position of the inter-commissural line (*X/Y*: 0/0 coordinate) is the source of two scalings: The same grid underlies each section and is continued along the right and upper sides of the drawings. This grid gives the actual dimensions of each histological section.

Another scale, indicated by numbers (also along the right and upper sides of the drawings), presents the calculated dimensions of the fixed brain, taking into account tissue shrinkage. The position of each section along the anterior-posterior extension of the brain (*Z* axis) is shown diagrammatically and also as (actual and calculated) distance with respect to the center of the anterior commissure (point zero). The diagrams depict most structures and subdivisions that can be detected on the accompa-

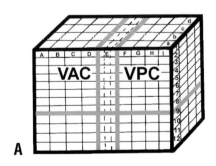 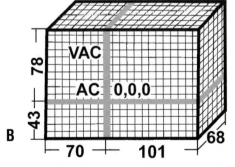

FIGURE 8 (**A**) Proportional grid system of Talairach *et al.* (1967, 1988). (**B**) Metrically defined grid system with standard dimensions. The topography of image data within the brain space is defined by (stereotaxic) coordinate points of *X*, *Y*, and *Z* coordinates. *X,Y,Z*-zero is located in the midpoint of the anterior commissure (AC). This grid model includes the advantage of (nonlinear) correlation of multiple image points because of metric scaling. (Abbreviations: AC-PC, distance between anterior and posterior commissure; F-AC, distance from frontal pole to the AC; ICL (intercommissural line), line defining the horizontal plane through the centers of the anterior and posterior commissures; L, lateralmost point of the parietotemporal cortex; ML (midline), interhemispheric saggital plane; O, posteriormostpoint of the occipital pole; T, lowest point of the temporal cortex; V, highest point of the parietal cortex; VCA, vertical through the AC; VCP, vertical through the PC.)

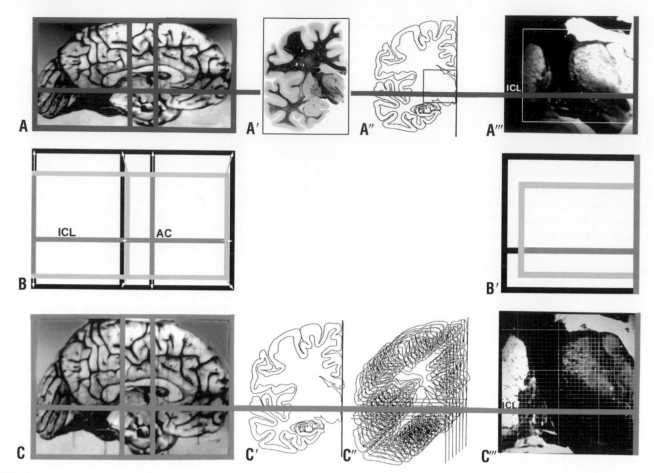

FIGURE 9 Standardization of the individual dimensions of the fixed brain and of the corresponding paraffin sections to the Talairach space. Left column: Standardization of the brain. (**A**) Photographs of each autopsy hemisphere overlaid with the individual orthogonal grid system (Talairach). The reference lines are the same as in the standard grid system. The metrical dimensions of the hemispheres were determined from the 1:1 scaled photographs of the median sagittal view (shown in **A**) and of the frontal view. (**B**) The individual orthogonal grid was then adjusted to the standard grid and the transformation factors for the anterior–posterior and the vertical dimension above and below the intercommissural line (IC) determined. The transformation factors for the mediolateral dimension (X coordinate) were derived from the 1:1 scaled photographs of the frontal view of the autopsy hemispheres. (**C**) Linear transformation into standard dimensions. For this step, the only point that was fixed was the center of the anterior commissure (**AC**). Remaining figures: Standardization of the paraffin sections. (**A′** to **A‴**) The position of each histological section is identified on the photographs showing the median sagittal view. This is provided by their serial number and their section thickness and in correspondence with the contours of sectioned structures. The median sagittal line was then positioned (symmetrical axis of the brain). The rectangular projections of the positions of the highest and lowest point on the section are marked on this median sagittal line. The relative position of the IC between these two points was then calculated from the corresponding relative position in the individual grid system at the position of the section. The IC was positioned at a right angle to the median sagittal line through this calculated point. The area encompassing the region of interest (ROI) was later delineated. (**B′**) Transformation of the individual dimensions of the ROI into standard dimensions. This step included the linear transformation parallel to the IC and parallel to the median sagittal line (x and y direction). The transformation factors were calculated from the transformation of the median and frontal views of the autopsy hemispheres to standard dimensions and the relative differences in height before and after dehydration and paraffin embedding of the macrotomic blocks (represented by the height of the actual histologic section and by the height of the hemisphere on the median photograph at the corresponding position). The degree of shrinkage of one block should be constant in all directions. The interindividual transformation factors differ from the vertical direction above the IC to the vertical direction below the IC and to the mediolateral direction. Therefore, each of these three factors must be multiplied by the constant paraffin shrinkage factor to obtain the correct transformation factors. (**C″**) Equal positions of the macroscopic and microscopic material, calculated from the Z coordinates of the standardized autopsy hemispheres and from the X and Y coordinates of the standardized histological sections, resulting in a metrically standardized three dimensional data set.

nying photograph; additionally, nuclear structures not evident on the photographs are represented. Because of the numerous cyto- and myeloarchitectonic studies that were previously performed on the represented brain (see p. 271) and the extent of available publications, the delineation of structures was problematic. As often as possible, we have used the original delineations provided by these earlier workers. In several instances we have changed original delineations, for example, when earlier interpretations were revised according to more recent immunohistochemical studies (thalamus, bed nucleus of the stria terminalis) or when the original drawings accentuated findings that were not typical either within the series or in different brains. Generally, the consistency of the drawings, section to section, was of higher importance than a precise correspondence between the photographs and the drawings.

To make it easier for the interested reader to correlate both sets of information, we have listed the section numbers presented in this atlas (Table 1). Since the Vogts and co-workers also regularly provide brain and section numbers, it is easy to compare the present delineations to those of earlier workers. Additionally, we have added drawings on which their most relevant delineations are included (pages 272–273).

2.2.6 Three-Dimensional Reconstructions

A series of 240 sequential sections through the region of the brain encompassing the basal ganglia was selected for 3-D analysis. In all of these sections the pial and ventricular surface contours, delineations of nuclei and their subdivisions (striatum, amygdala, basal nuclear complex, and thalamus), and some circumscribed fiber tracts (optic tract, anterior commissure) of one hemisphere were drawn. These drawings were necessary to align the sections according to the orthogonal coordinates of the brain, because no fiducial marks were made before sectioning. The "contour lines" defining pial and ventricular surfaces, as well as the borderlines around distinguished grisea ("iso lines"; see Mai *et al.,* 1984), were fitted with the neighboring sections. This process was repeated throughout the center of the brain. In structures selected for 3-D reconstruction the contour and iso lines were smoothed and the *X/Y* coordinates were used for the 3-D graphical representation according to the procedure described by Teckhaus *et al.* (1979). Reconstructions are not included in the printed version of the atlas.

2.2.7 Application of a Reference System (Topometry)

As stated earlier (Section 2.2.5.), every section—and thus every brain structure—was adjusted to a defined spatial coordinate system. Our atlas uses the reference system of Talairach *et al.* (1967, 1988), with the minor modification that the intercommissural line, ICL, passes through the centers of the anterior and posterior commissures.

However, with the advent of computer-aided image analysis and transformation routines, we find it advantageous not to apply proportional scaling, as proposed by Talairach, but to define the grid system metrically with standard dimensions (Sievert, 1992). In this model brain, space is defined metrically (cm,mm) with the point zero (= point 0/0/0) for all three dimensions in the center of the anterior commissure. The morphologic data of the hemispheres thus are handled as coordinate points in this 3-dimensional (metric)

grid as *X* (mediolateral), *Y* (vertical), and *Z* coordinates (fronto-occipital) (Fig. 8B). Scaling of the photographs and accompanying diagrams is therefore in metric coordinates.

2.2.8 Standardization

In application of a reference brain ("Model-Brain"), shrinkage artifacts and interindividual variability are the foremost variables that must be considered. To compensate for these influences, we used linear transformation routines. Both hemispheres were transformed to standard metric dimensions such that the space between the reference planes was defined metrically with point zero in the center of the AC.

Correction for shrinkage artifacts was based on correlating 1:1 scaled photographs of the fixed brain with the histologic sections (Sievert, 1992.) The degree of shrinkage was determined separately for each of the 12 partial volumes of the Talairach system. Transformation of the histological sections according to the shrinkage calculated for any of these volumes allowed fitting of the histological sections with the dimensions of the autopsy brain. We have not included such figures in this atlas because of the loss of resolution in reformatted images. Since the major obstacle in comparing brain morphology is not the problem of shrinkage but that of interindividual variability, we have directly transformed our image data into the Talairach dimensions.

Transformation of image data into the Talairach space (standard dimensions) was based on the 1:1 scaled photographs of the fixed brain (Fig. 9A). In this reformatted brain space the position and the expansion of every (histological) section had to be calculated. As in the procedure for determining shrinkage induced by paraffin embedding and sectioning, new (*X, Y, Z*) coordinates were calculated and fitted to the dimensions of the "standardized" hemispheres. (The *X* and *Y* coordinates for the mediolateral and vertical positions were derived from transformed histological sections. *Z* coordinates for the fronto-occipital positions were taken from standardized photographs of the autopsy brains.) The "standardized" histological sections were supplied

with a standard metric overlay (1-mm × 1-mm coordinates).

Standardized three-dimensional data set: The results of all these transformations were photographs of the fixed hemispheres and pictures of histological sections standardized to the same metric scale (dimensions). Equal positions in the macroscopic and microscopic material could be calculated. On pages 274–280 we present a series of simplified drawings from a standardized data set. In this way the scale of the histological sections can be directly correlated with *in vivo* sections.

Transformation of histological image data: The most important goal of our approach was the application and correlation of highly detailed architectonic images (histological sections) to a less detailed imagery from various kinds of tomograms. It became clear that sections (obtained from either MRI or anatomy) from different brains can (due to the high degree of interindividual variability) rarely be compared directly and must therefore be transformed. Another transformation procedure is necessary to compensate the artifacts induced by histological processing. In our opinion, the problems that derive from the high degree of variability between different brains are more severe than those engendered by paraffin embedding (Mai *et al.,* 1992).

If a model brain is developed, it will most likely be applied to the interpretation of MR images derived from singular brains. In our opinion, the ingredients of a model brain must derive from the thorough analysis of the distribution patterns of a single brain. This can be accomplished by various means of data transformation, relying on internal landmarks. Correlation between histomorphologic data and MRI seems to be feasible by the three-dimensional reconstruction of microscopic sections to *in vivo* conditions with compensation for the artifacts mentioned above. This correlation can be achieved by a transformation routine, which aids localization in the histologic material, providing standardized, topometrically defined data, and a correspondence between the topometry in the autopsy and the *in vivo* brain. For this application—the fine-grained (detailed) structural analysis of an individual brain—a probabilistic or statistical approach appears not appropriate because it lowers the spatial resolution of the images. According to this concept, to obtain a satisfactory prediction of the position of histo-anatomical structures (and their function) in patient images by overlay of the model brain, it is necessary to provide a model that consists of statistically evaluated distribution patterns of a large number of brains. All these brains must be mapped in the same model with the same dimensions. Therefore, the transformation mode also must be correct for interindividual variability.

2.3 REFERENCES

Assheuer, J., Lanta, L., Longerich, U., Sievert, T., and Mai, J. K.: Standardisierung der cerebralen Bilddarstellung in der Magnetresonanztomographie. *Röfo* **153**, 296-302 (1990).

Grösch, L., and Noack, F. NMR relaxation investigation of water mobility in aqueous bovine serum albumin solutions. Biochem. *Biophys. Acta* **453**, 218-232 (1976).

Kaiserling, C. Über Conservierung und Aufstellung pathologisch- anatomischer Präparate für die Schaund Lehrsammlungen. *Verh. Dt. Path. Ges.* **2**, 203-217 (1900).

Lange, H., and Thörner, G. *Zur Neuroanatomie und Neuropathologie des Corpus striatum, Globus pallidus und Nucleus subthalamicus beim Menschen,* Thesis, University Düsseldorf (1974).

Longerich, U. *MRI-Untersuchungen an in vivo und in vitro Gehirngewebe: Einfluß von Fixierung und Temperatur auf das Relaxationsverhalten, die Protonendichte und das Kontrastverhalten.* Thesis, University Düsseldorf (1989).

Mai, J. K., Stephens, P., Hopf A., and Cuello, A. C. Substance P in the human brain. *Neuroscience* **17**, 709-739 (1986).

Paxinos, G., and Watson, C. *The Rat Brain in Stereotaxic Coordinates.* Academic Press, Sydney (1982).

Paxinos, G., and Huang, X.-F. *Atlas of the Human Brainstem.* Academic Press, San Diego (1995).

Romeis, B. *Mikroskopische Technik.* R. Oldenbourg Verlag, München/Wien (1968).

Schulze, H. A. Zur individuellen cytoarchitektonischen Gestaltung der linken und rechten Hemisphäre des Lobulus parietalis inferior. *J. Hirnforsch.* **4**, 486-534 (1960).

Talairach, J., and Szikla, G. *Atlas d'Anatomie stereotaxique du Telencephale.* Masson & Cie., Paris (1967).

Talairach J., and Tournoux, P. *Co-planar Stereotaxic Atlas of the Human Brain.* G. Thieme, Stuttgart/New York (1988).

Teckhaus, L., Lübbers, D. W. and Rager, G. A new method of three-dimensional reconstruction of complicated structures by combining an automatic and interactive computer technique. *Microscopica Acta Suppl.* **3**, 235-240 (1979).

Vogt, O. Das Pantomikrotom des Neurobiologischen Laboratoriums. *J. Psychol. Neurol.* **6**, 121-125 (1905).

3 TOPOGRAPHIC AND TOPOMETRIC ATLAS

Horizontal Sections:

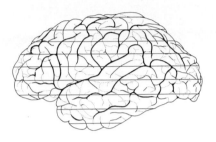

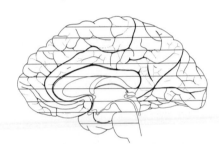

Coronal Sections:

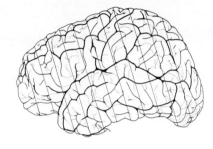

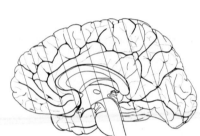

Sagittal Sections:

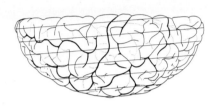

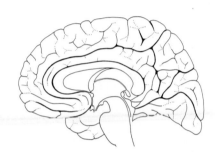

Presentation of the images

All anatomical head and brain slices (Sections 3.1 to 3.3) are mounted in the same way. Each series of sections begins with *in vitro* MR images of the head taken prior to sectioning. To provide a comprehensive view of the head, MR images are shown in all three orthogonal planes. This allows a better orientation in the three-dimensional space and helps in recognition of the topography of selected structures. The page following the MR images presents two surface views of the brain sectioned with the placement of sections indicated. The next page provides surface views of the brain with the most important gyri and sulci delineated. The midsagittal views depict the brain with the Talairach space. The main part of each topographic and topometric atlas presents anatomical head and brain slices. These are mounted to show every section from both sides. This allows the pursuit of any structure of interest throughout the series of sections. These presentations are accompanied by four MR images of the corresponding plane and (normally) two images showing the real section, the radiograph of the real section and/or the vasculatory territory within the brain section. MR images were performed from a healthy, 25-year-old volunteer. The MR images differ with respect to T_1, T_2, and proton density (N(H)) contrast.

Sagittal plane

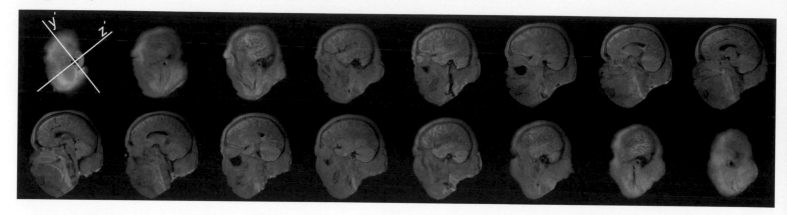

y´ direction

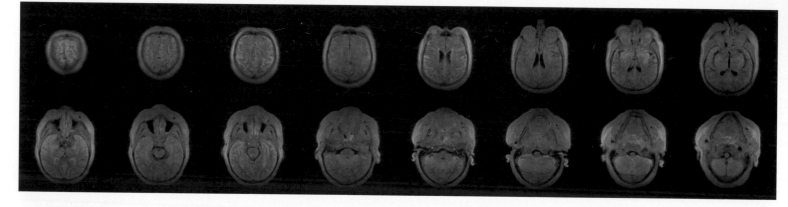

z´ direction

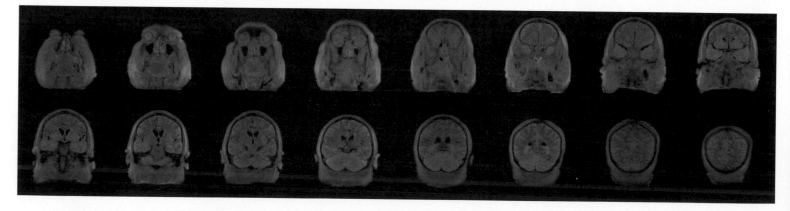

MR images of the head shown on the following pages.

The head whose horizontal sections are depicted on pages 24–54 was imaged before sectioning. Parameters: 0.15 Tesla, matrix 256×256, field of view 25 cm, multislice, slice thickness 5 mm, 4 excitations, sequence: 5000/40. The contrast of these images is poor since they are highly proton-density (N(H)) weighted. The top panel presents the sagittal MRIs and specifies the planes of sectioning of the middle and lower panel. Note that the angle of sectioning of the two latter panels is tilted about 45° from the plane of sectioning of the anatomic slices. This was intended to provide a more comprehensive view of the head.

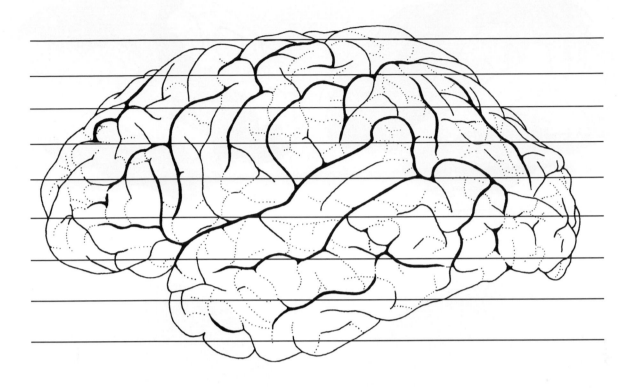

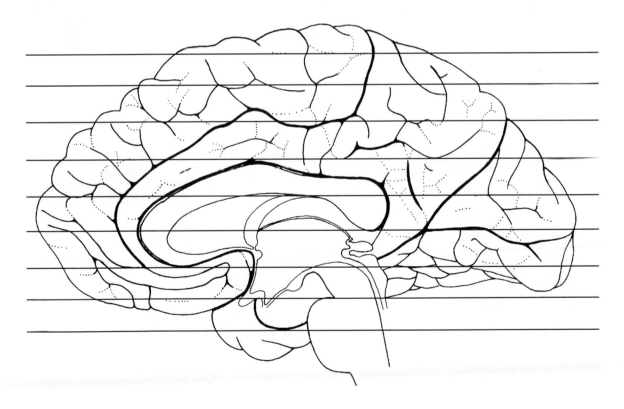

Surface views of the right hemisphere of the brain sectioned in the horizontal plane as indicated. The drawing of the lateral aspect is mirror-imaged to demonstrate the correspondence of section levels between convexity and midline structures.

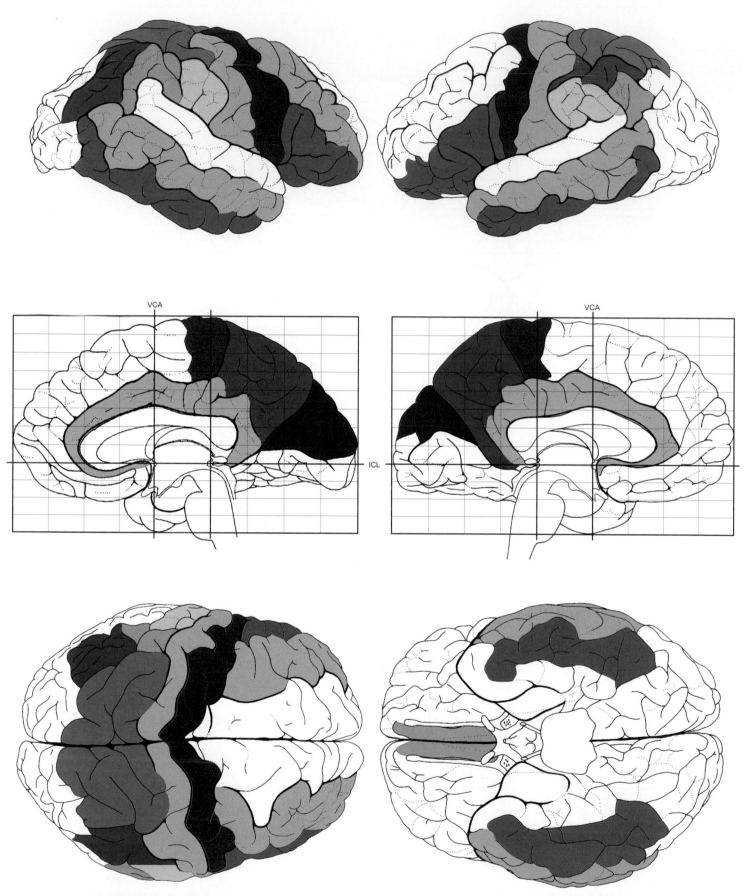

Surface views of the brain shown in the subsequent pages. The most important gyri are delineated. The midsagittal views depict the brain with the Talairach space (ICL, intercommissural line; VCA, plane vertical to the intercommissural line at the level of the anterior commissure).

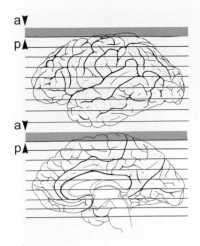

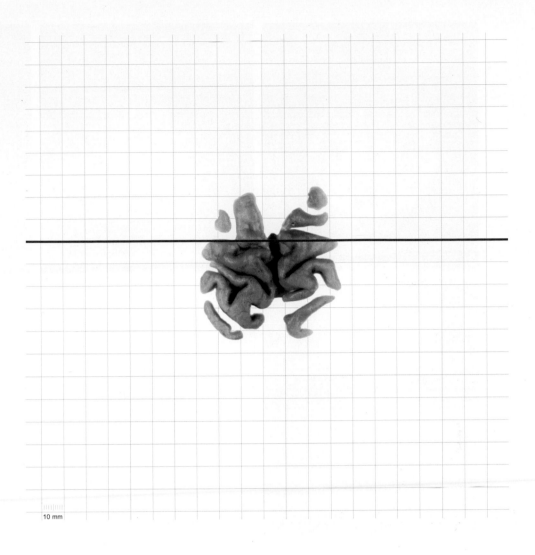

10 mm

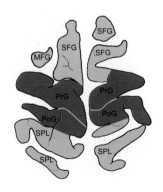

Section 1a:
anterior view of the section

sFG superior frontal gyrus
MFG medial frontal gyrus
PrG precentral gyrus
PoG postcentral gyrus
SPL superior parietal lobule

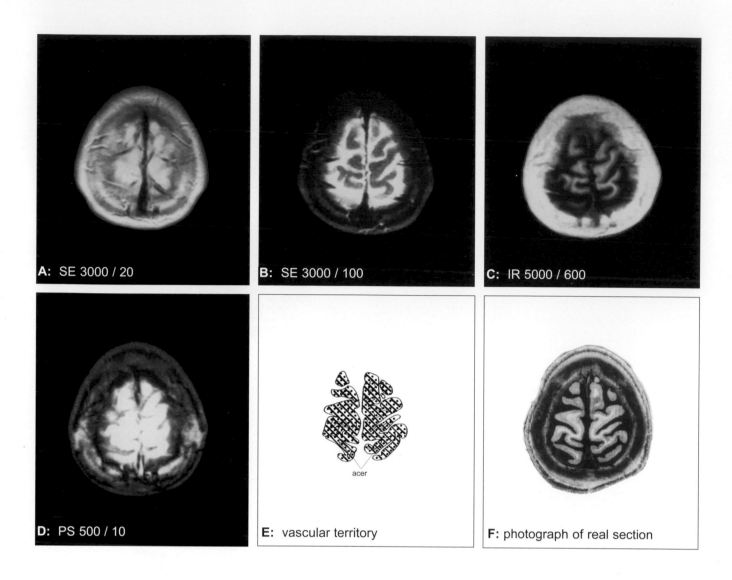

A: SE 3000 / 20

B: SE 3000 / 100

C: IR 5000 / 600

D: PS 500 / 10

E: vascular territory

acer

F: photograph of real section

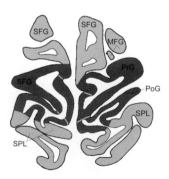

(A–D) Four MR images of different modalities from a 25-year-old volunteer, presenting the same plane as the anatomical sections. These MR images show different tissue contrast: N(H) (A), T_2 (B), T_1 (C), and T_1 with partial fat suppression (D). (E) Vasculatory territory within the brain section. (F) Posterior view of the anatomical section. The labeled diagram is based on the photograph of the real section. Photograph is the undersurface of the 1- cm-thick section whose top surface is shown on the previous page.

Section 1p: posterior view of the section

acer   anterior cerebral artery
SFG   superior frontal gyrus
MFG   medial frontal gyrus
PrG   precentral gyrus
PoG   postcentral gyrus
SPL   superior parietal lobule

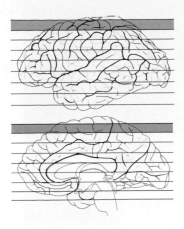

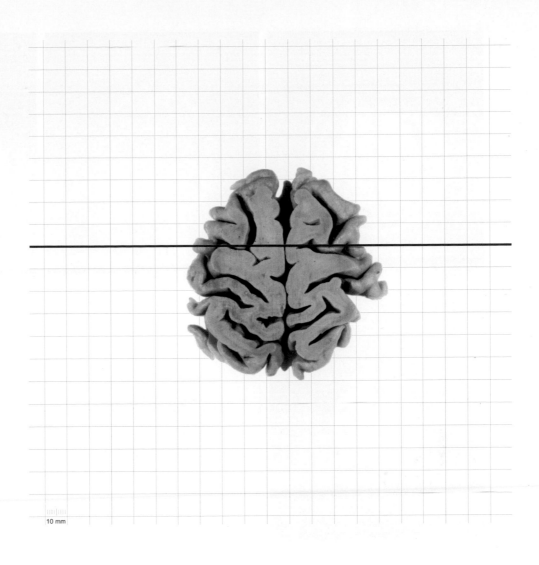

10 mm

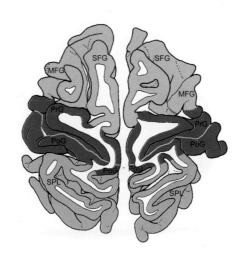

Section 2a:

MFG   medial frontal gyrus
PCL   paracentral lobule
PoG   postcentral gyrus
PrG   precentral gyrus
SFG   superior frontal gyrus
SPL   superior parietal lobule

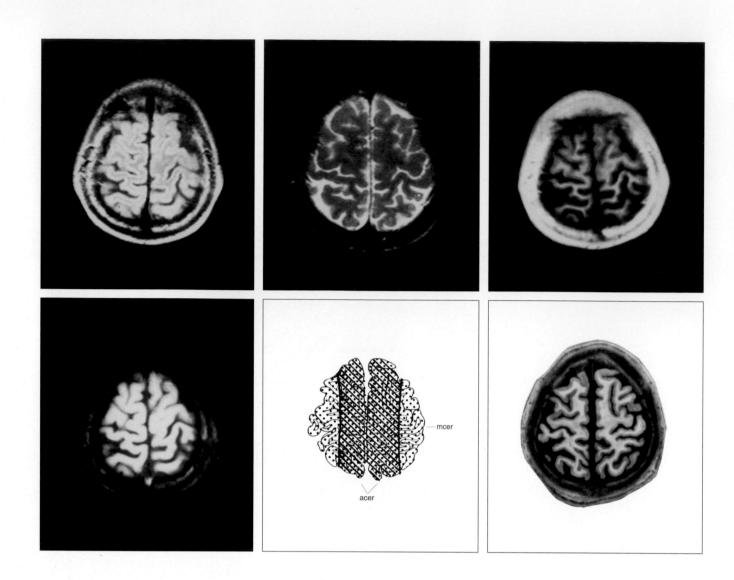

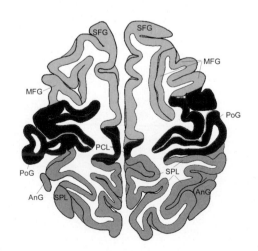

Section 2p:

acer	anterior cerebral artery
AnG	angular gyrus
mcer	middle cerebral artery
MFG	medial frontal gyrus
PCL	paracentral lobule
PoG	postcentral gyrus
PrG	precentral gyrus
SFG	superior frontal gyrus
SPL	superior parietal lobule

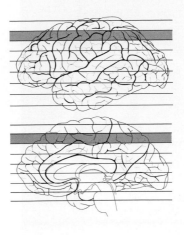

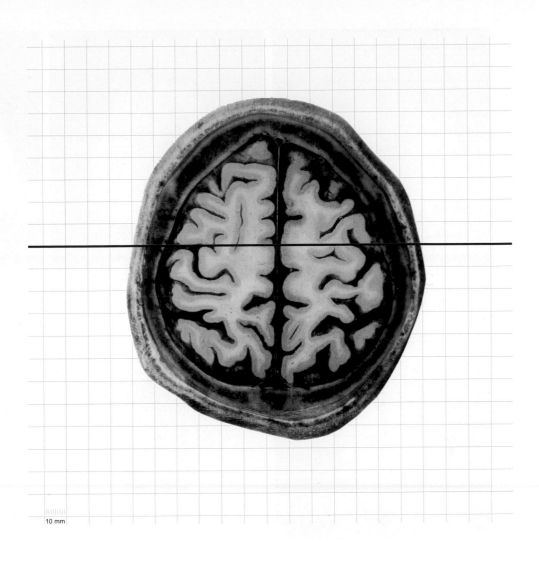

10 mm

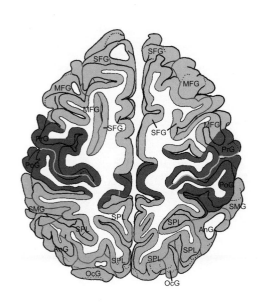

Section 3a:

AnG   angular gyrus
MFG   medial frontal gyrus
OcG   occipital gyri
PoG   postcentral gyrus
PrG   precentral gyrus
SFG   superior frontal gyrus
SMG   supramarginal gyrus
SPL   superior parietal lobule

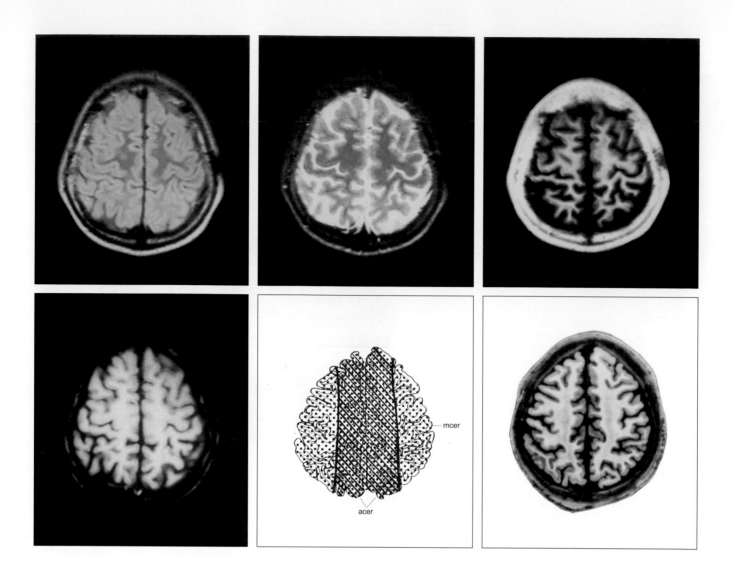

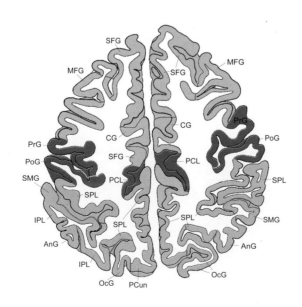

SFG

MFG

SFG

MFG

CG

PrG

PrG

CG

PoG

PoG

SFG

PCL

SMG

PCL

SPL

SPL

SPL

SPL

SPL

SMG

IPL

AnG

AnG

IPL

AnG

OcG

OcG

PCun

Section 3p:

acer   anterior cerebral artery
AnG   angular gyrus
CG   cingulate gyrus
IPL   inferior parietal lobule
mcer   middle cerebral artery
MFG   medial frontal gyrus
OcG   occipital gyri
PCL   paracentral lobule
PCun   precuneus
PoG   postcentral gyrus
PrG   precentral gyrus
SFG   superior frontal gyrus
SMG   supramarginal gyrus
SPL   superior parietal lobule

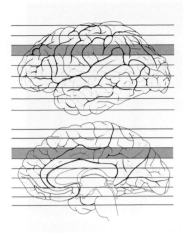

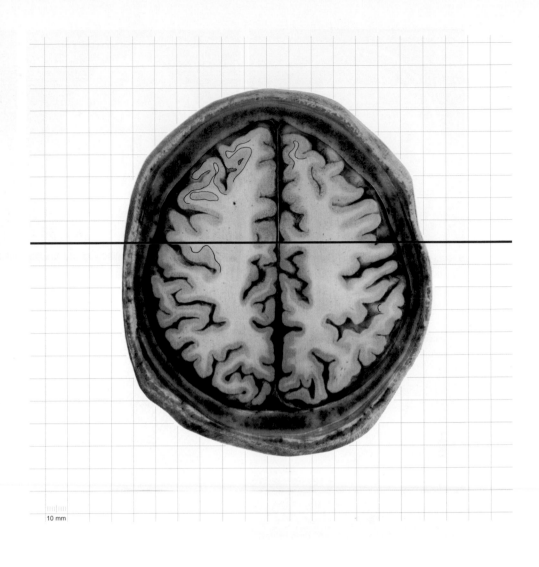

10 mm

Section 4a:

17	striate area
AnG	angular gyrus
CG	cingular gyrus
IFG	inferior frontal gyrus, opercular part
IPL	inferior parietal lobule
MFG	middle frontal gyrus
OcG	occipital gyri
PCL	paracentral lobule
PoG	postcentral gyrus
PrG	precentral gyrus
SFG	superior frontal gyrus
SMG	supramarginal gyrus
SPL	superior parietal lobule
STG	superior temporal gyrus

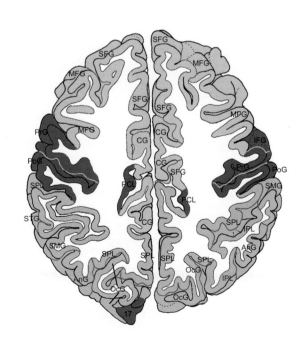

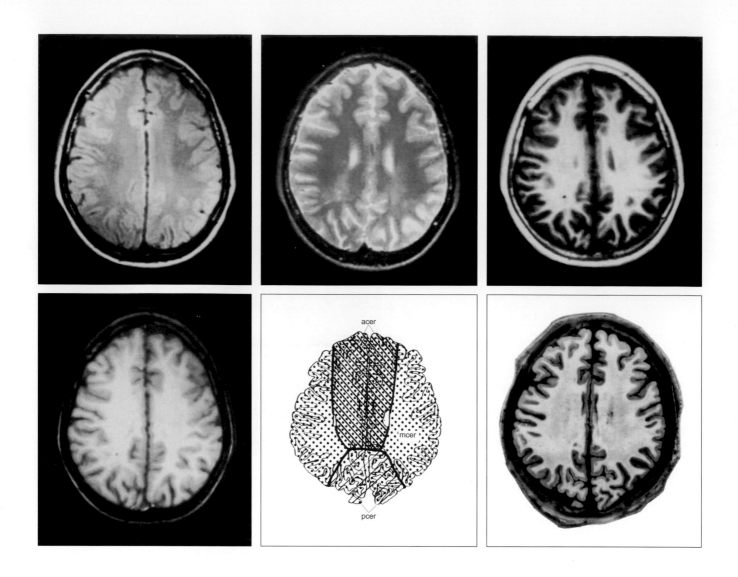

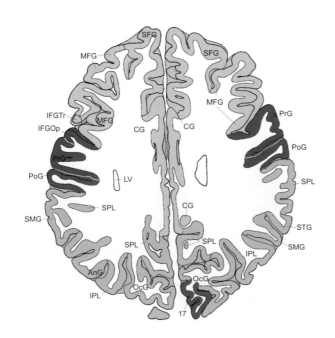

Section 4p:

17	striate cortex
acer	anterior cerebral artery
AnG	angular gyrus
CG	cingular gyrus
IFGOp	inferior frontal gyrus, opercular part
IFGTr	inferior frontal gyrus, triangular part
IPL	inferior parietal lobule
LV	lateral ventricle
mcer	middle cerebral artery
MFG	middle frontal gyrus
OcG	occipital gyri
pcer	posterior cerebral artery
PoG	postcentral gyrus
PrG	precentral gyrus
SFG	superior frontal gyrus
SMG	supramarginal gyrus
SPL	superior parietal lobule
STG	superior temporal gyrus

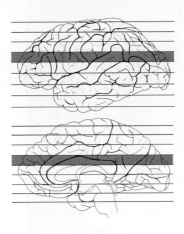

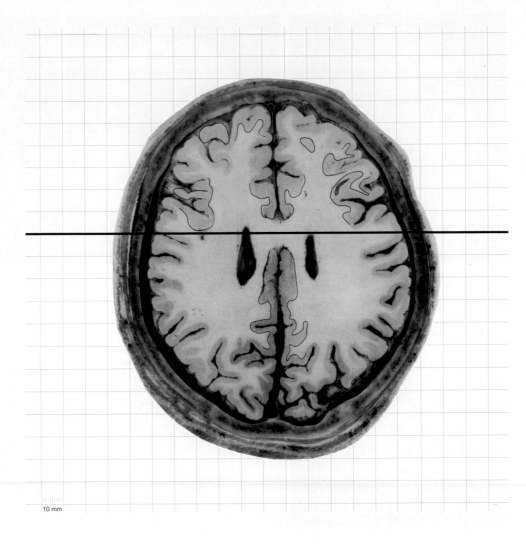

10 mm

Section 5a:

17	striate area
AnG	angular gyrus
CG	cingular gyrus
IFGOp	inferior frontal gyrus, opercular part
IFGTr	inferior frontal gyrus, triangular part
IPL	inferior parietal lobule
LV	lateral ventricle
MFG	middle frontal gyrus
MTG	middle temporal gyrus
OcG	occipital gyri
PoG	postcentral gyrus
PrG	precentral gyrus
SFG	superior frontal gyrus
SMG	supramarginal gyrus
SPL	superior parietal lobule
STG	superior temporal gyrus

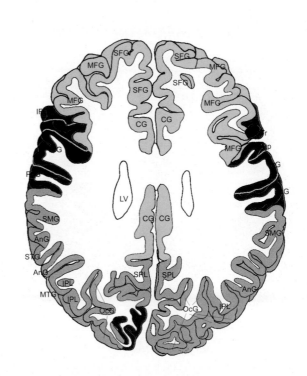

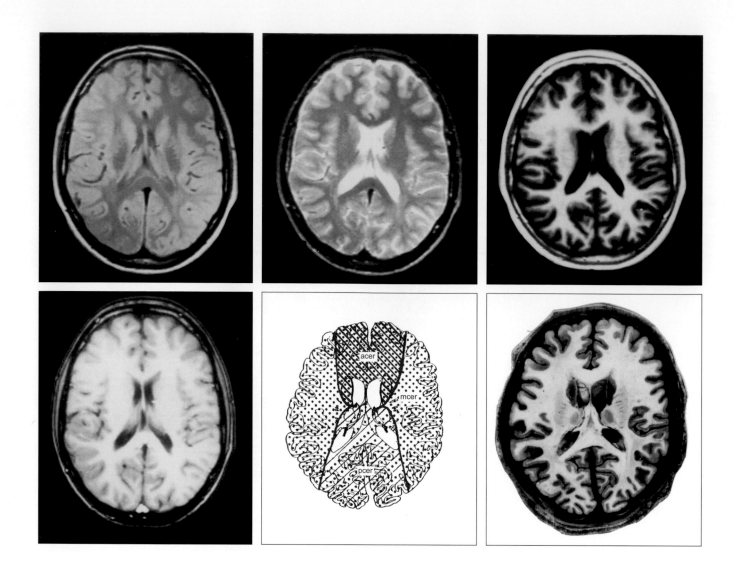

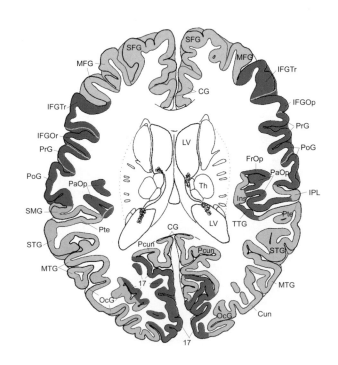

Section 5p:

17	striate cortex
acer	anterior cerebral artery
CG	cingular gyrus
Cun	cuneus
FrOp	frontal operculum
IFGOp	inferior frontal gyrus, opercular part
IFGOr	inferior frontal gyrus, orbital part
IFGTr	inferior frontal gyrus, triangular part
Ins	insula
IPL	inferior parietal lobule
LV	lateral ventricle
mcer	middle cerebral artery
MFG	middle frontal gyrus
MTG	middle temporal gyrus
OcG	occipital gyri
pcer	posterior cerebral artery
PaOp	parietal operculum
Pcun	precuneus
PoG	postcentral gyrus
PrG	precentral gyrus
Pte	planum temporale
SFG	superior frontal gyrus
SMG	supramarginal gyrus
STG	superior temporal gyrus
Th	thalamus
TTG	transverse temporal gyri

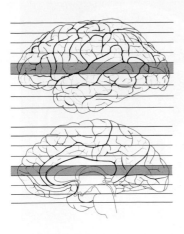

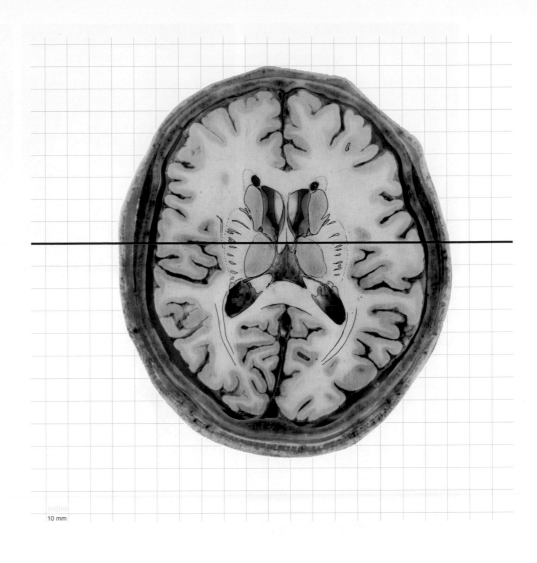

10 mm

Section 6a:

17	striate area
3V	third ventricle
CG	cingular gyrus
chp	choroid plexus
FLV	frontal horn of lateral ventricle
fmi	forceps minor of the corpus callosum
fmj	forceps major of the corpus callosum
FrOp	frontal operculum
fx	fornix
gcc	genu of the corpus callosum
HCd	head of caudate nucleus
IFGOp	inferior frontal gyrus, opercular part
IFGOr	inferior frontal gyrus, orbital part
IFGTr	inferior frontal gyrus, triangular part
Ins	insula
MFG	middle frontal gyrus
MTG	medial temporal gyrus.
OcG	occipital gyri
OLV	occipital horn of lateral ventricle
PCun	precuneus
PoG	postcentral gyrus
PrG	precentral gyrus
PTe	planum temporale
scc	splenium of the corpus callosum
SFG	superior frontal gyrus
SMG	supramarginal gyrus
sof	superior occipitofrontal fascicle
st	stria terminalis
STG	superior temporal gyrus
TCd	tail of caudate nucleus
TTG	transverse temporal gyri
Th	thalamus
tsv	thalamostriate vein

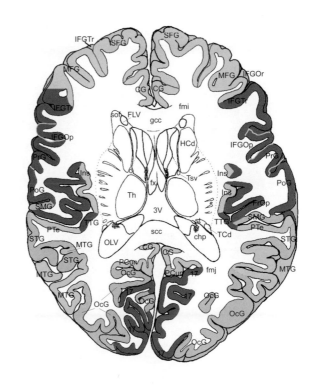

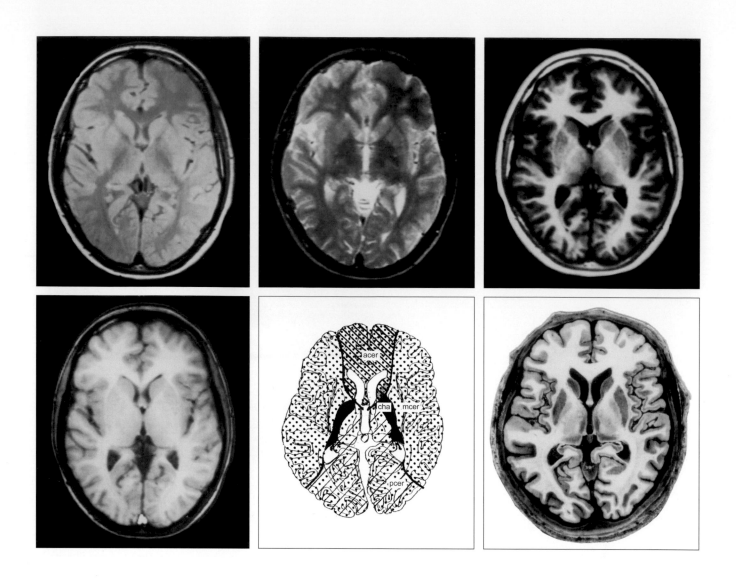

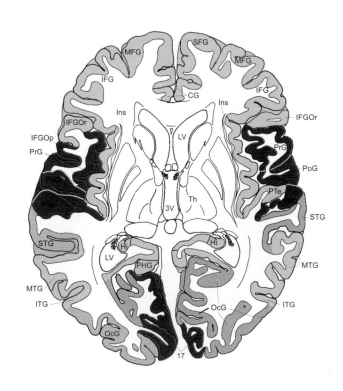

Section 6p:

17	striate cortex
3V	third ventricle
acer	anterior cerebral artery
CG	cingulate gyrus
cha	choroid artery
Hi	hippocampus
IFG	inferior frontal gyrus
IFGOp	inferior frontal gyrus, opercular part
IFGOr	inferior frontal gyrus, orbital part
Ins	insula
ITG	inferior temporal gyrus
LV	lateral ventricle
mcer	middle cerebral artery
MFG	middle frontal gyrus
MTG	middle temporal gyrus
OcG	occipital gyri
pcer	posterior cerebral artery
PHG	parahippocampal gyrus
PoG	postcentral gyrus
PrG	precentral gyrus
PTe	planum temporale
SFG	superior frontal gyrus
STG	superior temporal gyrus
Th	thalamus
TTG	transverse temporal gyri

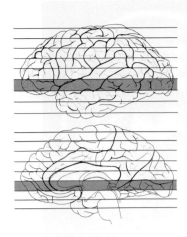

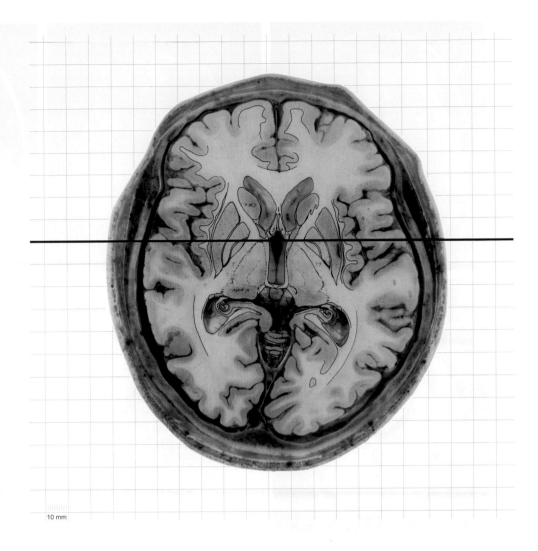

10 mm

Section 7a:

17	striate area
3V	third ventricle
aic	anterior limb of the internal capsule
ATh	anterior thalamus
CG	cingular gyrus
chp	choroid plexus
Cl	claustrum
ec	external capsule
exc	extreme capsule
fi	fimbria hippocampi
FLV	frontal horn of lateral ventricle
FuG	fusiform gyrus
fx	fornix
gcc	genu of the corpus callosum
gic	internal capsule, genu
GP	globus pallidus
Hb	habenular nuclei
HCd	head of caudate nucleus
Hi	hippocampus
IFG	inferior frontal gyrus
IFGOp	inferior frontal gyrus, opercular part
IFGOr	inferior frontal gyrus, orbital part
IFGTr	inferior frontal gyrus, triangular part
Ins	insula
ITG	inferior temporal gyrus
MFG	middle frontal gyrus
MTG	middle temporal gyrus
OcG	occipital gyri
OLV	occipital horn of lateral ventricle
or	optic radiation
PCun	precuneus
Pi	pineal gland
pic	posterior limb of the internal capsule
PoG	postcentral gyrus
PrG	precentral gyrus
PTe	planum temporale
Pu	putamen
Pul	pulvinar thalami
SFG	superior frontal gyrus
sm	stria medullaris of thalamus
st	stria terminalis
STG	superior temporal gyrus
TCd	tail of caudate nucleus
Th	thalamus
TTG	transverse temporal gyri
Ver	vermis of cerebellum

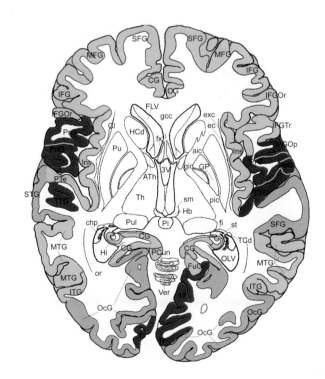

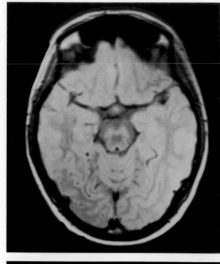
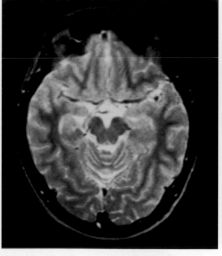
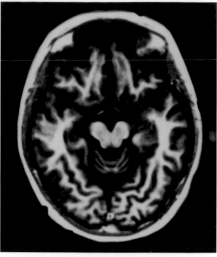

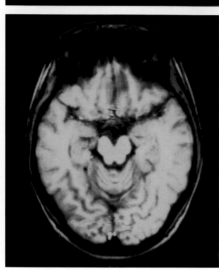
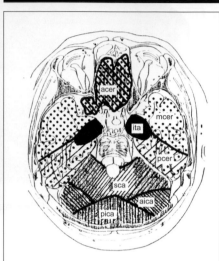
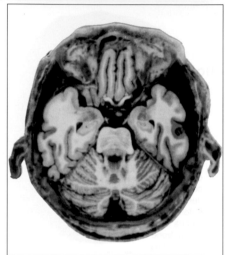

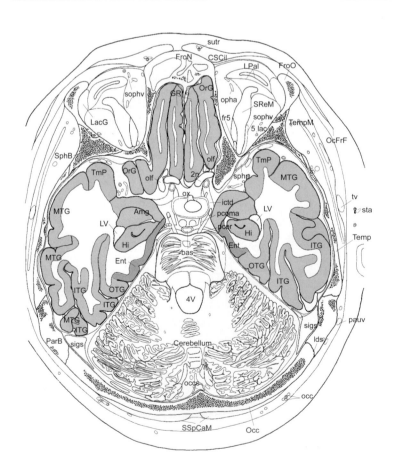

Section 8p:

2n	optic nerve
4V	fourth ventricle
5lac	lacrimal nerve
acer	anterior cerebral artery
aica	anterior inferior cerebellar artery
Amg	amygdala
bas	basilar artery
cha	choroid artery
CSCil	corrugator supercilii muscle
Ent	entorhinal cortex
fr5	frontal nerve
FroN	frontal bone (nasal spine)
FroO	frontal bone (orbital plate)
GR	gyrus rectus
Hi	hippocampus
ictd	internal carotid artery
ITG	inferior temporal gyrus
lac5	lacrimal nerve
LacG	lacrimal gland
LPal	levator palpebrae superioris muscle
LV	lateral ventricle
mcer	middle cerebral artery
MTG	middle temporal gyrus
Occ	occipital bone
occ	occipital artery, vein and nerve
occs	occipital sinus
OcFrF	occipito-frontal muscle, frontal belly
olf	olfactory tract
opha	ophthalmic artery
OrG	orbital gyrus
OTG	occipito-temporal gyrus
ox	optic chiasm
ParB	parietal bone
pauv	posterior auricularis vein
pcer	posterior cerebral artery
pcoma	posterior communicating artery
pica	posterior inferior cerebellar artery
sca	superior cerebellar artery
sigs	sigmoid sinus
sophv	superior ophthalmic vein
SphB	sphenoid bone
sphp	sphenoparietal sinus
SReM	superior rectus muscle
SSpCaM	semispinalis capitis muscle
sta	superficial temporal artery
sutr	supratrochlear artery, vein and nerve
Temp	temporal bone
TempM	temporalis muscle
TmP	temporal pole
tv	temporal vein

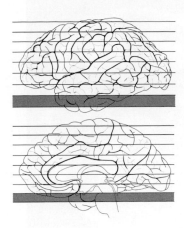

Section 9a:

2n	optic nerve
3 n	oculomotor nerve
4 n	trochlear nerve
4V	fourth ventricle
5 n	trigeminal nerve
Amg	amygdala
ang	angular vein
bas	basilar artery
cav	cavernous sinus
CCil	corrugator supercilii muscle
CGal	crista galli
Ci	cistern
Ent	entorhinal cortex
frn	frontal nerve
FroN	frontal bone, nasal part
FroO	frontal bone, orbital part
Hi	hippocampus
ictd	internal carotid artery
ITG	inferior temporal gyrus
LacG	lacrimal gland
ld	lambdoid suture
LPal	levator palpebrae superioris muscle
mmf	middle meningeal artery, frontal branch
MTG	middle temporal gyrus
nuf	nuchal fascia
Occ	occipital bone
occ/occv	occipital artery, occipital vein
occn	occipital nerve
OOM	orbicularis oculi muscle
opha	ophthalmic artery
ophv	ophthalmic vein
ophav	ophthalmic artery and vein
OrG	orbital gyrus
OTG	occipito-temporal gyrus
pauv	posterior auricular vein
Pit	pituitary gland
Pons	pons
RG	rectus gyrus
s4a/v	supratrochlear artery/vein
sigs	sigmoid sinus
SObM	superior oblique muscle
SphB	sphenoid bone
sphp	sphenoparietal sinus
sphzg	spheno-zygomatic suture
SReM	superior rectus muscle
SSpCaM	semispinalis capitis muscle
sta	superficial temporal artery
sutrn	supratrochlear nerve
sutrv	supratrochlear vein
Temp	temporal bone
TempM	temporal muscle
tf	temporal fascia
TLV	temporal horn of lateral ventricle
TmP	temporal pole
tv	temporal vein

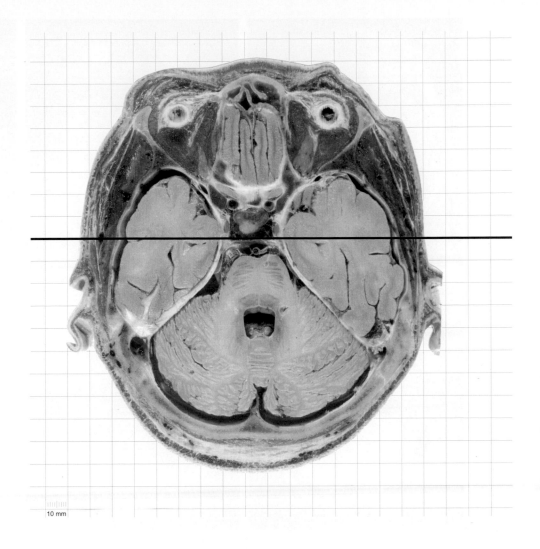

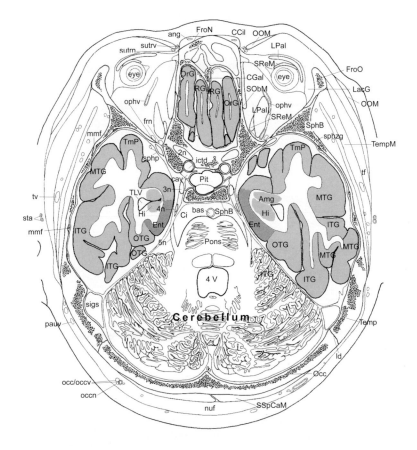

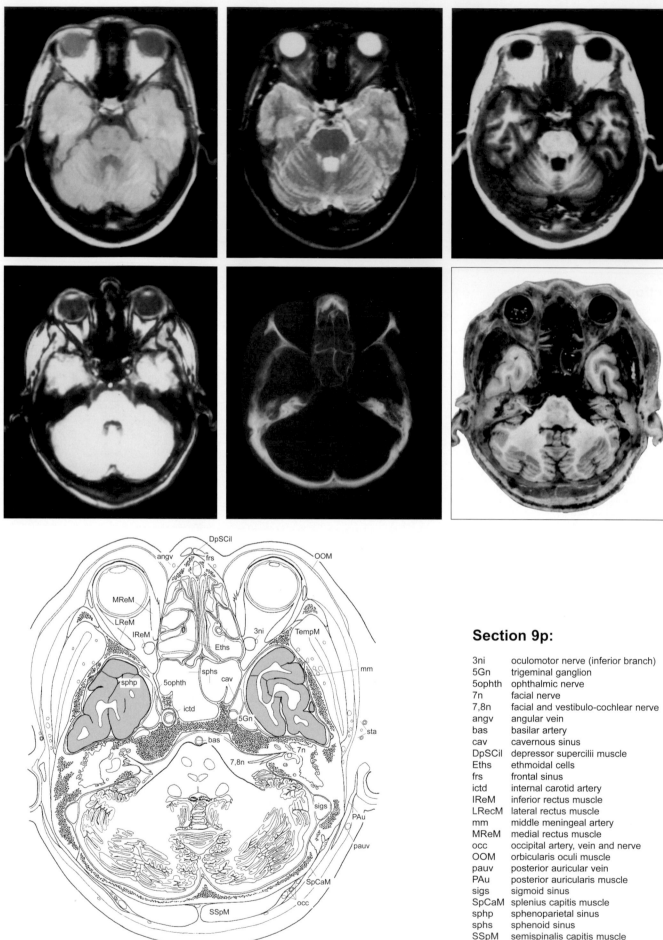

Section 9p:

3ni	oculomotor nerve (inferior branch)
5Gn	trigeminal ganglion
5ophth	ophthalmic nerve
7n	facial nerve
7,8n	facial and vestibulo-cochlear nerve
angv	angular vein
bas	basilar artery
cav	cavernous sinus
DpSCil	depressor supercilii muscle
Eths	ethmoidal cells
frs	frontal sinus
ictd	internal carotid artery
IReM	inferior rectus muscle
LRecM	lateral rectus muscle
mm	middle meningeal artery
MReM	medial rectus muscle
occ	occipital artery, vein and nerve
OOM	orbicularis oculi muscle
pauv	posterior auricular vein
PAu	posterior auricularis muscle
sigs	sigmoid sinus
SpCaM	splenius capitis muscle
sphp	sphenoparietal sinus
sphs	sphenoid sinus
SSpM	semispinalis capitis muscle
sta	superficial temporal artery
TempM	temporalis muscle

(**A–D**) MR images showing different tissue contrast: N(H) (**A**), T_2 (**B**), T_1 (**C**), and T_1 with partial fat suppression (**D**). (**E**) Radiograph of the real section. (**F**) Posterior view of the undersurface of the 1-cm-thick section whose top surface is shown on the previous page.

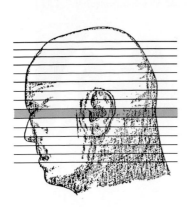

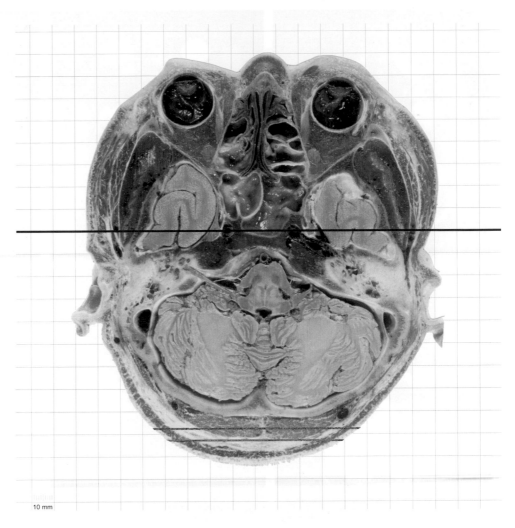

10 mm

Section 10a:

3n	oculomotor nerve (inferior branch)
4V	fourth ventricle
5Gn	trigeminal ganglion (Gasseri)
5mx	maxillary nerve
5ophth	ophthalmic nerve
7n	facial nerve
8n	vestibulo-cochlear nerve
ang	angular artery and vein
bas	basilar artery
BasCi	basilar cistern
CAnT	common anular tendon
CilM	ciliaris muscle
DpSCil	depressor supercilii muscle
emi	emissary vein
EthS	ethmoidal sinus (cells)
eye	eyeball
gocn	greater occipital nerve
gpetn	greater petrosal nerve
ictd	internal carotid artery
ipets	inferior petrosal sinus
IReM	inferior rectus muscle
lacv	lacrimal vein
LRecM	lateral rectus muscle
mm	middle meningeal artery
MReM	medial rectus muscle
Na	nasal bone
nuf	nuchal fascia
Occ	occipital bone
occ	occipital artery and vein
ocm	occipito-mastoid suture
OOM	orbicularis oculi muscle
ophv	ophthalmic vein
pauv	posterior auricular vein
sca	superior cerebellar artery
sigs	sigmoid sinus
SpCaM	splenius capitis muscle
SphB	sphenoid bone
sphp	spheno-parietal sinus
sphpe	spheno-petrosal suture
sphs	sphenoid sinus
SSpCaM	semispinalis capitis muscle
sta	superficial temporal artery and vein
TempM	temporalis muscle
TempP	temporal bone, petrosal part
TempS	temporal bone, squamous part
tf	temporal fascia
TL	temporal lobe
tv	temporal veins
TyC	tympanic cavity
ZygB	zygomatic bone

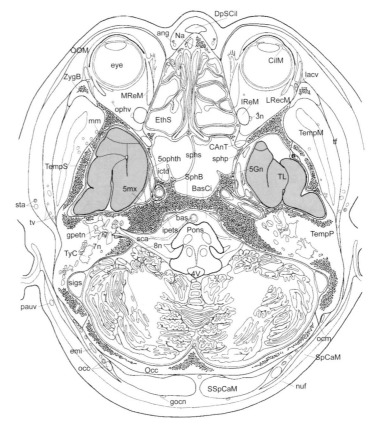

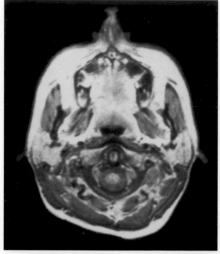
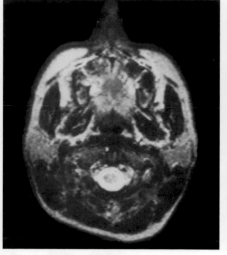
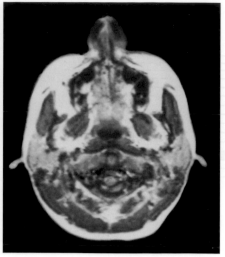
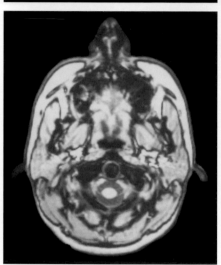
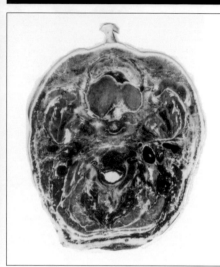
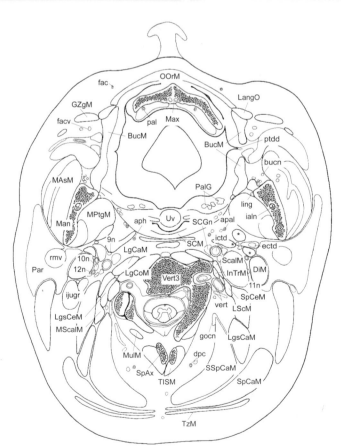

Section 13p:

9n	glossopharyngeal nerve
10n	vagus nerve
11n	accessory nerve
12n	hypoglossal nerve
apal	ascending palatine artery
aph	ascending pharyngeal artery
BucM	buccinator muscle
bucn	buccal nerve
DiM	digastic muscle
dpc	deep cervical artery and vein
ectd	external carotid artery
fac	facial artery
facv	facial vein
gocn	greater occipital nerve
GZgM	greater zygomatic muscle
ialn	inferior alveolar artery
ictd	internal carotid artery
ijugr	internal jugular vein
InTrM	intertransversarii muscles
LangO	levator anguli oris muscle
LgCaM	longus capitis muscle
LgCoM	longus colli muscle
LgsCaM	longissimus capitis muscle
LgsCeM	longissimus cervicis muscle
ling	lingual nerve
LScM	levator scapulae muscle
Man	mandible
MAsM	masseter muscle
Max	maxilla
MPtgM	medial pterygoideus muscle
MScalM	medial scalenus muscle
MulM	multifidus muscle
OOrM	orbicularis oris muscle
pal	palatine artery
PalG	palatine glands
Par	parotid gland
ptdd	parotid duct
rmv	retromandibular vein
ScalM	scalenus muscle
SCGn	superior cervical ganglion
SCM	superior constrictor of the pharynx
SpAx	spinous process of axis
SpCaM	splenius capitis muscle
SpCeM	splenius cervicis muscle
SSpCaM	semispinalis capitis muscle
TISM	tendon of interspinalis muscle
TempT	tendon of temporalis muscle
TzM	trapezius muscle
Uv	uvula
vert	vertebral artery
Vert3	vertebra 3
*	styloglossus, stylohyoideus, stylo pharyngeus muscle

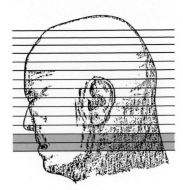

Sections 14a, 15a:

10n	vagus nerve
11n	accessory nerve
12n	hypoglossal nerve
9n	glossopharyngeal nerve
all	anterior longitudinal ligament
apal	ascending palatine artery
aph	ascending pharyngeal artery
Axis	axis
BucM	buccinator muscle
bucn	buccal nerve
DiM	digastric muscle
dpc	deep cervical artery and vein
ectd	external carotid artery
fac	facial artery
facv	facial vein
GZgM	greater zygomatic muscle
HyGl	hyoglossus muscle
ialv	inferior alveolar artery, vein and nerve
ictd	internal carotid artery
ijugv	internal jugular vein
IncC	incisive canal with nasopalatine artery
InTrM	intertransversarii muscles
ISM	interspinalis muscle
LAngO	levator anguli oris muscle
LgCa	longus capitis muscle
LgCo	longus colli muscle
LgsCa	longissimus capitis muscle
LgsCe	longissimus cervicis muscle
LgsCeT	tendon of longissimus cervicis muscle
LScM	levator scapulae muscle
Man	mandible
MasM	masseter muscle
Max	maxilla
MPtgM	medial pterygoid muscle
Mult	multifidus muscle
MyHy	mylohyoid muscle
nuf	nuchal fascia
occ	occipital artery
OOrM	orbicularis oris muscle
pal	palatine artery
papx	parotid plexus
Par	parotid gland
Plat	platysma
PlGl	palatoglossus muscle
SCM	superior constrictor of the pharynx
S/MCM	superior and middle constrictor of the pharynx
ScalM	scalenus muscle
SCGn	superior cervical ganglion
sln	superior laryngeal nerve
SMG	submandibular gland
SpCa	splenius capitis muscle
SpCe	splenius cervicis muscle
sphn	superior pharyngeal nerve
SpM	spinalis muscle
SSpCa	semispinalis capitis muscle
SSpCe	semispinalis cervicis muscle
StM	sternomastoid muscle
StyGl	styloglossus muscle
StyHy	stylohyoid muscle
StyPh	stylopharyngeus muscle
Symp	sympathetic trunk
TzM	trapezius muscle
Uv	uvula
v	veins
vert	vertebral artery
Vert3	third cervical vertebra
Vert4	fourth cervical vertebra

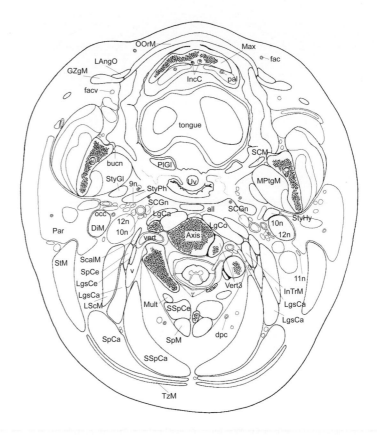

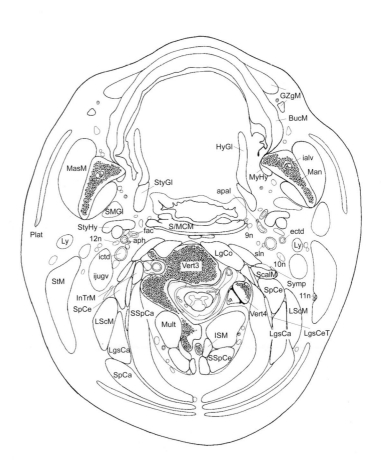

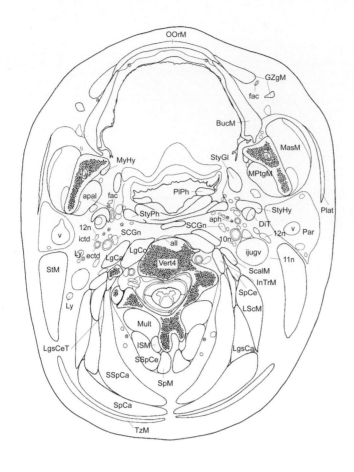

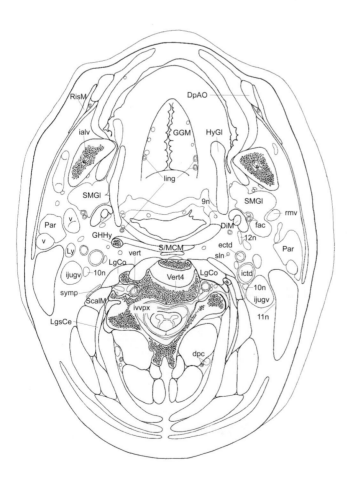

Sections 14p, 15p:

10n	vagus nerve
11n	accessory nerve
12n	hypoglossal nerve
9n	glossopharyngeal nerve
all	allocortex
apal	ascending palatine artery
aph	ascending pharyngeal artery
BucM	buccinator muscle
bucn	buccal nerve
DiM	digastric muscle
DiT	digastric muscle, tendon
DpAO	depressor anguli oris muscle
dpc	deep cervical artery and vein
ectd	external carotid artery
fac	facial artery and glandular branches
GGM	genioglossus muscle
GHHy	greater horn of hyoid bone
GZgM	greater zygomatic muscle
HyGl	hyoglossus muscle
ialv	inferior alveolar artery and nerve
ictd	internal carotid artery
ijugv	internal jugular vein
InTrM	intertransversarii muscles
ISM	interspinalis muscle
ivvpx	internal vertebral venous plexus
LgCa	longus capitis muscle
LgCo	longus colli muscle
LgsCa	longissimus capitis muscle
LgsCe	longissimus cervicis muscle
LgsCeT	longissimus cervicis muscle, tendon
ling	lingual artery
LScM	levator scapulae muscle
Ly	lymph node
MasM	masseter muscle
MPtgM	medial pterygoid muscle
Mult	multifidus muscle
MyHy	mylohyoid muscle
OOrM	orbicularis oris muscle
Par	parotid gland
Plat	platysma
PlPh	palatopharyngeus muscle
RisM	risorius muscle
rmv	retromandibular vein
S/MCM	superior and middle constrictor of the pharynx
ScalM	scalenus muscle
SCGn	superior cervical ganglion
sln	superior laryngeal nerve
SMGl	submandibular gland
SpCa	splenius capitis muscle
SpCe	splenius cervicis muscle
SpM	spinalis muscle
SSpCa	semispinalis capitis muscle
SSpCe	semispinalis cervicis muscle
StM	sternomastoid muscle
StyGl	styloglossus muscle
StyHy	stylohyoid muscle
StyPh	stylopharyngeus muscle
symp	sympathetic trunk
TzM	trapezius muscle
v	vein
vert	vertebral artery
Vert3	third cervical vertebra
Vert4	fourth cervical vertebra

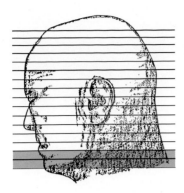

Sections 16a, 17a:

10n	vagus nerve
11n	accessory nerve
ancer	ansa cervicalis
BucM	buccinator muscle
cctd	common carotid artery
cern	cervical nerve
cplx	carotid plexus
DiM	digastric muscle
DiT	digastric muscle (tendon)
DpAO	depressor anguli oris muscle
dpc	deep cervical artery and vein
ectd	external carotid artery
fac	facial artery
GGM	genioglossus muscle
GHHy	greater horn of hyoid bone
glda	glandular branches of facial artery
HyGl	hyoglossus muscle
ICM	inferior constrictor of the pharynx
ictd	Internal carotid artery
ijugv	internal jugular vein
ilab	inferior labial artery and vein
ISM	interspinalis muscle
LgCa	longus capitis muscle
LgCo	longus colli muscle
LgsCa	longissimus capitis muscle
LgsCe	longissimus cervicis muscle
ling	lingual artery
LgGl	anterior lingual gland
LScM	levator scapulae muscle
Ly	lymph node
Man	mandible
MCM	middle constrictor of the pharynx
Mult	multifidus muscle
MyHy	mylohyoid muscle
myhy	mylohyoid nerve
OOrM	orbicularis oris muscle
Plat	platysma
RisM	risorius muscle
S/MCM	superior and middle constrictor of the pharynx
ScalM	scalenus muscle
SHThC	superior horn of thyroid cartilage
SLGl	sublingual gland
sln	superior laryngeal nerve
smd	submandibular duct
SMGl	submandibular gland
SpCa	splenius capitis muscle
SpCe	splenius cervicis muscle
SpM	spinalis muscle
SSpCa	semispinalis capitis muscle
SSpCe	semispinalis cervicis muscle
sthy	superior thyroid artery
StM	sternomastoid muscle
StyHy	stylohyoid muscle
Symp	sympathetic trunk
ThHy	thyrohyoid muscle
ThHyMe	thyrohyoid membrane
TzM	trapezius muscle
v	vein
vert	vertebral artery
Vert3	third cervical vertebra
Vert4	fourth cervical vertebra

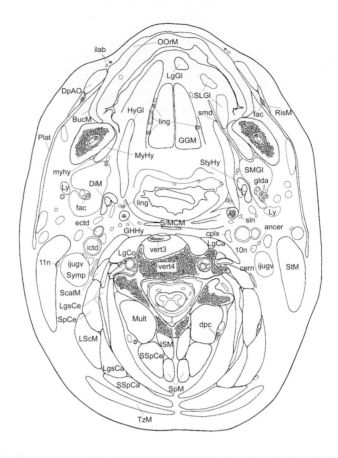

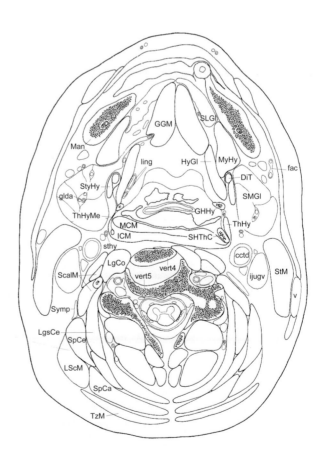

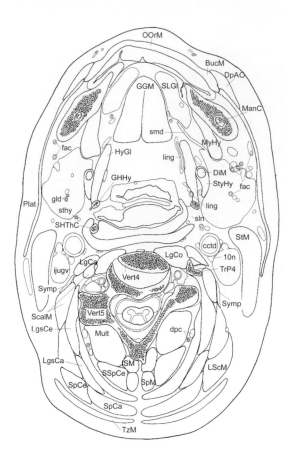

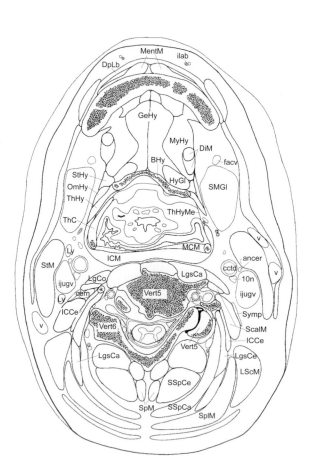

Sections 16p, 17p:

10n	vagus nerve
ancer	ansa cervicalis
BHy	body of hyoid bone
BucM	buccinator muscle
cctd	common carotid artery
cern	cervical nerve
DiM	digastric muscle
DpAO	depressor anguli oris muscle
dpc	deep cervical artery and vein
DpLb	depressor labii inferioris muscle
fac	facial artery
facv	facial vein
GeHy	geniohyoid muscle
GGM	genioglossus muscle
GHHy	greater horn of hyoid bone
gld	glandular branches of facial artery
HyGl	hyoglossus muscle
ICCe	iliocostalis cervicis muscle
ICM	inferior constrictor of the pharynx
ijugv	internal jugular vein
ilab	inferior labial artery and vein
ISM	interspinalis muscle
LgCa	longus capitis muscle
LgCo	longus colli muscle
LgsCa	longissimus capitis muscle
LgsCe	longissimus cervicis muscle
ling	lingual artery
LScM	levator scapulae muscle
Ly	lymph node
ManC	mandibular canal with inferior alveolar artery and nerve
MasM	masseter muscle
MCM	middle constrictor of the pharynx
MentM	mentalis muscle
Mult	multifidus muscle
MyHy	mylohyoid muscle
OmHy	omohyoideus muscle
OOrM	orbicularis oris muscle
Plat	platysma
ScalM	scalenus muscle
SHThC	superior horn of thyroid cartilage
SLGl	sublingual gland
sln	superior laryngeal nerve
smd	submandibular duct
SMGl	submandibular gland
SpCa	splenius capitis muscle
SpCe	splenius cervicis muscle
SplM	splenius capitis and cervicis muscle
SpM	spinalis muscle
SSpCa	semispinalis capitis muscle
SSpCe	semispinalis cervicis muscle
sthy	superior thyroid artery
StM	sternomastoid muscle
StyHy	stylohyoid muscle
Symp	sympathetic trunk
ThC	thyroid cartilage
ThHy	thyrohyoid muscle
ThHyMe	thyrohyoid membrane
TrP4	transverse process of fourth vertebra
TzM	trapezius muscle
vert	vertebral artery
Vert4	fourth cervical vertebra
Vert5	fifth cervical vertebra
Vert6	sixth cervical vertebra

Sagittal plane

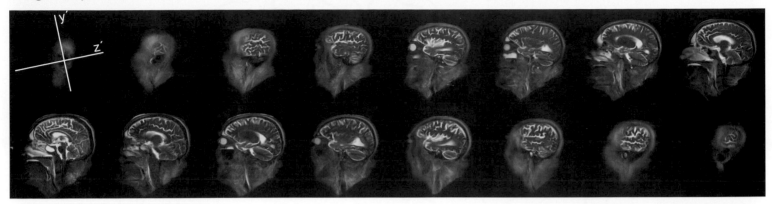

y´ direction

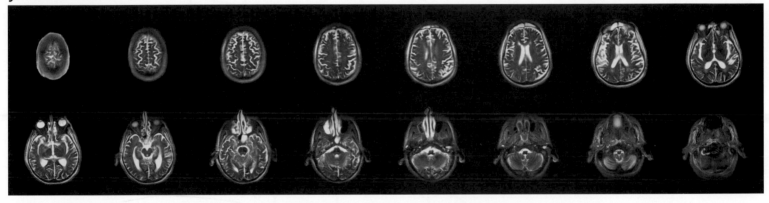

z´ direction

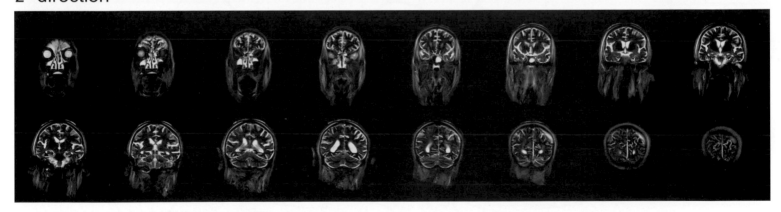

MR images of the head presented on the following pages.

The head whose sections are depicted on the following pages was imaged in three orthgonal planes using the following parameters: 0.15 Tesla, matrix 256 × 256, field of view 25 cm, multi-slice, slice thickness 5 mm, 4 excitations, sequence: 5000/160. These heavy T_2-weighted images highlight fluid-containing structures. Note that artificial fluid collections are visible in the nasal and paranasal cavities. The top panel presents the sagittal MRIs and specifies the planes of sectioning of the middle and lower panel. Orientation of these MRIs was based on the brainstem axis. Therefore the orientation of the coronal MRIs in the lower panel corresponds to the plane of cryosectioning of the head and direct comparisons can be made with photographs and diagrams of the following pages. The middle panel presents the horizontal MRIs from top to bottom.

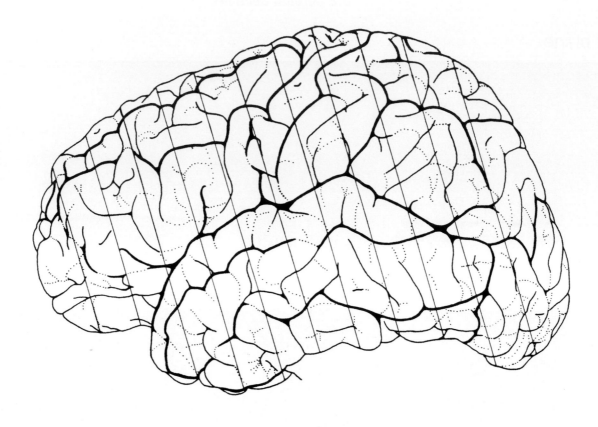

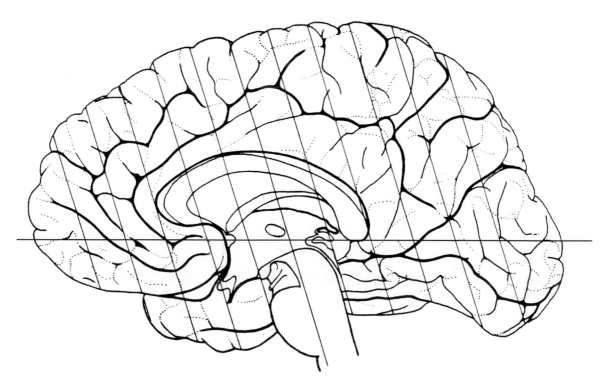

Surface views of the left hemisphere of the brain sectioned in the coronal plane (-20° angulation) as indicated. The drawing of the midsagittal view is mirror-imaged to help identify structures that lie in the same plane of sectioning as the lateral and median views.

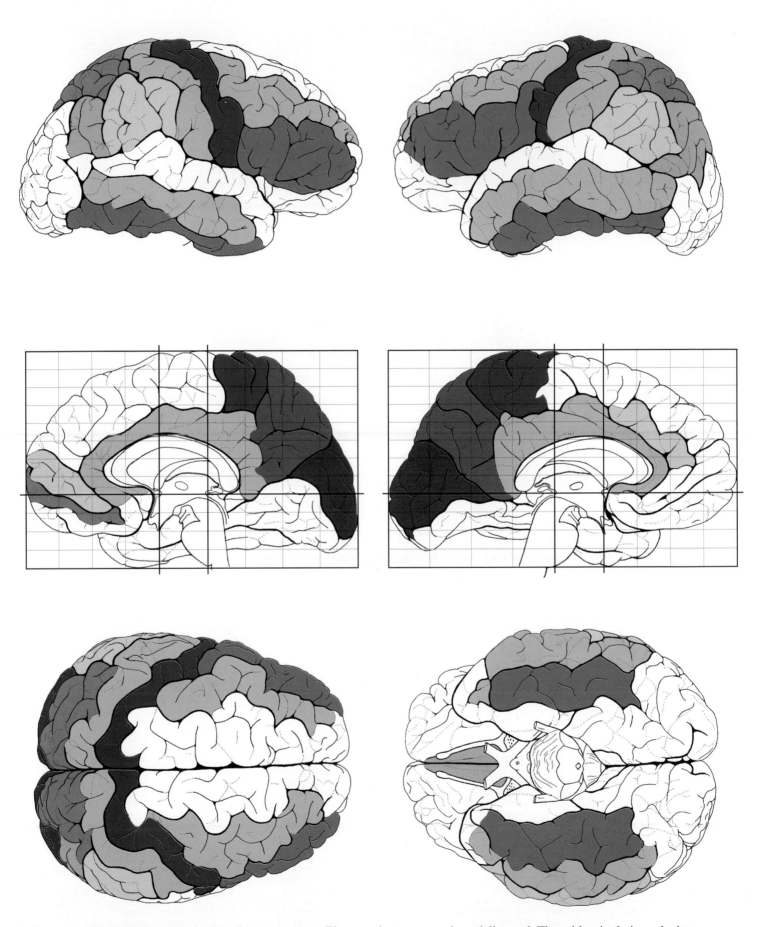

Surface views of the brain shown in the subsequent pages. The most important gyri are delineated. The midsagittal views depict the brain with the Talairach space.

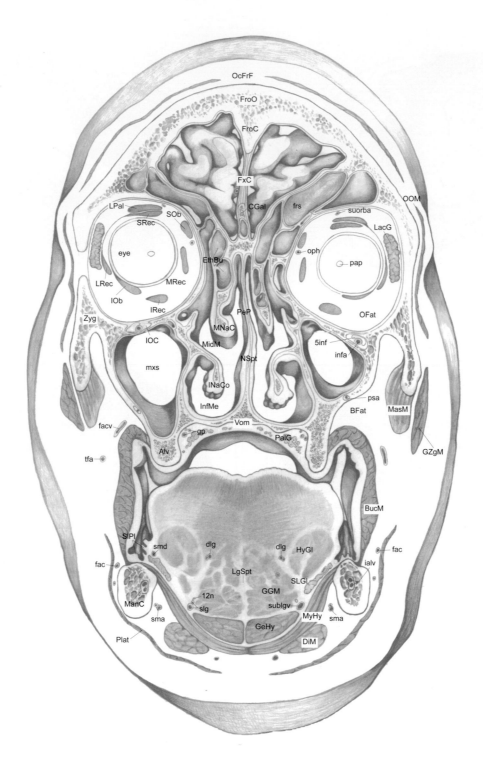

Section 4a:

12n	hypoglossal nerve (lingual branch)	GeHy	geniohyoid muscle	LPal	levator palpebrae superioris muscle	PeP	perpendicular plate
5inf	infraorbital nerve	GGM	genioglossus muscle	LRec	lateral rectus muscle	Plat	platysma
Alv	alveolar process of maxilla	gp	greater palatine artery	ManC	mandibular canal	psa	posterior superior alveolar artery
BFat	buccal fat pad	gpa	greater palatine artery, vein and	MasM	masseter muscle	slg	sublingual artery and vein
BucM	buccinator muscle		nerve	MidM	middle meatus of nasal cavity	SLGl	sublingual gland and duct
CGal	crista galli	GZgM	greater zygomatic muscle	MNaC	middle nasal concha	SlPl	sublingual plica
DiM	digastric muscle, ant. belly	HyGl	hyoglossus muscle	MRec	medial rectus muscle	sma	submental artery
dlg	deep lingual artery and vein	ialv	inferior alveolar artery and nerve	mxs	maxillary sinus	smd	submandibular duct
EthBu	ethmoidal bulla	INaCo	inferior nasal concha	MyHy	mylohyoid muscle	SOb	superior oblique muscle
eye	eye	infa	infraorbital artery	NSpt	nasal septum	SRec	superior rectus muscle
fac	facial artery	InfMe	inferior meatus of nasal cavity	OcFrF	occipito-frontal muscle, frontal belly	sublgv	sublingual vein
facv	facial vein	IOb	inferior oblique muscle	OFat	orbital fat pad	suorba	supraorbital artery
FroC	frontal bone, crest	IOC	infraorbital canal	OOM	orbicularis oculi muscle	tfa	transverse facial artery
FroO	frontal bone, orbital part	IRec	inferior rectus muscle	oph	ophthalmic artery	Vom	vomer
frs	frontal sinus	LacG	lacrimal gland	PalG	palatine glands	Zyg	zygomatic bone
FxC	falx cerebri	LgSpt	lingual septum	pap	optic papilla		

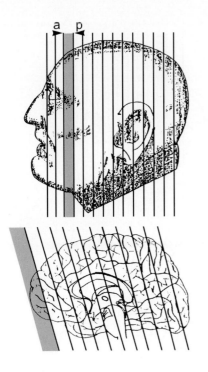

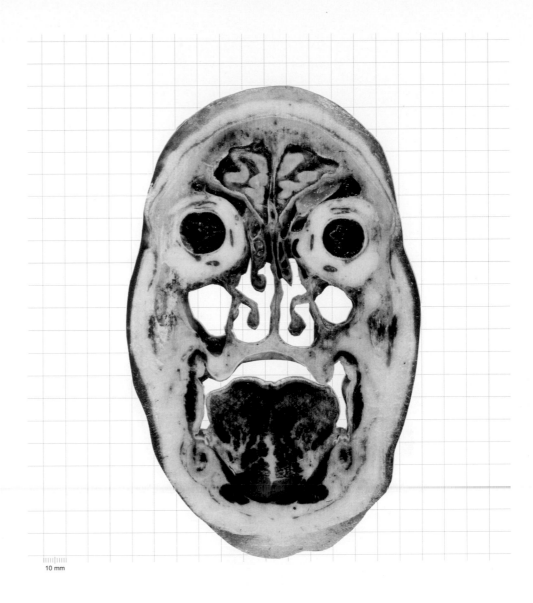

10 mm

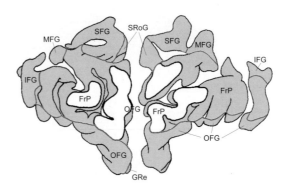

Section 4a:

FrP   frontopolar cortex
GRe   gyrus rectus
IFG   inferior frontal gyrus
MFG   medial frontal gyrus
OFG   orbitofrontal gyri
SFG   superior frontal gyrus
SRoG   superior rostral gyrus

MRI of the anterior surface of the 1-cm-thick section (see shaded areas in the upper inset). The labeled diagram (bottom) presents the brain contained in this section. The posterior side of the same 1-cm-thick tissue block is shown on the following page. The labeled diagram on the facing page is based on the photograph of the real section shown on this page.

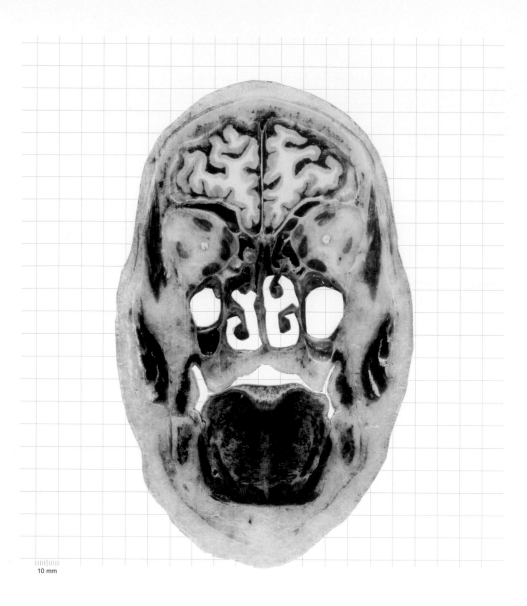

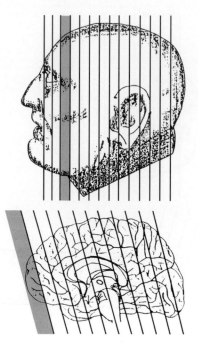

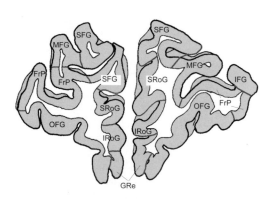

Opposite page: The four top panels depict MRIs of a 25-year-old volunteer presenting the same plane as the facing anatomical sections. Images present different proton-density, T_1, and T_2 contrast. The lower left panel is the radiograph of the anatomical section; the lower right panel shows the vasculature territory of the cerebral arteries in the brain slice contained in this section.

Section 4p:

FrP	frontopolar cortex
GRe	gyrus rectus
IFG	inferior frontal gyrus
IRoG	inferior rostral gyrus
MFG	medial frontal gyrus
OFG	orbitofrontal gyri
SFG	superior frontal gyrus
SRoG	superior rostral gyrus

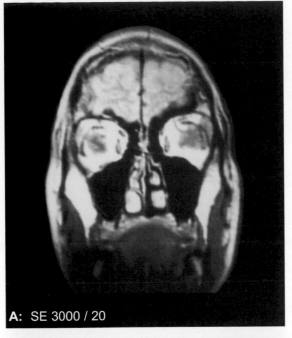

A: SE 3000 / 20

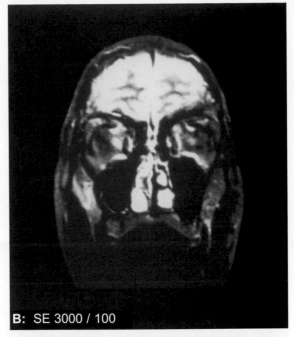

B: SE 3000 / 100

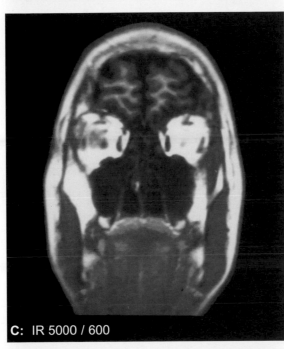

C: IR 5000 / 600

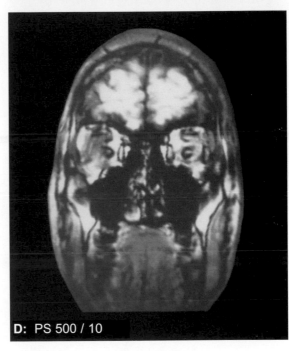

D: PS 500 / 10

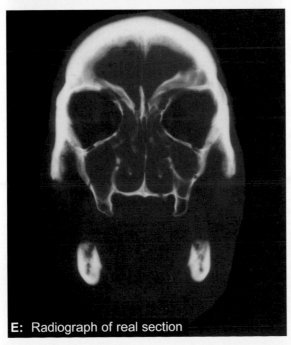

E: Radiograph of real section

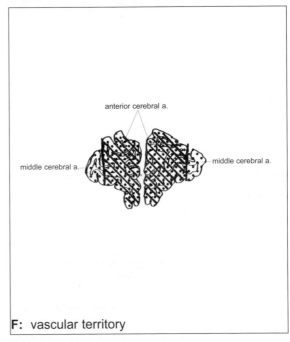

anterior cerebral a.

middle cerebral a.

middle cerebral a.

F: vascular territory

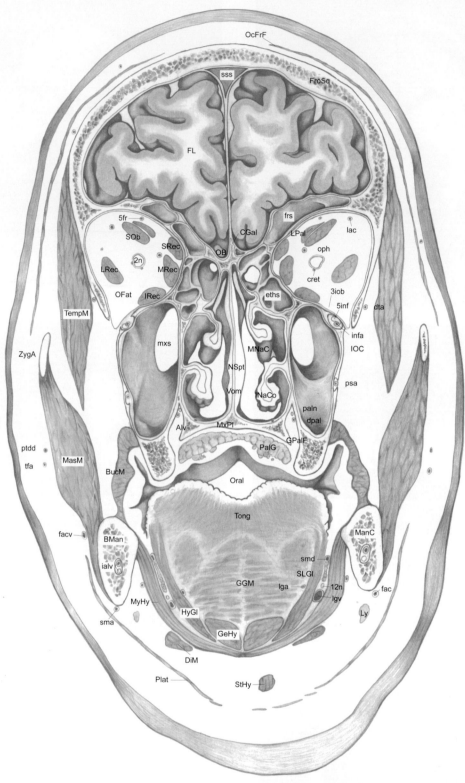

Section 5a:

12n	hypoglossal nerve or its root	FL	frontal lobe	LRec	lateral rectus muscle		
2n	optic nerve	FroSq	frontal bone, squamosal part	Ly	submental lymph node	Plat	platysma
3iob	oculomotor nerve, branches to inf. oblique muscle	frs	frontal sinus	ManC	mandibular canal	psa	posterior superior alveolar artery
		GeHy	geniohyoid muscle	MasM	masseter muscle	ptdd	parotid duct
5fr	frontal nerve of trigeminus	GGM	genioglossus muscle	MNaC	middle nasal concha	SLGl	sublingual gland
5inf	infraorbital nerve	GPalF	greater palatine foramen	MRec	medial rectus muscle	sma	submental artery
Alv	alveolar process of maxilla	HyGl	hyoglossus muscle	MxPl	maxilla, palatine process	smd	submandibular duct
BMan	body of mandible	ialv	inferior alveolar artery, vein and nerve	mxs	maxillary sinus	SOb	superior oblique muscle
BucM	buccinator muscle	INaCo	inferior nasal concha	MyHy	mylohyoid muscle	SRec	superior rectus muscle
CGal	crista galli	infa	infraorbital artery	NSpt	nasal septum	sss	superior sagittal sinus
cret	central artery of retina	IOb	inferior oblique muscle	OB	olfactory bulb	StHy	sternohyoid muscle
DiM	digastric muscle, ant. belly	IOC	infraorbital canal	OcFrF	occipito-frontal muscle, frontal belly	TempM	temporalis muscle
dpal	descending palatine artery	IRec	inferior rectus muscle	OFat	orbital fat	tfa	transverse facial artery
dta	deep temporal artery (arteries)	lac	lacrimal artery	oph	ophthalmic artery	Tong	intrinsic muscles of the tongue
eths	ethmoidal sinus (cells)	lga	lingual artery	Oral	oral cavity	Vom	vomer
fac	facial artery	lgv	lingual vein	PalG	palatine glands	ZygA	zygomatic arch
facv	facial vein	LPal	levator palpebrae superioris muscle	paln	palatine nerve (s)		

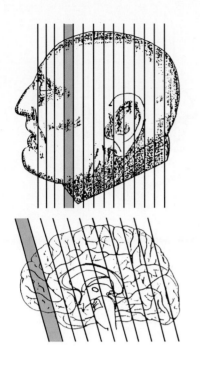

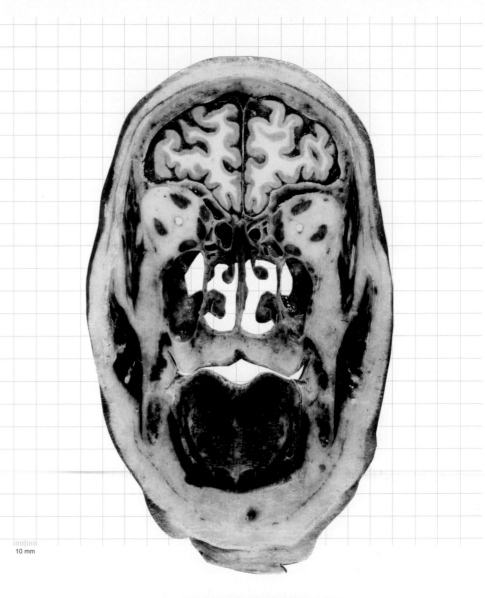

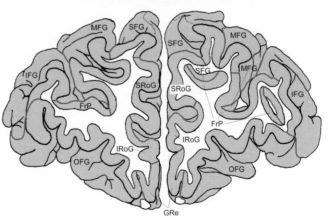

Section 5a:

FrP	frontopolar cortex
GRe	gyrus rectus
IFG	inferior frontal gyrus
IRoG	inferior rostral gyrus
MFG	medial frontal gyrus
OFG	orbitofrontal gyri
SFG	superior frontal gyrus
SRoG	superior rostral gyrus

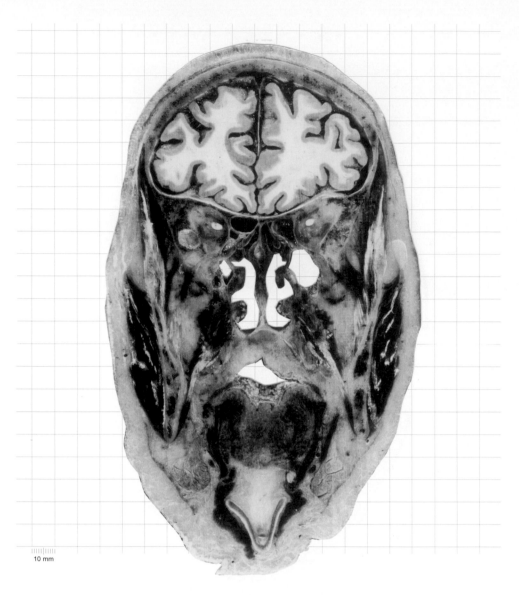

10 mm

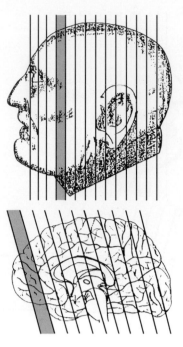

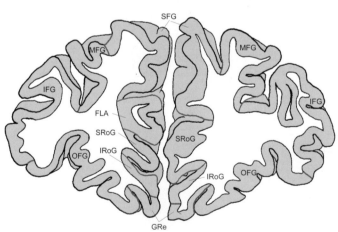

Section 5p:

FLA	frontal limbic area
IFG	inferior frontal gyrus
MFG	medial frontal gyrus
OFG	orbitofrontal gyri
GRe	gyrus rectus
IRoG	inferior rostral gyrus
SFG	superior frontal gyrus
SRoG	superior rostral gyrus

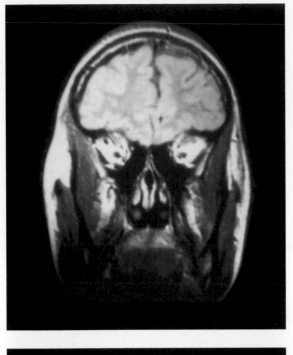

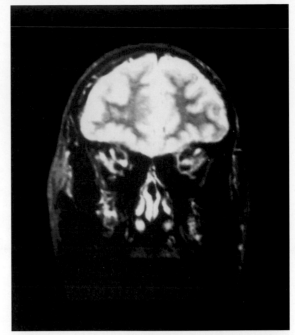

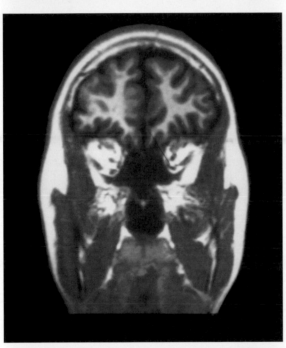

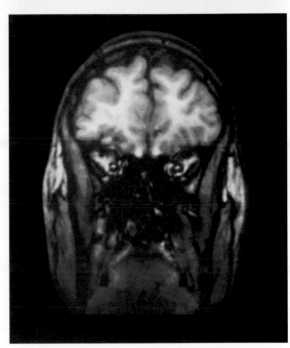

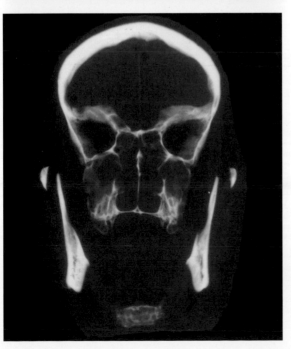

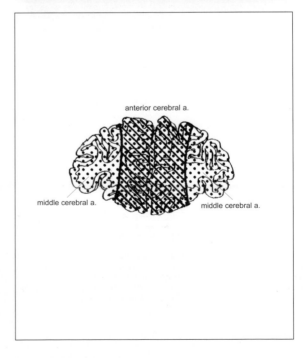

anterior cerebral a.

middle cerebral a.

middle cerebral a.

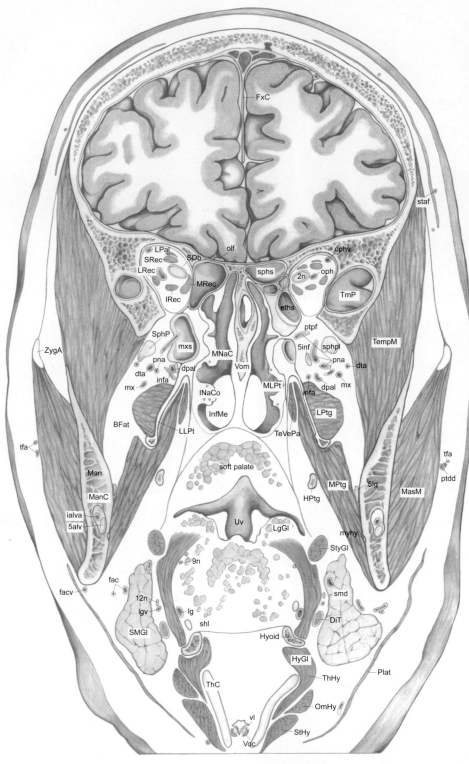

Section 6a:

12n	hypoglossal nerve or its root	ialva	inferior alveolar artery	MRec	medial rectus muscle	sphs	sphenoid sinus
2n	optic nerve	INaCo	inferior nasal concha	mx	maxillary artery	SRec	superior rectus muscle
5alv	inferior alveolar nerve	infa	infraorbital artery	mxs	maxillary sinus	staf	superior temporal artery, frontal
5lg	lingual nerve	InfMe	inferior meatus of nasal cavity	myhy	mylohyoid nerve		branch
5inf	infraorbital nerve	IRec	inferior rectus muscle	olf	olfactory tract	StHy	sternohyoid muscle
9n	glossopharyngeal nerve	lg	lingual artery	OmHy	omohyoid muscle	StyGl	styloglossus muscle
BFat	buccal fat pad	LgGl	lingual gland	oph	ophthalmic artery	TempM	temporalis muscle
DiT	digastric muscle, tendon	lgv	lingual vein	ophv	ophthalmic vein	TeVePa	tensor veli palatini muscle
dpal	descending palatine artery	LLPt	lateral lamina of pterygoid process	Plat	platysma	tfa	transverse facial artery and vein
dta	deep temporal artery (arteries)	LPal	levator palpebrae superioris muscle	pna	posterior nasal artery	ThC	thyroid cartilage
eths	ethmoidal sinus (labyrinth and air cells)	LPtg	lateral pterygoid muscle	ptdd	parotid duct	ThHy	thyrohyoid muscle
fac	facial artery	LRec	lateral rectus muscle	ptpf	pterygopalatine fossa	TmP	temporal pole
facv	facial vein	Man	mandible	shl	stylohyoid ligament	Uv	uvula
FxC	falx cerebri	ManC	mandibular canal	smd	submandibular duct	vl	vocal ligament
HPtg	pterygoid hamulus see hamulus of	MasM	masseter muscle	SMGl	submandibular gland	Voc	vocalis muscle
	the pterygoid bone	MLPt	medial lamina of pterygoid process	SOb	superior oblique muscle	Vom	vomer
HyGl	hyoglossus muscle	MNaC	middle nasal concha	SphP	sphenopalatine ganglion	ZygA	zygomatic arch
Hyoid	hyoid bone	MPtg	medial pterygoid muscle	sphpl	sphenopalatine artery		

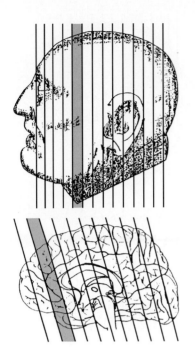

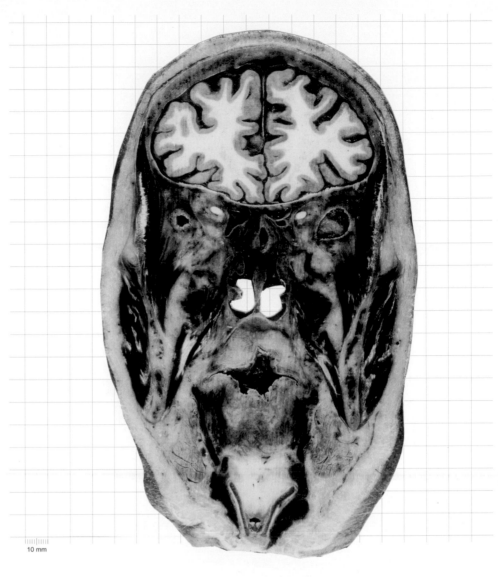

10 mm

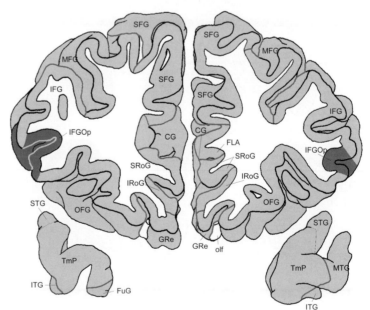

Section 6a:

CG	cingulate gyrus
GRe	gyrus rectus
IFG	inferior frontal gyrus
IFGOp	inferior frontal gyrus, opercular part
IRoG	inferior rostral gyrus
ITG	inferior temporal gyrus
FLA	frontal limbic area
FuG	fusiform gyrus
MFG	medial frontal gyrus
MTG	medial temporal gyrus
OFG	orbitofrontal gyri
olf	olfactory tract
SFG	superior frontal gyrus
SRoG	superior rostral gyrus
STG	superior temporal gyrus
TmP	temporal pole

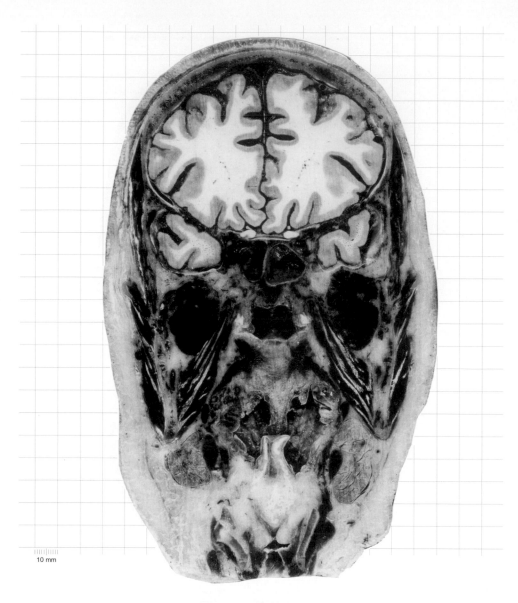

10 mm

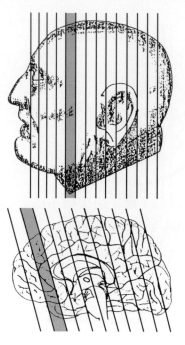

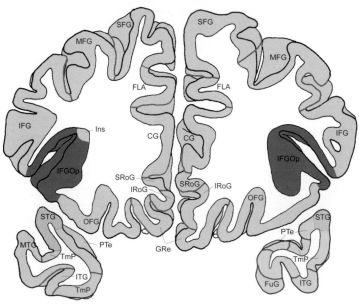

Section 6p:

CG	cingulate gyrus
FLA	frontal limbic area
FuG	fusiform gyrus
GRe	gyrus rectus
IFG	inferior frontal gyrus
IFGOp	inferior frontal gyrus, opercular part
IRoG	inferior rostral gyrus
Ins	insula
ITG	inferior temporal gyrus
MFG	medial frontal gyrus
MTG	medial temporal gyrus
OFG	orbitofrontal gyri
PTe	planum temporale
SFG	superior frontal gyrus
SRoG	superior rostral gyrus
STG	superior temporal gyrus
TmP	temporal pole

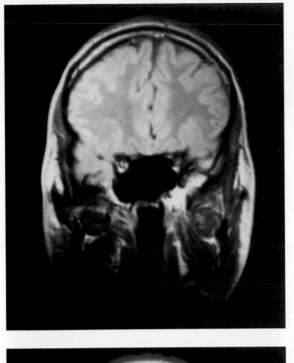

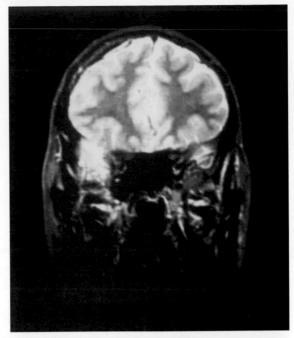

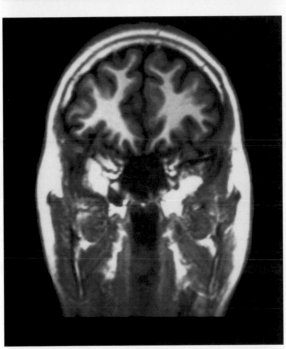

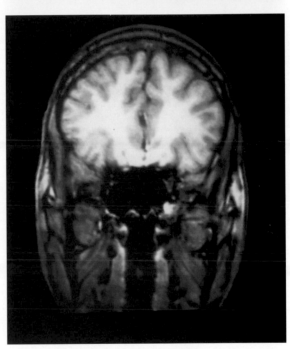

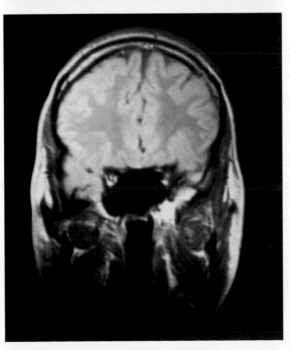

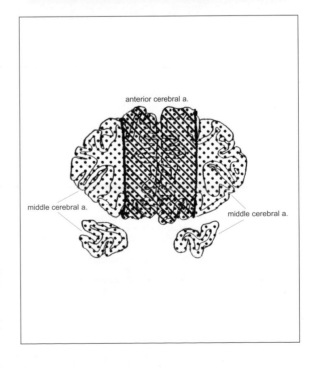

anterior cerebral a.

middle cerebral a.   middle cerebral a.

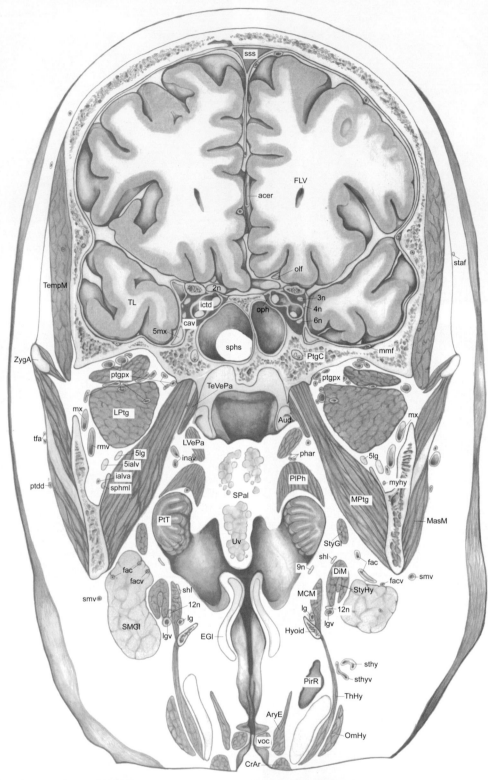

Section 7a:

12n	hypoglossal nerve or its root	facv	facial vein	olf	olfactory tract	
2n	optic nerve	FLV	frontal horn of lateral ventricle	OmHy	omohyoid muscle	
3n	oculomotor nerve or its root	Hyoid	hyoid bone	oph	ophthalmic artery	sss superior sagittal sinus
4n	trochlear nerve or its root	ialva	inferior alveolar artery	phar	pharyngeal branches	staf superficial temporal artery, frontal root
5ialv	inferior alveolar nerve	ictd	internal carotid artery	PirR	piriform recess	sthy superior thyroid artery
5lg	lingual nerve	lg	lingual artery	PlPh	palatopharyngeus muscle	sthyv superior thyroid vein
5mx	maxillary nerve of the trigeminal	lgv	lingual vein	ptdd	parotid duct	StyGl styloglossus muscle
6n	abducens nerve or its root	LPtg	lateral pterygoid muscle	PtgC	pterygoid canal	StyHy stylohyoid muscle
9n	glossopharyngeal nerve	LVePa	levator veli palatini muscle	ptgpx	pterygoid plexus	TempM temporalis muscle
acer	anterior cerebral artery	MasM	masseter muscle	PtT	palatine tonsil	TeVePa tensor palatini muscle
AryE	aryepiglotticus muscle	MCM	medial constrictor muscle of pharynx	rmv	retromandibular vein	tfa transverse facial artery and vein
Aud	auditory tube			shl	stylohyoid ligament	ThHy thyrohyoid muscle
cav	cavernous sinus	mmf	middle meningeal artery, frontal branch	SMGl	submandibular gland	TL temporal lobe
CrAr	cricoarytenoid muscle, lat. portion			smv	submental vein	Uv uvula
DiM	digastric muscle, post belly	MPtg	medial pterygoid muscle	SPal	soft palate	voc vocalis muscle
EGl	epiglottis	mx	maxillary artery	sphml	sphenomandibular ligament	ZygA zygomatic arch
fac	facial artery	myhy	mylohyoid nerve	sphs	sphenoid sinus	

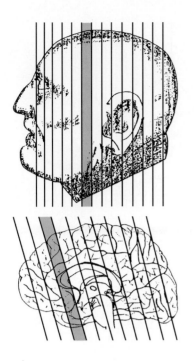

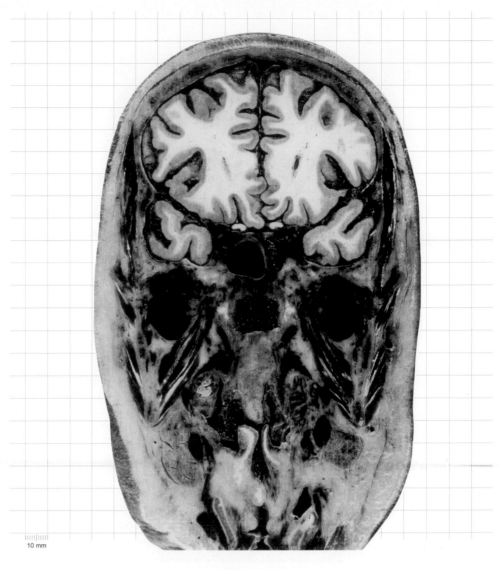

10 mm

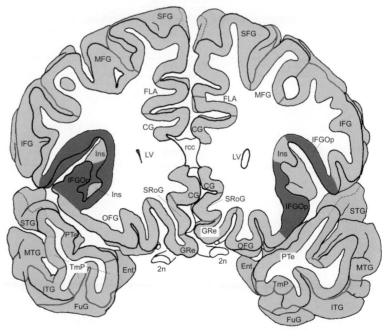

Section 7a:

2n	optic nerve
CG	cingulate gyrus
Ent	entorhinal cortex
FLA	frontal limbic area
FuG	fusiform gyrus
GRe	gyrus rectus
IFG	inferior frontal gyrus
IFGOp	inferior frontal gyrus, opercular part
Ins	insula
ITG	inferior temporal gyrus
LV	lateral ventricle
MFG	medial frontal gyrus
MTG	medial temporal gyrus
OFG	orbitofrontal gyri
PTe	planum temporale
rcc	rostrum of corpus callosum
SFG	superior frontal gyrus
SRoG	superior rostral gyrus
STG	superior temporal gyrus
TmP	temporal pole

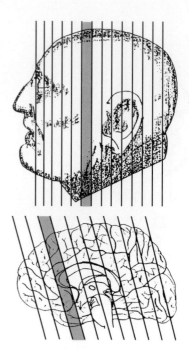

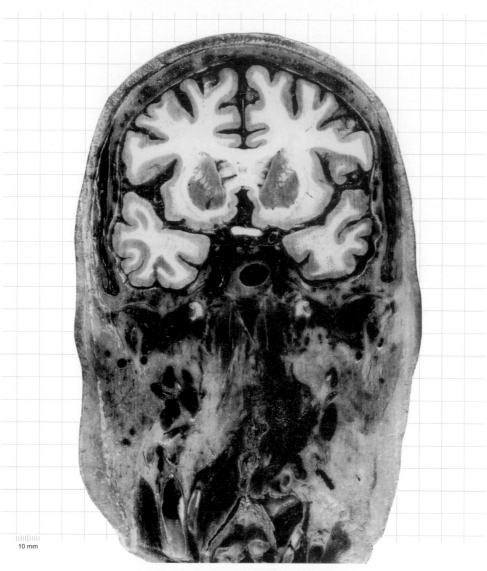

10 mm

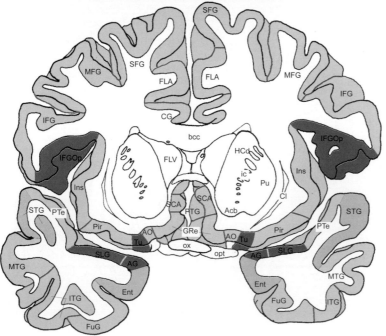

Section 7p:

Acb	accumbens nucleus
AG	ambiens gyrus
AO	anterior olfactory nucleus
bcc	body of corpus callosum
CG	cingulate gyrus
Cl	claustrum
Ent	entorhinal cortex
FLA	frontal limbic area
FLV	frontal horn of lateral ventricle
FuG	fusiform gyrus
GRe	gyrus rectus
HCd	head of caudate nucleus
ic	internal capsule
IFG	inferior frontal gyrus
IFGOp	inferior frontal gyrus, opercular part
Ins	insula
ITG	inferior temporal gyrus
MFG	medial frontal gyrus
MTG	medial temporal gyrus
opt	optic tract
ox	optic chiasm
Pir	piriform cortex
PTe	planum temporale
PTG	paraterminal gyrus
Pu	putamen
SCA	subcallosal area
SFG	superior frontal gyrus
SLG	semilunar gyrus
STG	superior temporal gyrus
Tu	olfactory tubercle

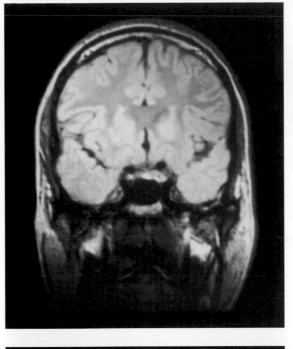

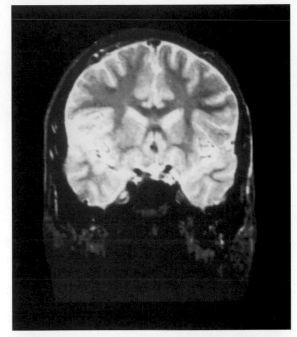

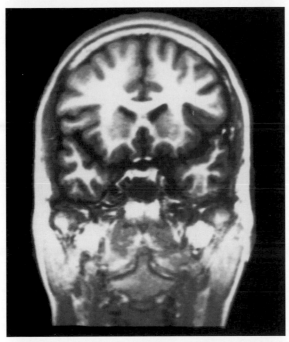

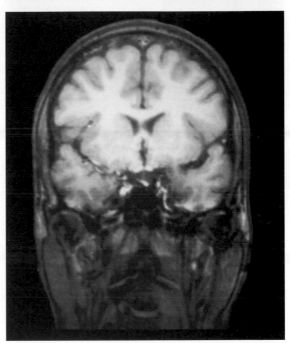

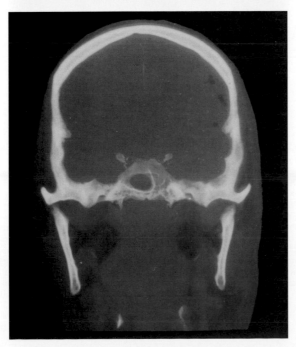

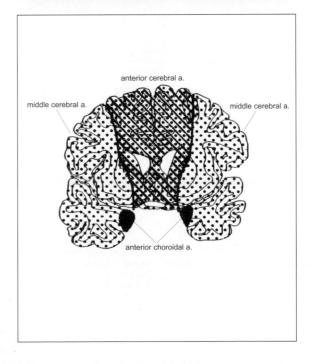

anterior cerebral a.

middle cerebral a.

middle cerebral a.

anterior choroidal a.

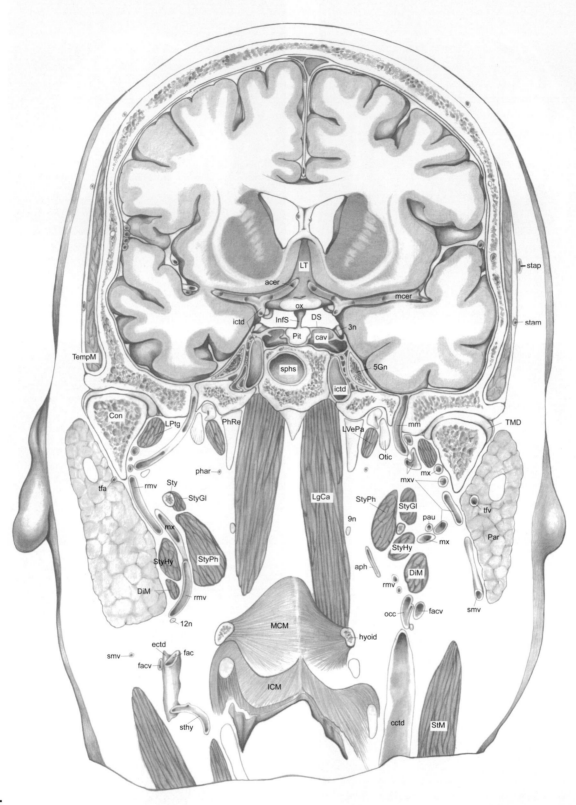

Section 8a:

12n	hypoglossal nerve or its root	facv	facial vein	mx	maxillary artery	stam	superficial temporal artery, median root
3n	oculomotor nerve or its root	ICM	inferior constrictor muscle of pharynx	mxv	maxillary vein		
5Gn	trigeminal ganglion			occ	occipital artery	stap	superficial temporal artery, parietal root
9n	glossopharyngeal nerve	ictd	internal carotid artery	Otic	otic ganglion		
acer	anterior cerebral artery	InfS	infundibular stalk	ox	optic chiasm	sthy	superior thyroid artery
aph	ascending pharyngeal artery	LgCa	longus capitis muscle	Par	patotid gland	StM	sternomastoid muscle
cav	cavernous sinus	LPtg	lateral pterygoid muscle	pau	posterior auricular artery	Sty	styloid process
cctd	common carotid artery	LT	lamina terminalis	phar	pharyngeal branches	StyGl	styloglossus muscle
Con	condylar process of mandible	LVePa	levator veli palatini muscle	PhRe	pharyngeal recess	StyHy	stylohyoid muscle
DiM	digastric muscle, post belly	mcer	middle cerebral artery	Pit	pituitary gland	StyPh	stylopharyngeus muscle
DS	diaphragma sellae	MCM	medial constrictor muscle of pharynx	rmv	retromandibular vein	TempM	temporalis muscle
ectd	external carotid artery			smv	submental vein	tfa	transverse facial artery
fac	facial artery	mm	middle meningeal artery	sphs	sphenoid sinus	tfv	transverse facial vein
						TMD	temporomandibular disc

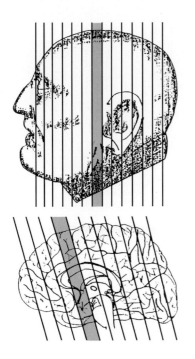

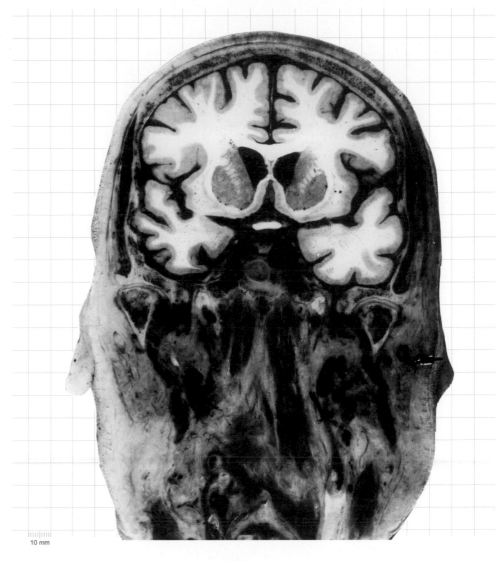

10 mm

Section 8a:

AG   ambiens gyrus
bcc   body of corpus callosum
CG   cingulate gyrus
Cl   claustrum
DB   diagonal band nucleus
ec   external capsule
Ent   entorhinal cortex
ex   extreme capsule
FLA   frontal limbic area
FLV   frontal horn of lateral ventricle
FuG   fusiform gyrus
HCd   head of caudate nucleus
IFG   inferior frontal gyrus
IFGOp   inferior frontal gyrus, opercular part
Ins   insula
ITG   inferior temporal gyrus
MFG   middle frontal gyrus
MTG   middle temporal gyrus
ox   optic chiasm
Pir   piriform cortex
PTe   planum temporale
PTG   paraterminal gyrus
Pu   putamen
SFG   superior frontal gyrus
SLG   semilunar gyrus
SptP   septum pellucidum
STG   superior temporal gyrus
Tu   olfactory tubercle
Un   uncus

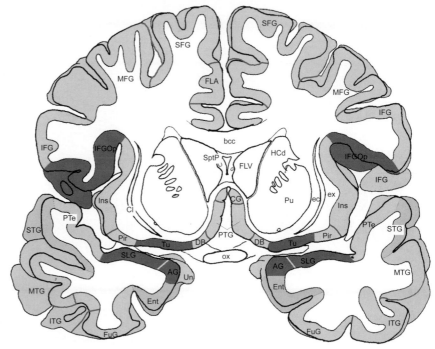

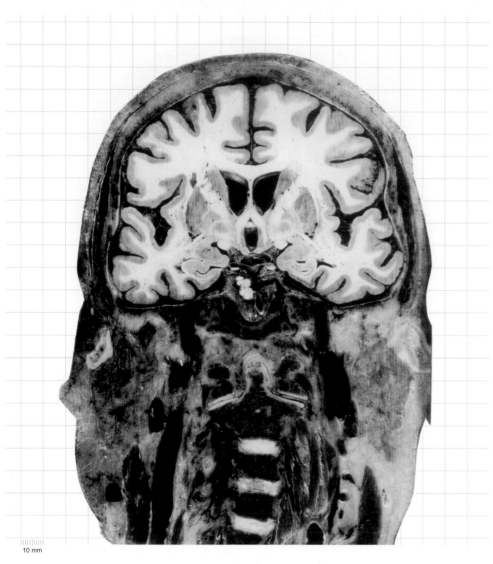

10 mm

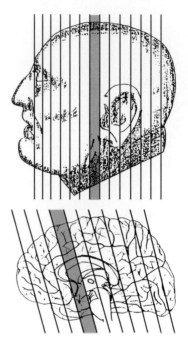

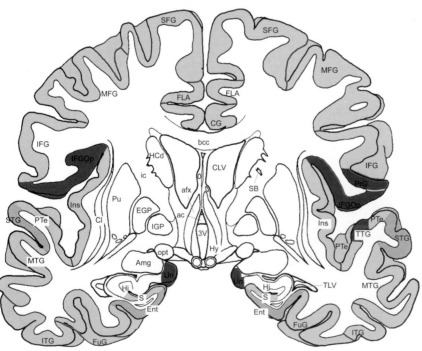

Section 8p:

3V	third ventricle
ac	anterior commissure
afx	anterior column of fornix
Amg	amygdala
bcc	body of corpus callosum
CG	cingulate gyrus
Cl	claustrum
CLV	central part of lateral ventricle
EGP	external globus pallidus
Ent	entorhinal cortex
FLA	frontal limbic area
FuG	fusiform gyrus
HCd	head of caudate nucleus
Hi	hippocampus
Hy	hypothalamus
ic	internal capsule
IFG	inferior frontal gyrus
IFGOp	inferior frontal gyrus, opercular part
IGP	internal globus pallidus
Ins	insula
ITG	inferior temporal gyrus
MFG	middle frontal gyrus
MTG	middle temporal gyrus
opt	optic tract
PrG	precentral gyrus
PTe	planum temporale
Pu	putamen
S	subiculum
SB	striatal cell bridges
SFG	superior frontal gyrus
STG	superior temporal gyrus
TLV	temporal horn of lateral ventricle
TTG	transverse temporal gyri
Un	uncus

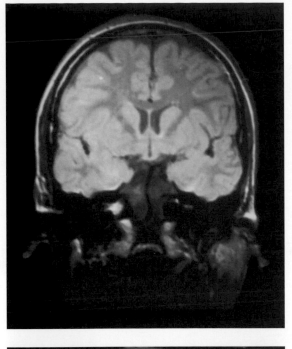

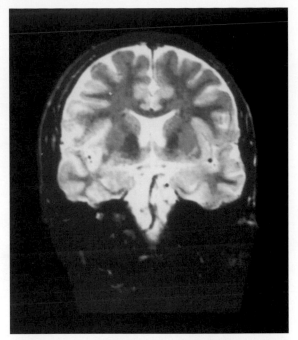

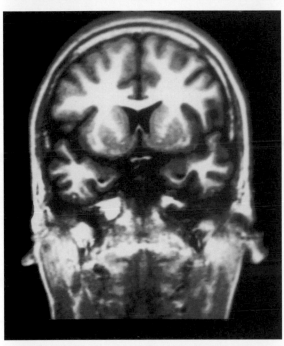

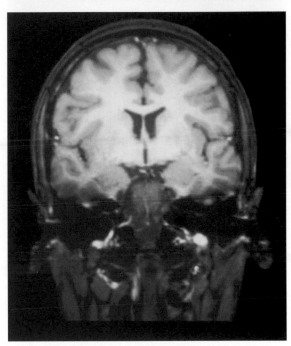

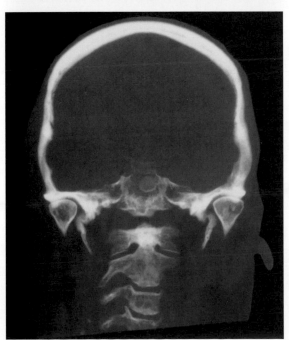

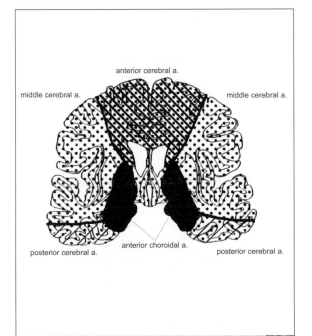

anterior cerebral a.

middle cerebral a.   middle cerebral a.

posterior cerebral a.   anterior choroidal a.   posterior cerebral a.

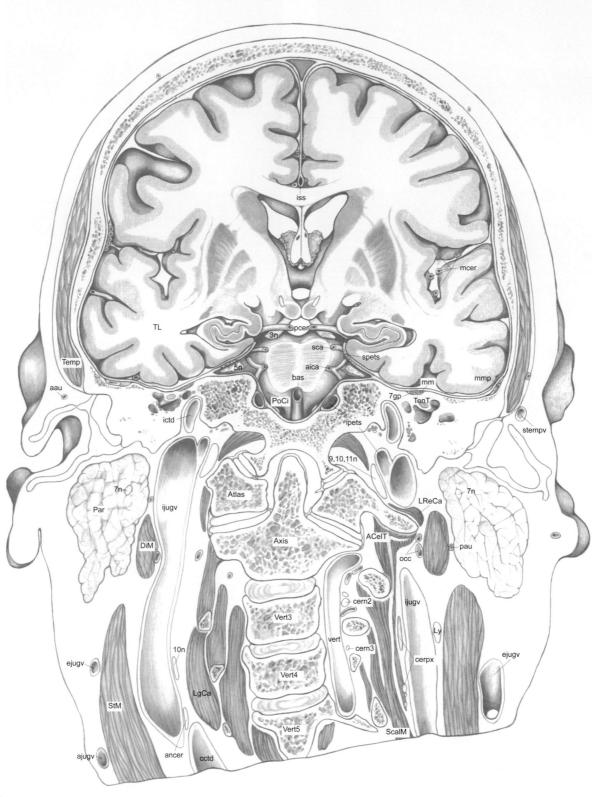

Section 9a:

10n	vagus nerve	Atlas	atlas (C1 vertebra)	LgCa	longus capitis muscle	PoCi	pontine cistern
3n	oculomotor nerve or its root	Axis	axis (C2 vertebra)	LReCa	lateral rectus capitis muscle	sca	superior cerebellar artery
5n	trigeminal nerve	bas	basilar artery	Ly	lymph node	ScalM	scalenus muscle
7gp	greater petrosal nerve	cctd	common carotid artery	mcer	middle cerebral artery (silvian	spets	superior petrosal sinus
7n	facial nerve	cern2	cervical nerve 2		branches in insular cistern)	stempv	superficial temporal vein
9,10,11n	glossopharyngeal, vagus and	cern3	cervical nerve 3	mm	middle meningeal artery,	StM	sternomastoid muscle
	accessory nerves	cerpx	cervical plexus		petrosal branch	Temp	temporal bone
aau	anterior auricular artery	DiM	digastric muscle, post belly	mmp	middle meningeal artery, parietal	TenT	tensor tympani muscle
ACeIT	anterior cervical	ejugv	external jugular vein		branch	TL	temporal lobe
	intertransversarii muscle	ictd	internal carotid artery	occ	occipital artery	vert	vertebral artery
aica	anterior inferior cerebellar artery	ijugv	internal jugular vein	Par	parotid gland	Vert3	vertebra 3
ajugv	anterior jugular vein	ipets	inferior petrosal sinus	pau	posterior auricular artery	Vert4	vertebra 4
ancer	ansa cervicalis	iss	inferior sagittal sinus	pcer	posterior cerebral artery	Vert5	vertebra 5

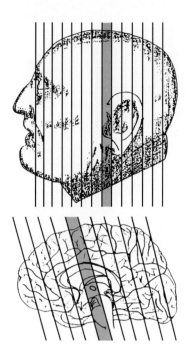

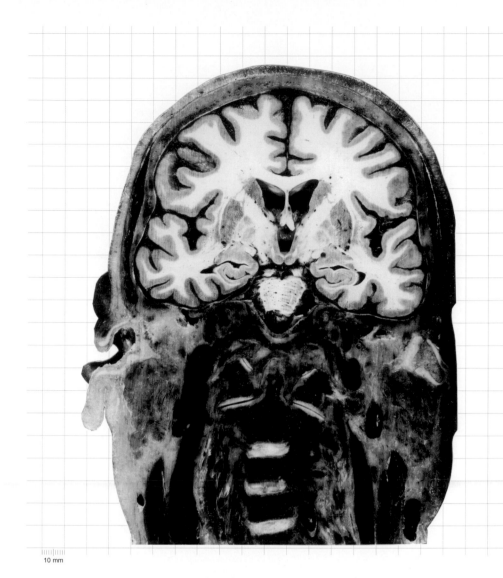

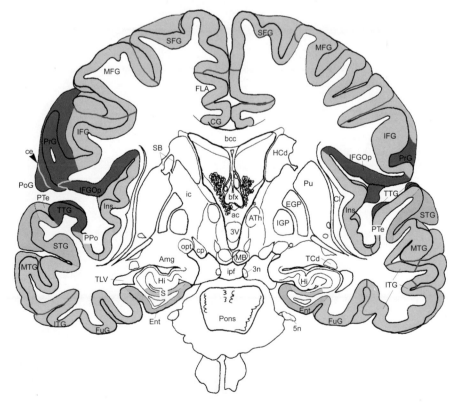

Section 9a:

3n	oculomotor nerve
3V	third ventricle
5n	trigeminal nerve
ac	anterior commissure
Amg	amygdala
ATh	anterior thalamic nucleus
bcc	body of corpus callosum
bfx	body of fornix
ce	central sulcus
CG	cingulate gyrus
Cl	claustrum
cp	cerebral peduncle
EGP	external globus pallidus
Ent	entorhinal cortex
FLA	frontal limbic area
FuG	fusiform gyrus
HCd	head of caudate nucleus
Hi	hippocampus
ic	internal capsule
IFG	inferior frontal gyrus
IFGOp	inferior frontal gyrus, opercular part
IGP	internal globus pallidus
Ins	insula
ipf	interpeduncular fossa
ITG	inferior temporal gyrus
MB	mammillary body
MFG	middle frontal gyrus
MTG	middle temporal gyrus
opt	optic tract
PoG	postcentral gyrus
Pons	pons
PPo	planum polare
PrG	precentral gyrus
PTe	planum temporale
Pu	putamen
S	subiculum
SB	striatal cell bridges
SFG	superior frontal gyrus
STG	superior temporal gyrus
TCd	tail of caudate nucleus
TLV	temporal horn of lateral ventricle
TTG	transverse temporal gyri

10 mm

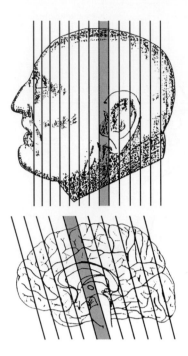

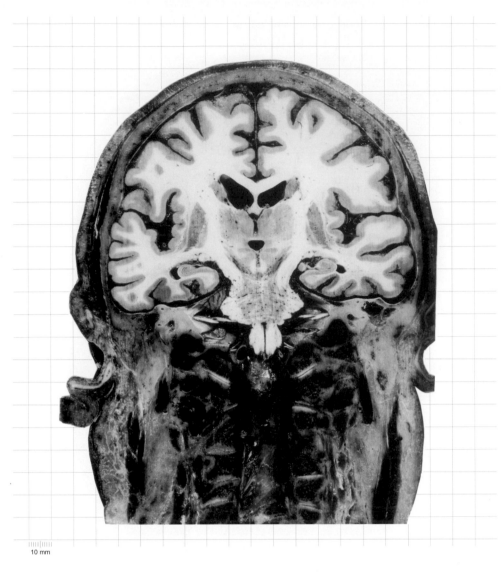

10 mm

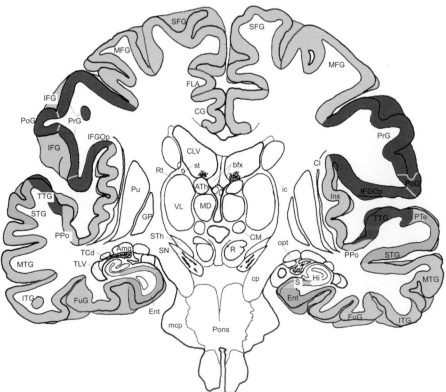

Section 9p:

Amg	amygdala
ATh	anterior thalamic nucleus
bfx	body of fornix
CG	cingulate gyrus
Cl	claustrum
CLV	central part (body) of lateral ventricle
CM	central medial thalamic nucleus
cp	cerebral peduncle
Ent	entorhinal cortex
FLA	frontal limbic area
FuG	fusiform gyrus
GP	globus pallidus
Hi	hippocampus
ic	internal capsule
IFG	inferior frontal gyrus
Ins	insula
ITG	inferior temporal gyrus
ITGOp	inferior frontal gyrus, opercular part
mcp	middle cerebellar peduncle
MD	medial dorsal thalamic nucleus
MFG	medial frontal gyrus
MTG	medial temporal gyrus
opt	optic tract
PoG	postcentral gyrus
Pons	pons
PPo	planum polare
PrG	precentral gyrus
PTe	planum temporale
Pu	putamen
R	red nucleus
Rt	reticular thalamic nucleus
S	subiculum
SFG	superior frontal gyrus
SN	substantia nigra
st	stria terminalis
STG	superior temporal gyrus
STh	subthalamic nucleus
TCd	tail of caudate nucleus
TLV	temporal horn of lateral ventricle
TTG	transverse temporal gyri
VL	ventral lateral thalamic nucleus

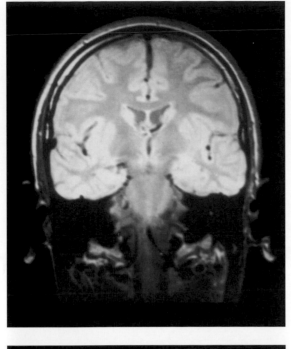

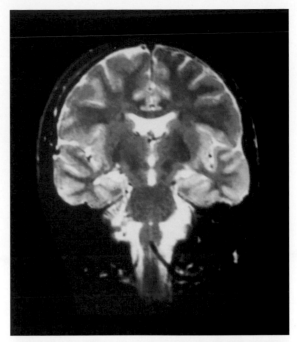

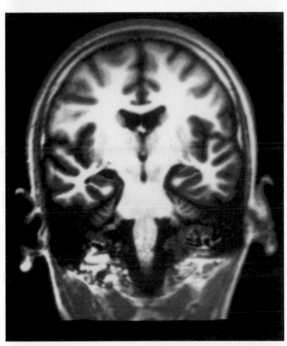

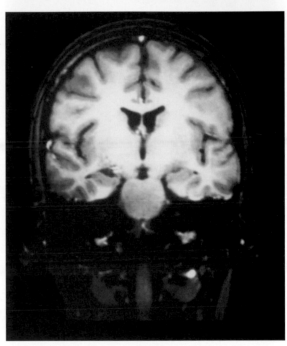

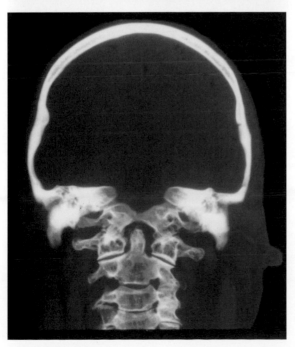

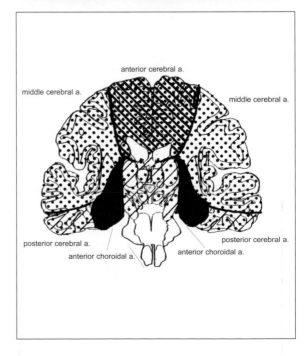

anterior cerebral a.

middle cerebral a.

middle cerebral a.

posterior cerebral a.

posterior cerebral a.

anterior choroidal a.

anterior choroidal a.

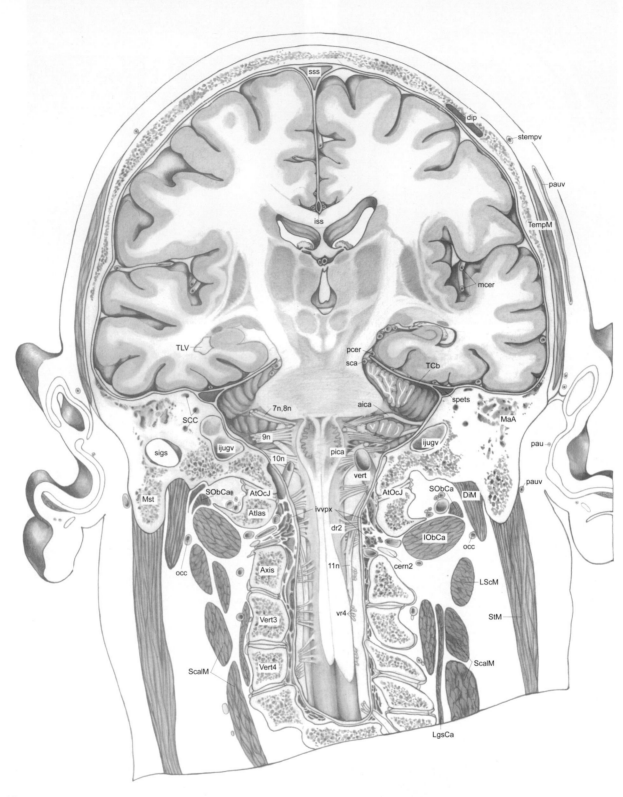

Section 10a:

10n	vagus nerve	dr2	dorsal root (C2)	occ	occipital artery and vein		
11n	spinal accessory nerve	ijugv	internal jugular vein, bulbus	pau	posterior auricular artery		
7n	facial nerve or its root	IObCa	inferior oblique capitis muscle	pauv	posterior auricular vein	sss	superior sagittal sinus
8n	vestibulocochlear nerve	iss	inferior sagittal sinus	pcer	posterior cerebral artery	stempv	superficial temporal vein
9n	glossopharyngeal nerve	ivvpx	internal vertebral venous plexus	pica	posterior inferior cerebellar	StM	sternomastoid muscle
aica	anterior inferior cerebellar artery	LgsCa	longissimus capitis muscle		artery	TCb	tentorium cerebelli
Atlas	atlas (C1 vertebra)	LScM	levator scapulae muscle	sca	superior cerebellar artery	TempM	temporalis muscle
AtOcJ	atlanto occipital joint	MaA	mastoid antrum	ScalM	scalenus muscle	TLV	temporal horn of lateral ventricle
Axis	axis (C2 vertebra)	mcer	middle cerebral artery (silvian	SCC	semicircular canals	vert	vertebral artery
cern2	cervical nerve 2		branches in insular cistern)	sigs	sigmoid sinus	Vert3	vertebra 3
DiM	digastric muscle, post belly	Mst	mastoid process of temporal	SObCa	superior oblique capitis muscle	Vert4	vertebra 4
dip	diploic vein		bone	spets	superior petrosal sinus	vr4	ventral root (C4)

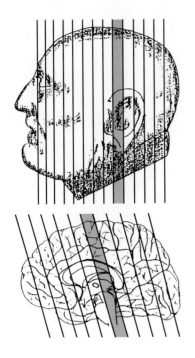

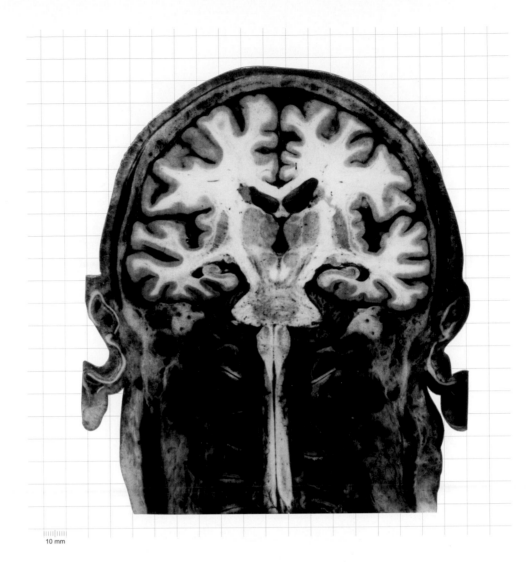

10 mm

Section 10a:

Amg	amygdala
3V	third ventricle
bfx	body of fornix
cc	corpus callosum
CG	cingulate gyrus
CH	cerebellar hemisphere
chp	choroid plexus
CLV	central part of lateral ventricle
cp	cerebral peduncle
Cl	claustrum
CM	central medial thalamic nucleus
Ent	entorhinal cortex
FuG	fusiform gyrus
GP	globus pallidus
Hi	hippocampus
ic	internal capsule
IFG	inferior frontal gyrus
IFGOp	inferior frontal gyrus, opercular part
Ins	insular gyri
IO	inferior olive
ITG	inferior temporal gyrus
LD	lateral dorsal thalamic nucleus
mcp	middle cerebellar peduncle
MD	medial dorsal thalamic nucleus
MFG	middle frontal gyrus
MTG	middle temporal gyrus
opt	optic tract
PoG	postcentral gyrus
PrG	precentral gyrus
Pons	pons
PTe	planum temporale
Pu	putamen
py	pyramidal tract
R	red nucleus
Rt	reticular thalamic nucleus
S	subiculum
SB	striatal cell bridges
SFG	superior frontal gyrus
SN	substantia nigra
STG	superior temporal gyrus
STh	subthalamic nucleus
TCd	tail of caudate nucleus
TLV	temporal horn of lateral ventricle
TTG	transverse temporal gyri
VL	ventral lateral thalamic nucleus

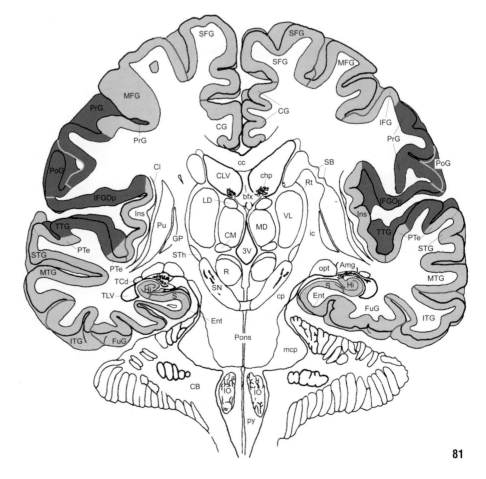

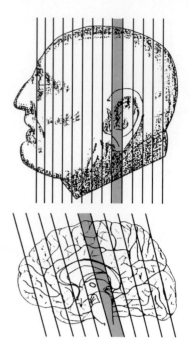

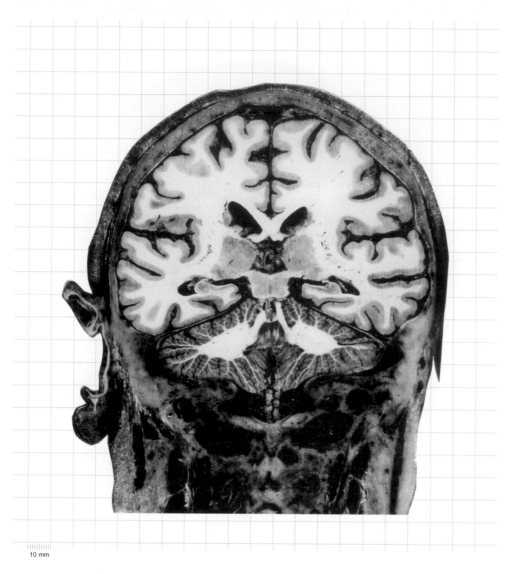

10 mm

82

Section 10p:

3V	third ventricle
4V	fourth ventricle
bcc	body of corpus callosum
BCd	body of caudate nucleus
bfx	body of fornix
CH	cerebellar hemisphere
CG	cingulate gyrus
Ent	entorhinal cortex
FuG	fusiform gyrus
Hi	hippocampus
IFGOp	inferior frontal gyrus, opercular part
Ins	insula
ITG	inferior temporal gyrus
LV	lateral ventricle
MFG	medial frontal gyrus
MTG	medial temporal gyrus
OcG	occipital gyrus
Pi	pineal gland
PoG	postcentral gyrus
PrG	precentral gyrus
PTe	planum temporale
Pul	pulvinar thalami
Rt	reticular thalamic nucleus
SB	striatal cell bridges
scp	superior cerebellar peduncle
SFG	inferior frontal gyrus
SMV	superior medullary velum
STG	superior temporal gyrus
TCd	tail of caudate nucleus
Tec	tectum
TLV	temporal horn of lateral ventricle
tsv	thalamostriate vein
TTG	transverse temporal gyri
Ver	vermis of cerebellum

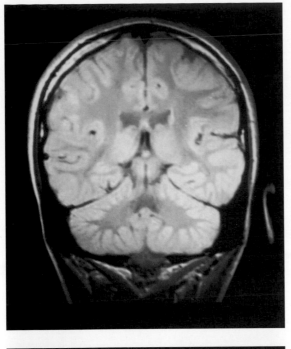

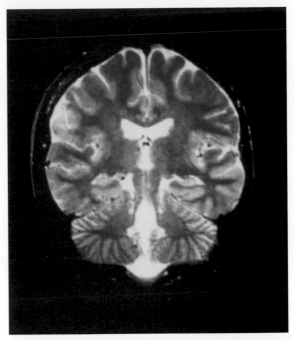

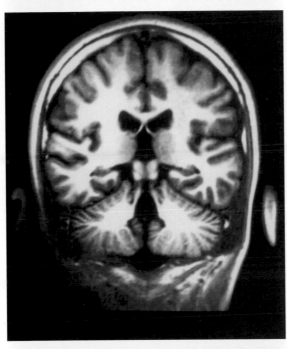

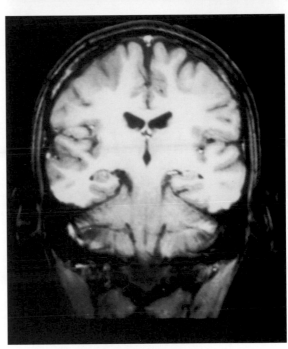

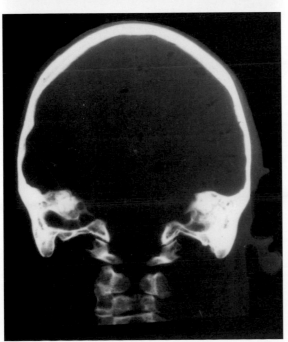

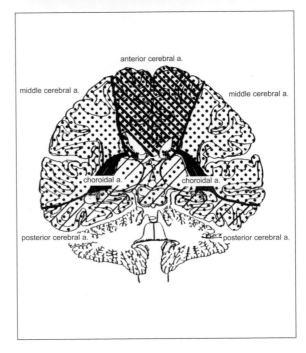

anterior cerebral a.

middle cerebral a.   middle cerebral a.

choroidal a.   choroidal a.

posterior cerebral a.   posterior cerebral a.

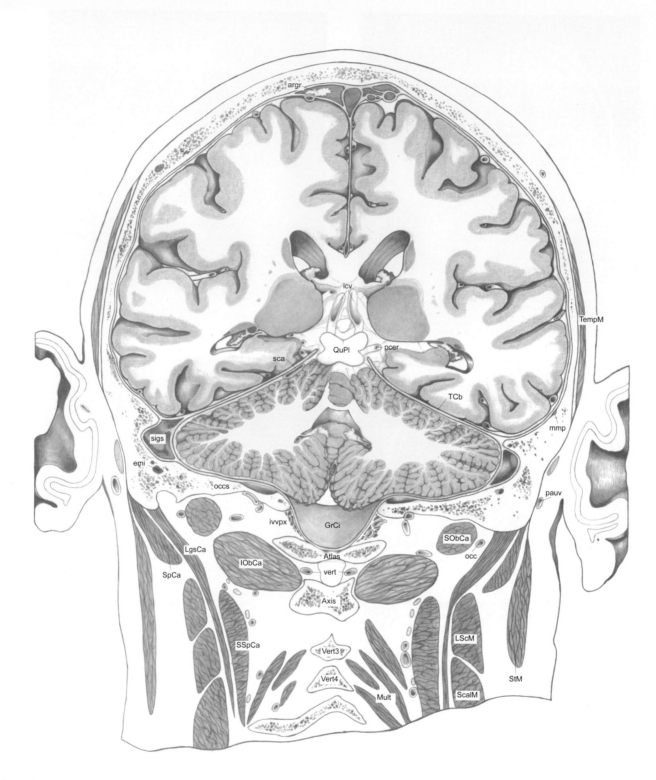

Section 11a:

argr	arachnoid granulations	ivvpx	internal vertebral venous plexus	pauv	posterior auricular vein
Atlas	atlas (C1 vertebra)	LgsCa	longissimus capitis muscle	pcer	posterior cerebral artery
Axis	axis (C2 vertebra)	LScM	levator scapulae muscle	QuPl	quadrigeminal plate
emi	emissary vein, (mastoid)	mmp	middle meningeal artery, parietal	ScalM	scalenus muscle
GrCi	great (cerebellomedullary)		branch	sigs	sigmoid sinus
	cistern	Mult	multifidus muscle	SObCa	superior oblique capitis muscle
icv	internal cerebral vein	occ	occipital artery	SpCa	splenius capitis muscle
IObCa	inferior oblique capitis muscle	occs	occipital sinus	SSpCa	semispinal capitis muscle

StM	sternomastoid muscle
TCb	tentorium cerebelli
TempM	temporalis muscle
vert	vertebral artery
Vert3	vertebra 3
Vert4	vertebra 4

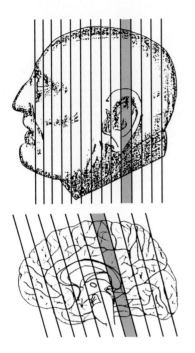

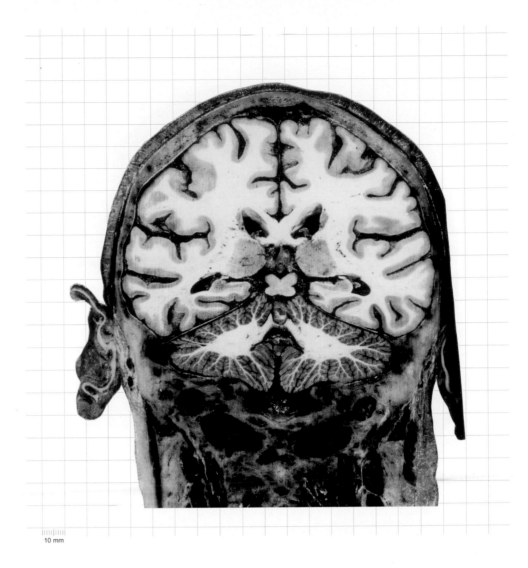

10 mm

Section 11a:

CG — cingulate gyrus
CH — cerebellar hemisphere
Ent — entorhinal cortex
FuG — fusiform gyrus
fx — fornix
Hi — hippocampus
IFGOp — inferior frontal gyrus, opercular part
Ins — insula
ITG — inferior temporal gyrus
LV — lateral ventricle
MFG — medial frontal gyrus
MTG — medial temporal gyrus
OcG — occipital gyri
PCL — paracentral lobule
Pi — pineal gland
PoG — postcentral gyrus
PrG — precentral gyrus
PTe — planum temporale
Pul — pulvinar thalami
QuPl — quadrigeminal plate
Rt — reticular thalamic nucleus
S — subiculum
scc — splenium of corpus callosum
SFG — superior frontal gyrus
st — stria terminalis
STG — superior temporal gyrus
TCd — tail of caudate nucleus
TLV — temporal horn of lateral ventricle
TTG — transverse temporal gyri

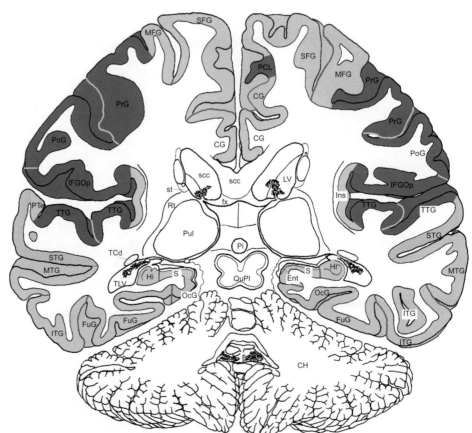

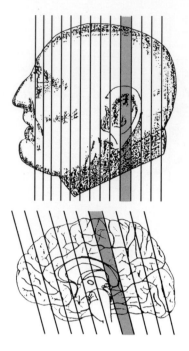

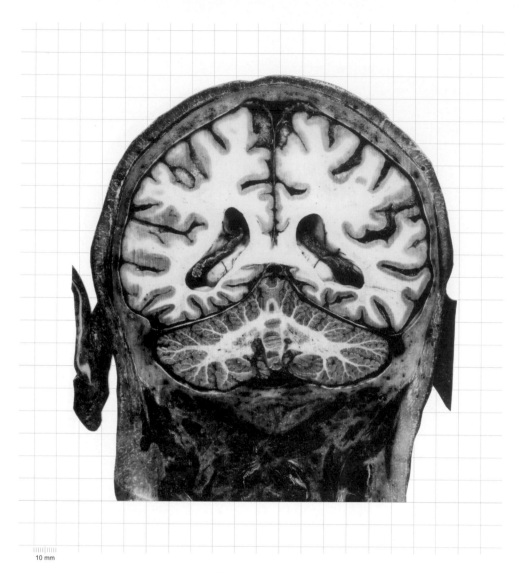

10 mm

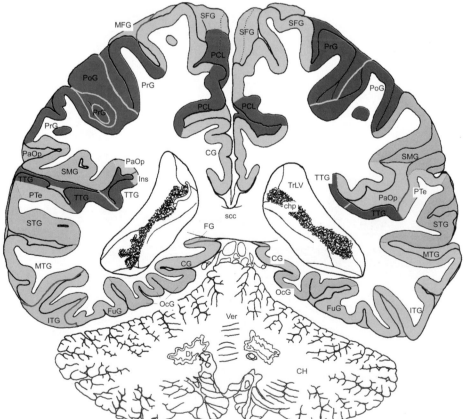

Section 11p:

CG   cingulate gyrus
CH   cerebellar hemisphere
chp   choroid plexus
Dt   dentate nucleus
FG   fasciolar gyrus
FuG   fusiform gyrus
Ins   insula
ITG   inferior temporal gyrus
MFG   medial frontal gyrus
MTG   medial temporal gyrus
OcG   occipital gyri
PaOp   parietal operculum
PCL   paracentral lobule
PoG   postcentral gyrus
PrG   precentral gyrus
PTe   planum temporale
scc   splenium of corpus callosum
SFG   superior frontal gyrus
SMG   supramarginal gyrus
STG   superior temporal gyrus
TrLV   trigone of lateral ventricle
TTG   transverse temporal gyri
Ver   vermis of cerebellum

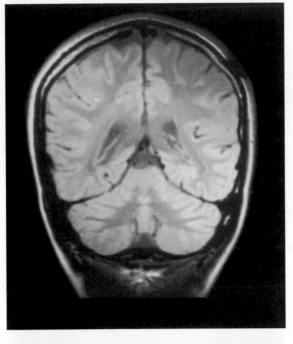

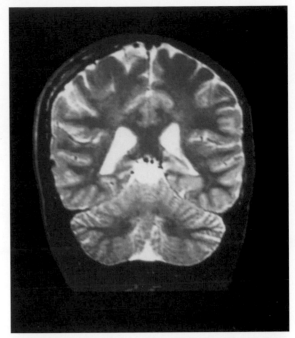

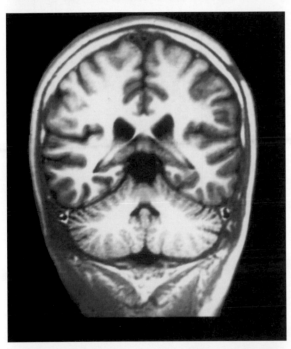

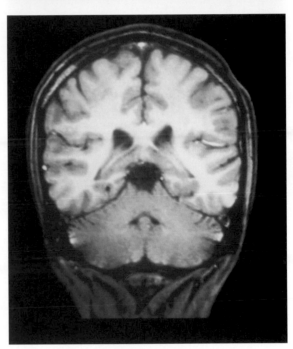

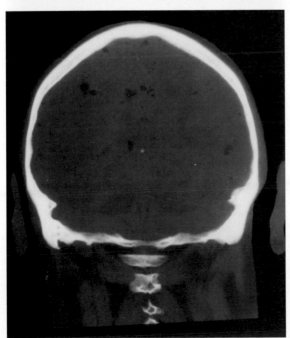

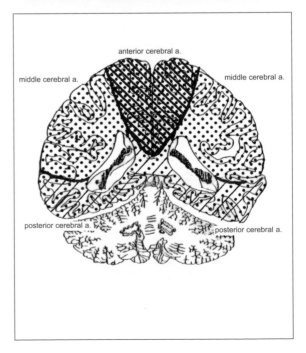

anterior cerebral a.

middle cerebral a.   middle cerebral a.

posterior cerebral a.   posterior cerebral a.

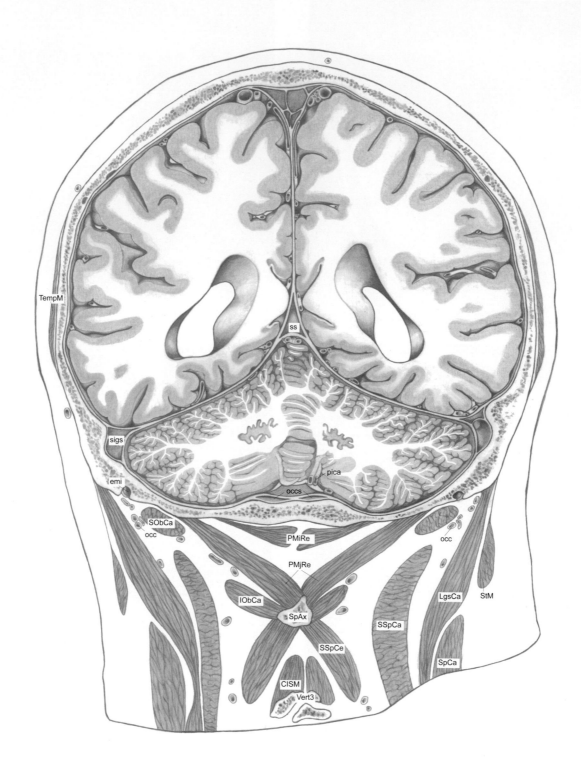

Section 12a:

CISM	cervical interspinal muscle	pica	posterior inferior cerebellar	sigs	sigmoid sinus		
emi	emissary vein, (mastoid)		artery	SObCa	superior oblique capitis muscle		
IObCa	inferior oblique capitis muscle	PMiRe	posterior minor rectus capitis	SpAx	spinous process of axis	SSpCe	semispinal cervicis muscle
LgsCa	longissimus capitis muscle		muscle	SpCa	splenius capitis muscle	StM	sternomastoid muscle
occ	occipital artery	PMjRe	posterior major rectus capitis	ss	straight sinus	TempM	temporalis muscle
occs	occipital sinus		muscle	SSpCa	semispinal capitis muscle	Vert3	vertebra

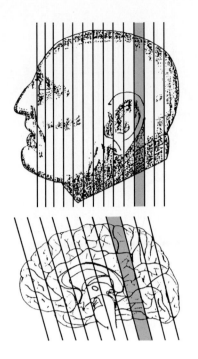

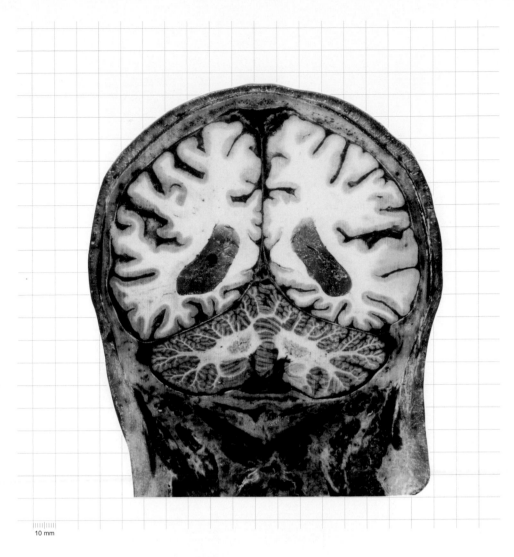

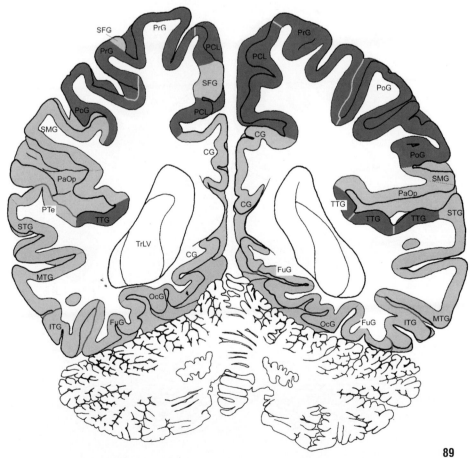

Section 12a:

CG   cingulate gyrus
FuG   fusiform gyrus
ITG   inferior temporal gyrus
MTG   medial temporal gyrus
OcG   occipital gyri
PaOp   parietal operculum
PCL   paracentral lobule
PoG   postcentral gyrus
PrG   precentral gyrus
PTe   planum temporale
SFG   superior frontal gyrus
SMG   supramarginal gyrus
STG   superior temporal gyrus
TrLV   trigone of lateral ventricle
TTG   transverse temporal gyrus (1,2,3)

10 mm

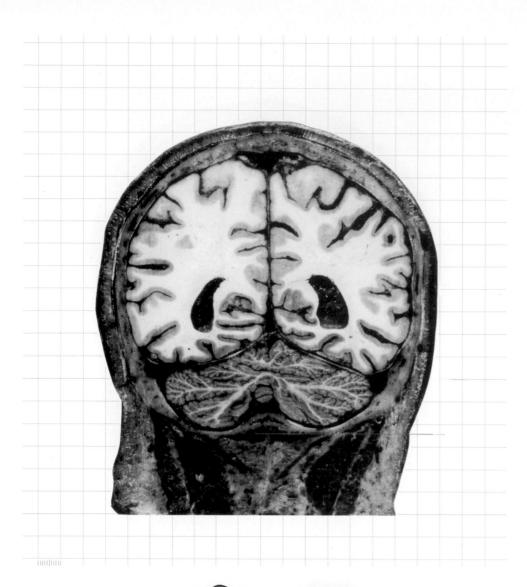

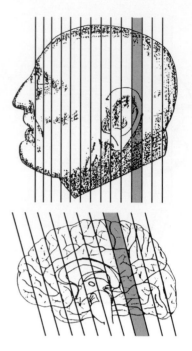

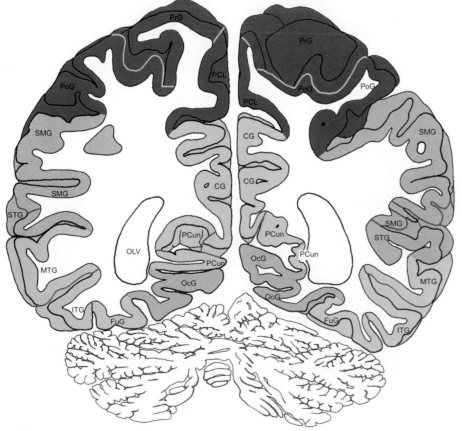

Section 12p:

CG	cingulate gyrus
Cun	cuneus
FuG	fusiform gyrus
ITG	inferior temporal gyrus
MTG	medial temporal gyrus
OcG	occipital gyri
OLV	occipital horn of lateral ventricle
PCL	paracentral lobule
PCun	precuneus
PoG	postcentral gyrus
PrG	precentral gyrus
SMG	supramarginal gyrus
STG	superior temporal gyrus

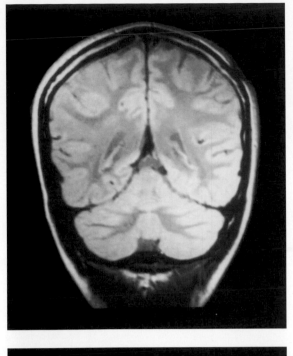

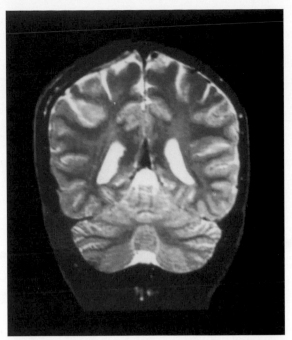

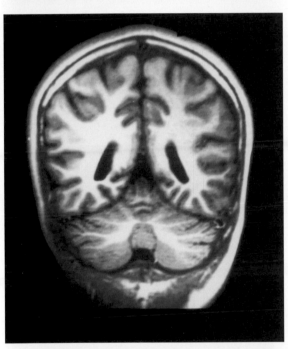

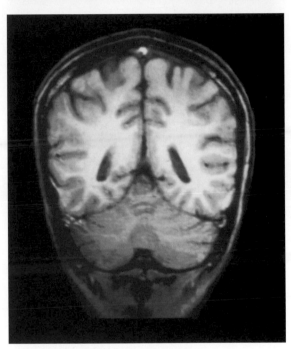

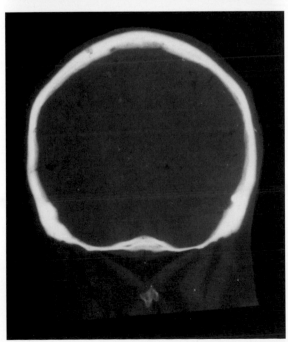

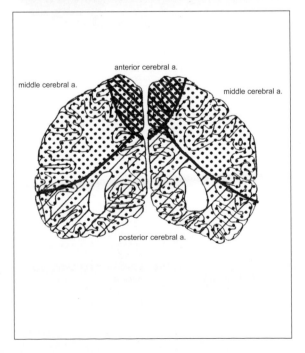

middle cerebral a.

anterior cerebral a.

middle cerebral a.

posterior cerebral a.

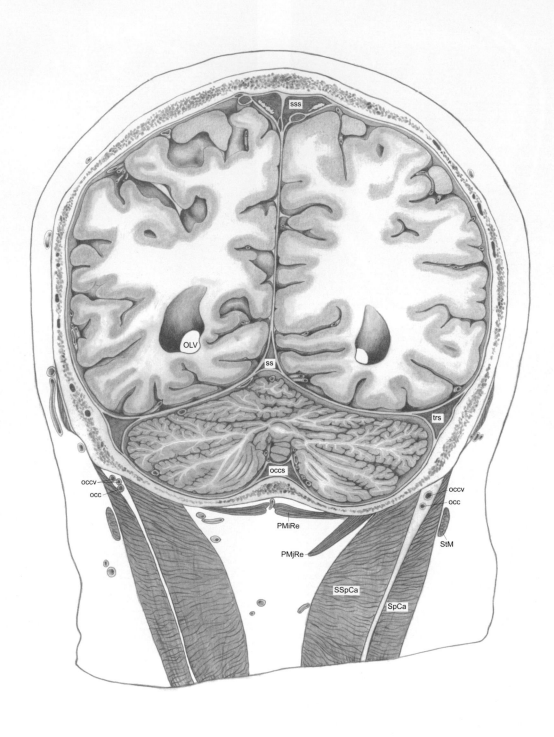

Section 13a:

occ	occipital artery	PMiRe	posterior minor rectus capitis muscle	SpCa	splenius capitis muscle		
occs	occipital sinus			ss	straight sinus	StM	sternomastoid muscle
occv	occipital vein	PMjRe	posterior major rectus capitis muscle	SSpCa	semispinal capitis muscle	trs	transverse sinus
OLV	occipital horn of lateral ventricle			sss	superior sagittal sinus		

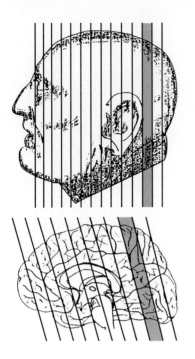

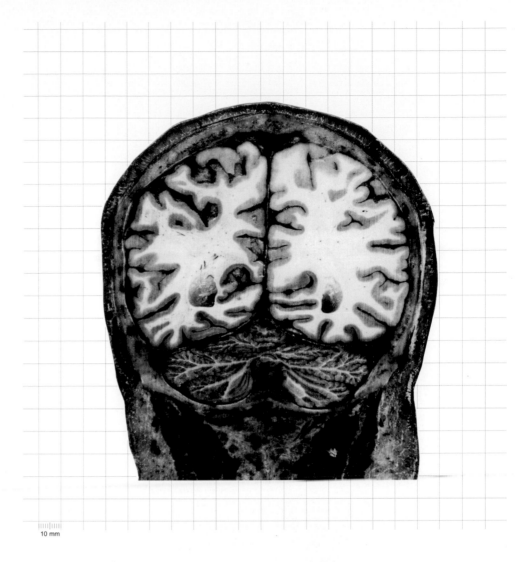

10 mm

Section 13a:

Ang   angular gyrus
CG   cingulate gyrus
Cun   cuneus
FuG   fusiform gyrus
ITG   inferior temporal gyrus
MTG   medial temporal gyrus
OcG   occipital gyri
OLV   occipital horn of lateral ventricle
PCL   paracentral lobule
PCun   precuneus
PoG   postcentral gyrus
PrG   precentral gyrus
SMG   supramarginal gyrus
SPL   superior parietal lobule
STG   superior temporal gyrus

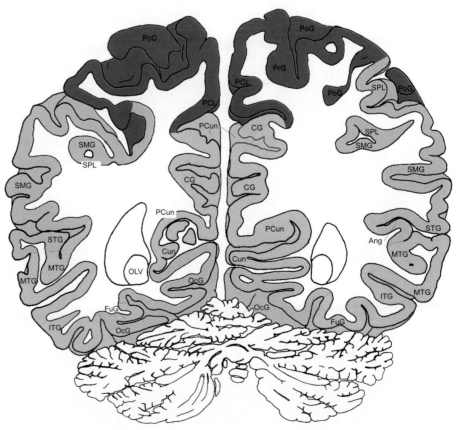

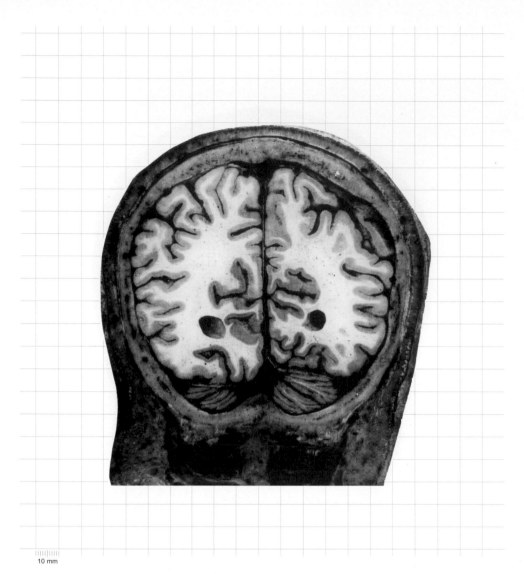

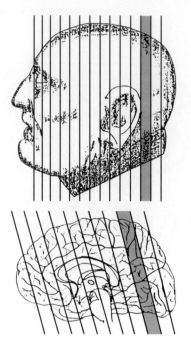

10 mm

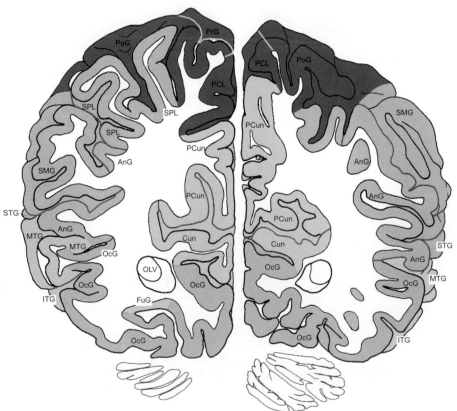

Section 13p:

AnG	angular gyrus
Cun	cuneus
FuG	fusiform gyrus
ITG	inferior temporal gyrus
MTG	medial temporal gyrus
OcG	occipital gyri
OLV	occipital horn of lateral ventricle
PCL	paracentral lobule
PCun	precuneus
PoG	postcentral gyrus
PrG	precentral gyrus
SMG	supramarginal gyrus
SPL	superior parietal lobule
STG	superior temporal gyrus

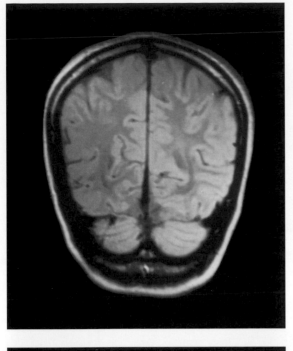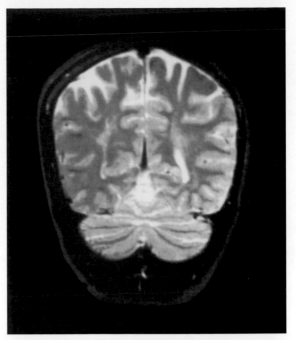

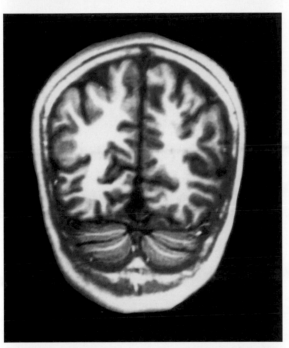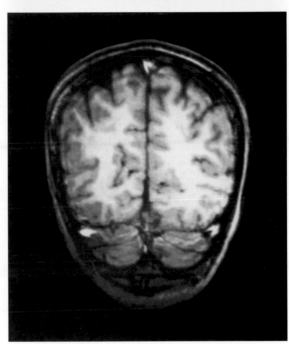

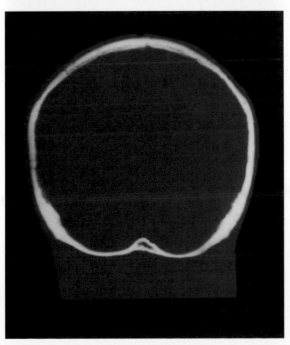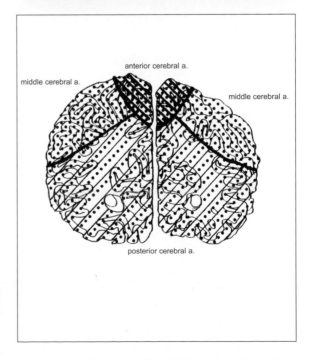

anterior cerebral a.

middle cerebral a.

middle cerebral a.

posterior cerebral a.

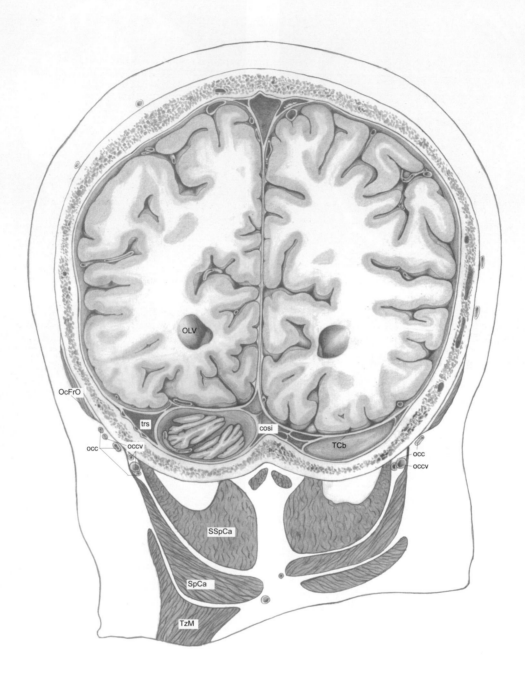

Section 14a:

cosi	confluence of sinuses	SpCa	splenius capitis muscle
occ	occipital artery	SSpCa	semispinal capitis muscle
occv	occipital vein	TCb	tentorium cerebelli
OcFrO	occipito-frontal muscle, occipital belly	trs	transverse sinus
OLV	occipital horn of lateral ventricle	TzM	trapezius muscle

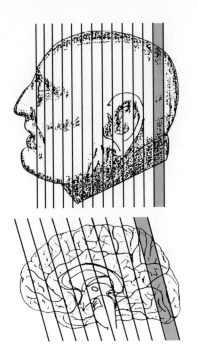

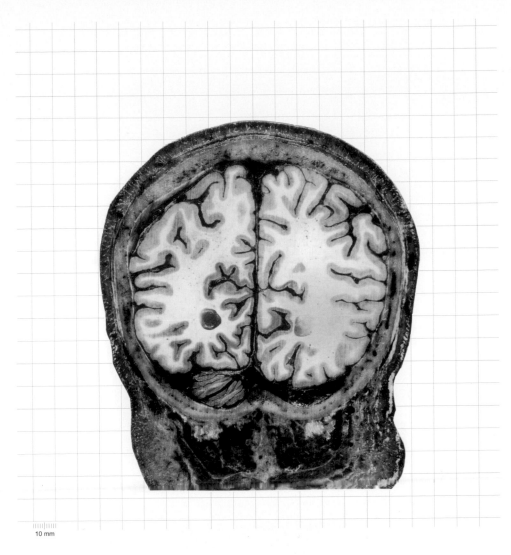

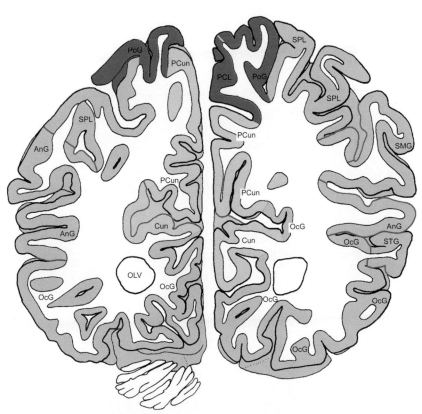

Section 14a:

AnG	angular gyrus
Cun	cuneus
OcG	occipital gyri
OLV	occipital horn of lateral ventricle
PCL	paracentral lobule
PCun	precuneus
PoG	postcentral gyrus
SMG	supramarginal gyrus
SPL	superior parietal lobule
STG	superior temporal gyrus

10 mm

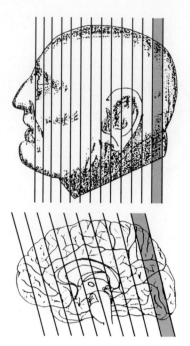

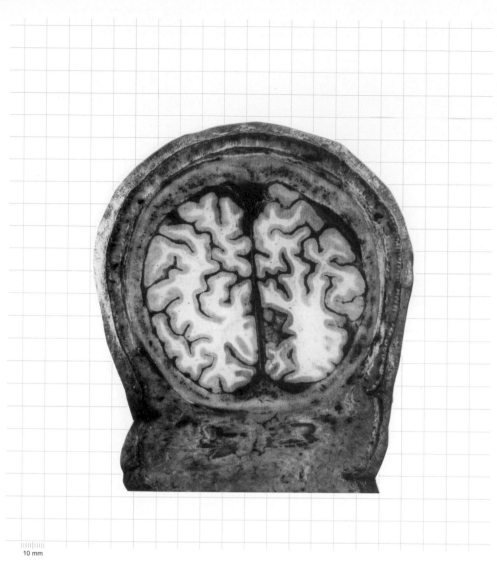

10 mm

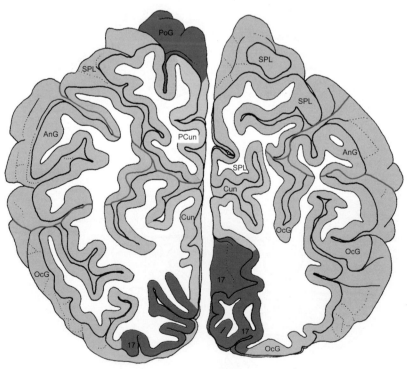

Section 14p:

17	striate cortex
AnG	angular gyrus
Cun	cuneus
OcG	occipital gyri
PCun	precuneus
PoG	postcentral gyrus
SPL	superior parietal lobule

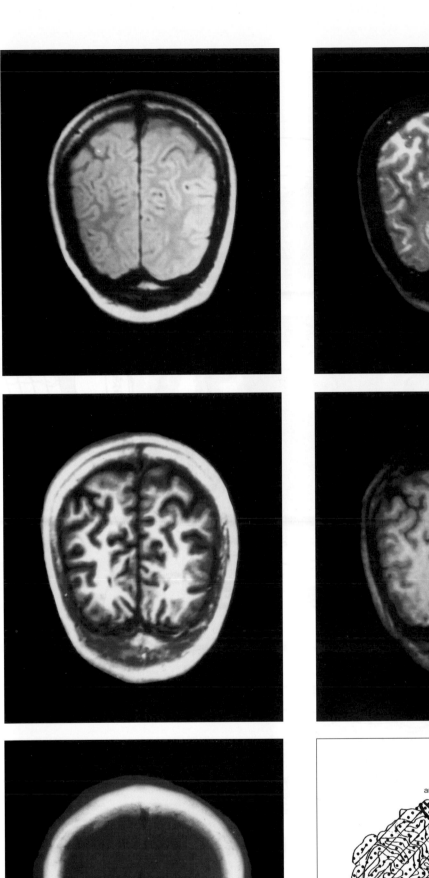
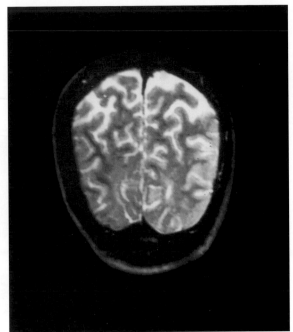
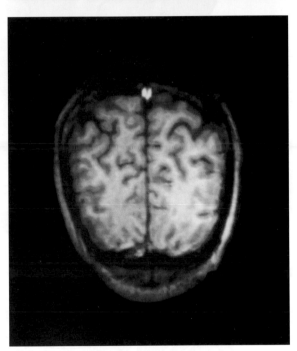
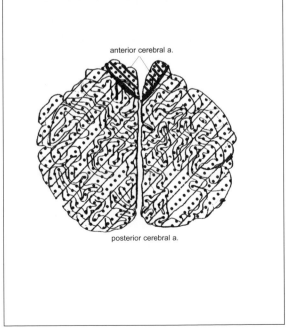

anterior cerebral a.

posterior cerebral a.

Sagittal plane

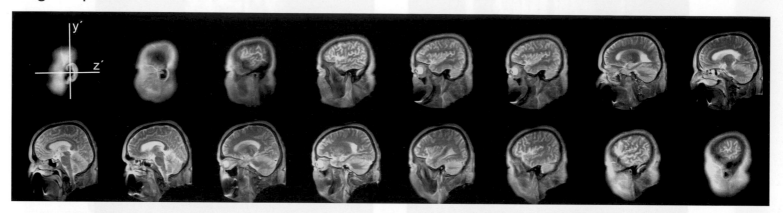

y´ direction

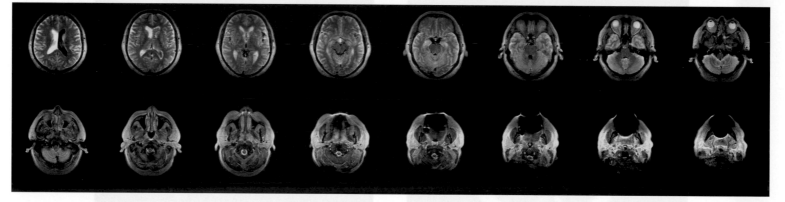

10 mm

z´ direction

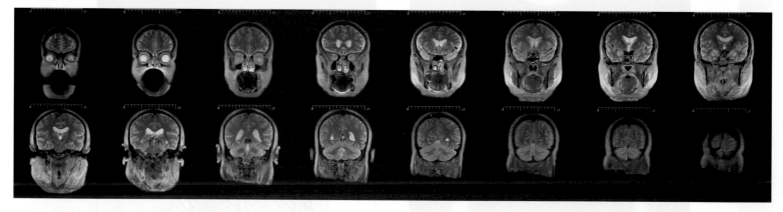

MR sequences of the head in three planes from which one hemisphere is shown on the following pages.

Parameters: 0.15 Tesla, matrix 256 X 256, field of view 25 cm, multislice, slice thickness 5 mm, 4 excitations, sequence: 5000/160. These heavy T_2 weighted images highlight fluid-containing structures; uneven fluid collections (see lateral ventricles) are therefore visible. Note also that a dental prosthesis caused single void and deviation artifacts. The top panel presents the sagittal MRIs and specifies the planes of sectioning of the middle and lower panels. Orientation of these MRIs was based on the intercommissural line. Therefore, the orientation of the horizontal MRIs in the middle panel corresponds to the plane of cryosectioning of the head shown in Section 3.1. Direct comparisons can be made with *in vivo* MRIs that accompany that series of sections. The lower panel presents the coronal MRIs.

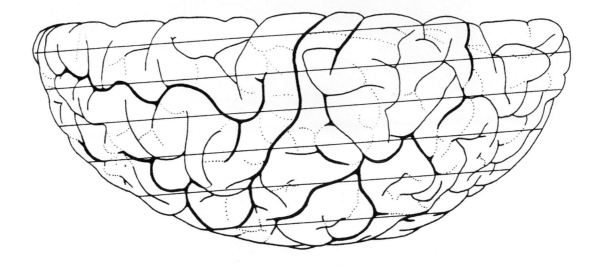

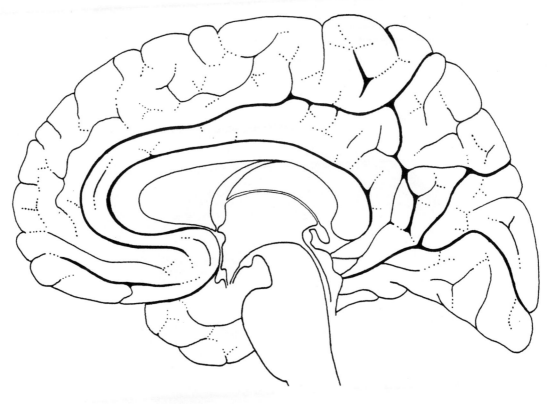

Surface views of the left hemisphere of the brain is sectioned in the sagittal plane as indicated. The drawing of the midsagittal view is mirror-imaged.

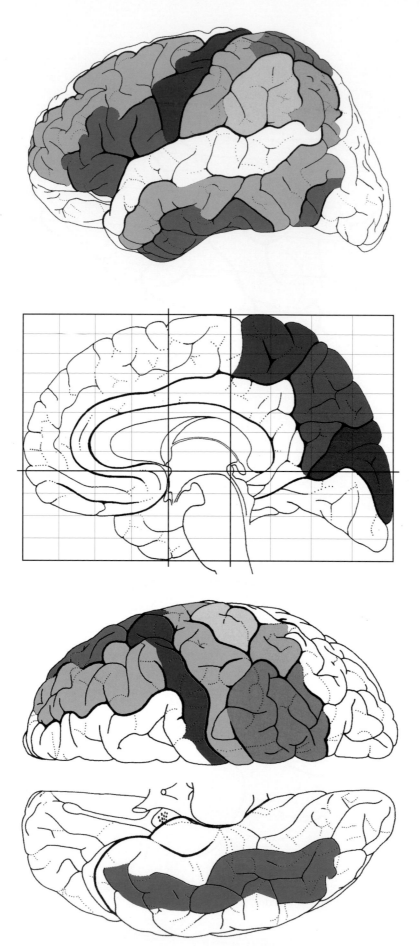

Surface views of the left hemisphere shown in the subsequent pages. The drawings of the hemisphere are arranged to show the same anterior–posterior orientation. The most important gyri are delineated. The midsagittal view depicts the hemisphere with the Talairach space.

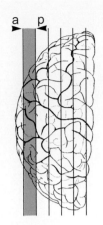

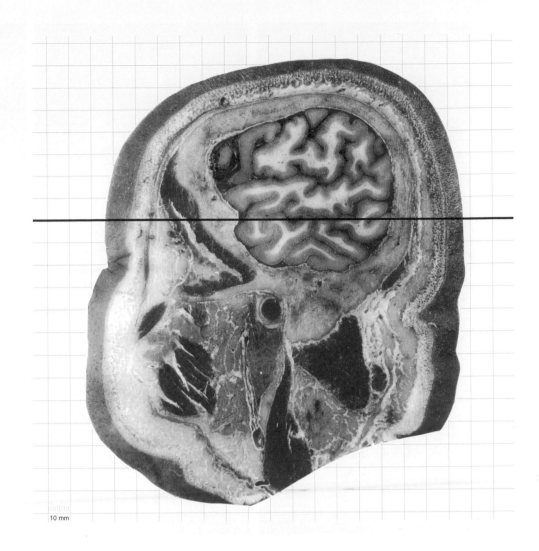

Section 3a:
(lateral surface)

Cerebral structures:

AnG	angular gyrus
IFG	inferior frontal gyrus
ITG	inferior temporal gyrus
MTG	medial temporal gyrus
PoG	postcentral gyrus
PrG	precentral gyrus
PTe	planum temporale
SMG	supramarginal gyrus
STG	superior temporal gyrus
TTG	transverse temporal gyri (I-II)

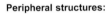
10 mm

Peripheral structures:

7n	facial nerve
EAM	external auditory meatus
ejug	external jugular vein
GZgM	greater zygomatic muscle
MasM	masseter muscle
Mst	mastoid process of temporal bone
MstC	mastoid cells
occv	occipital vein
OcFrF	occipito-frontal muscle, frontal belly
OcFrO	occipito-frontal muscle, occipital belly
OOM	orbicularis oculi muscle
Par	parotid gland
Plat	platysma
ptdd	parotid duct
rmv	retromandibular vein
SpCa	splenius capitis muscle
sta	superficial temporal artery
StM	sternomastoid muscle
TempM	temporalis muscle
TempT	temporalis muscle, tendon
ZygA	zygomatic arch

Photograph of the lateral surface of the 1-cm-thick sagittal section (see shaded area in the inset in the upper left) and corresponding diagram. Cerebral and extracerebral structures are indexed separately. The photograph and diagram of the medial side of the same section are presented on the next page.

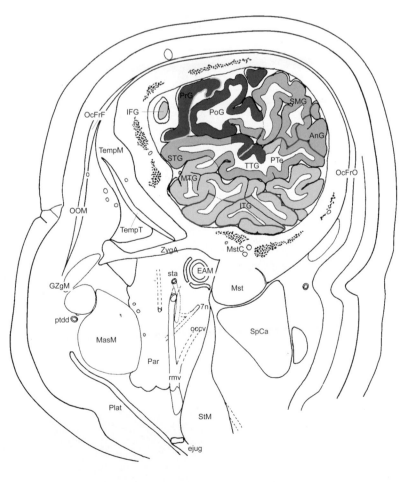

107

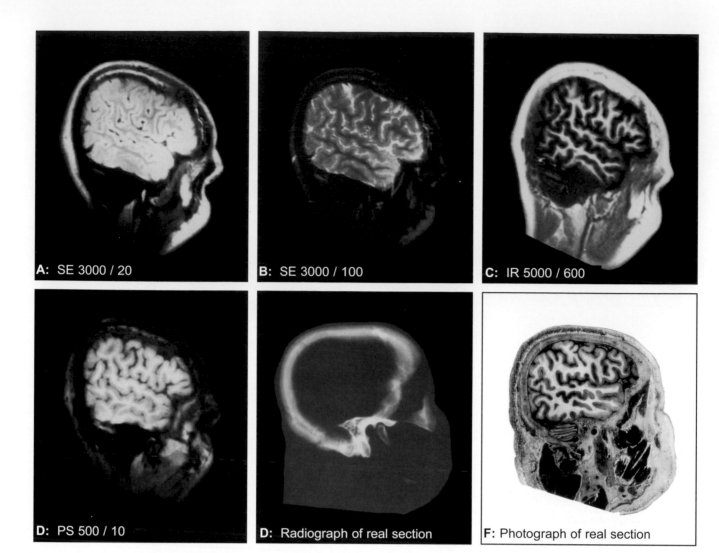

A: SE 3000 / 20

B: SE 3000 / 100

C: IR 5000 / 600

D: PS 500 / 10

D: Radiograph of real section

F: Photograph of real section

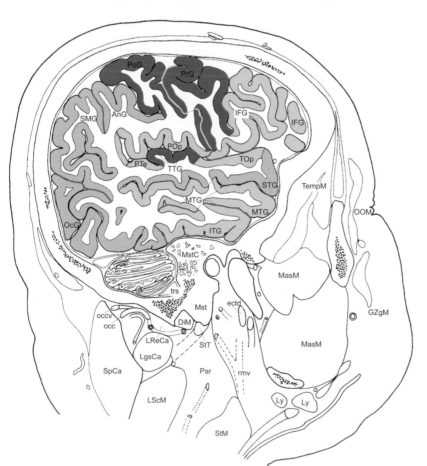

Section 3p
(medial surface, this page),
Section 4a
(lateral surface, facing page):

Cerebral structures:

AnG	angular gyrus
FuG	fusiform gyrus
IFG	inferior frontal gyrus
ITG	inferior temporal gyrus
MTG	medial temporal gyrus
OcG	occipital gyri
PoG	postcentral gyrus
POp	parietal operculum
PrG	precentral gyrus
PTe	planum temporale
SMG	supramarginal gyrus
STG	superior temporal gyrus
TOp	temporal operculum
TTG	transverse temporal gyri (I-II)

(**A-D**) MRIs of a 25-year-old volunteer showing the same plane as the facing anatomical sections. Images present different contrast: (**A**) proton-density, (**B**) T_2, (**C**) T_1, (**D**) T_1 with partial fat suppression. (**E**) Vascular territories of the cerebral arteries in the brain slice contained in this section. (**F**) Radiograph of the anatomical section. The index of cerebral and extracerebral structures refers to both diagrams on the facing pages representing the medial surface of the foregoing and the lateral surface of the following section.

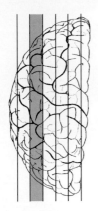

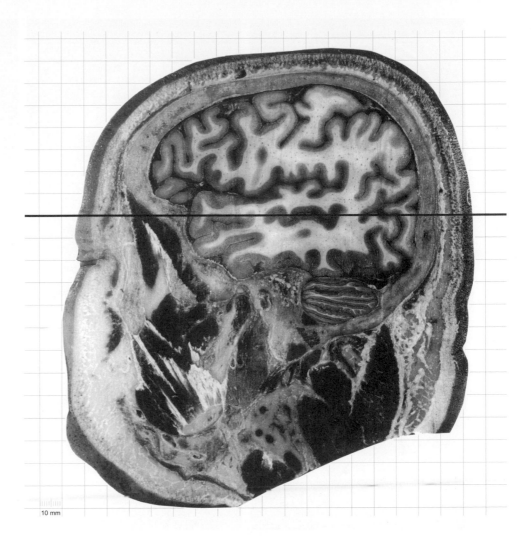

10 mm

Sections 3p, 4a:

Peripheral structures:

EAM	external auditory meatus
ATub	articular tubercle
DiM	digastric muscle
Disc	disk of temporo mandibular joint
ectd	external carotid artery
fac	facial artery
facv	facial vein
FroC	frontal bone, crest
GZgM	greater zygomatic muscle
ijugv	internal jugular vein
LgsCa	longissimus capitis muscle
LReCa	lateral rectus capitis muscle
LScM	levator scapulae muscle
Man	mandible
ManF	mandibular fossa
MasM	masseter muscle
Mst	mastoid process of temporal bone
MstC	mastoid cells
OcFrF	occipito-frontal muscle, frontal belly
OcFrO	occipito-frontal muscle, occipital belly
OOM	orbicularis oculi muscle
Par	parotid gland
Plat	platysma
ptdd	parotid duct
ptgpx	pterygoid plexus
rmv	retromandibular vein
sigs	sigmoid sinus
SMGl	submandibular gland
SpCa	splenius capitis muscle
SphGW	sphenoid, greater wing
StM	sternomastoid muscle
StT	sternomastoid muscle, tendon
TempM	temporalis muscle
TempT	temporalis muscle, tendon
trs	transverse sinus
Zyg	zygomatic bone
Ly	lymph node

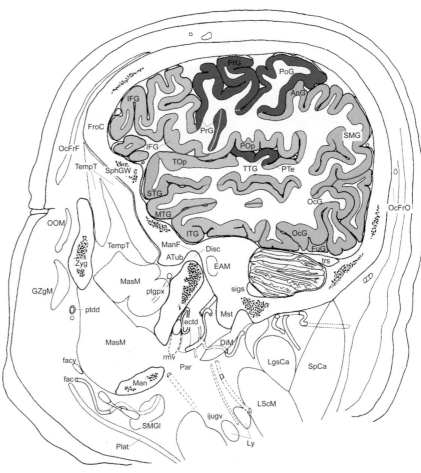

109

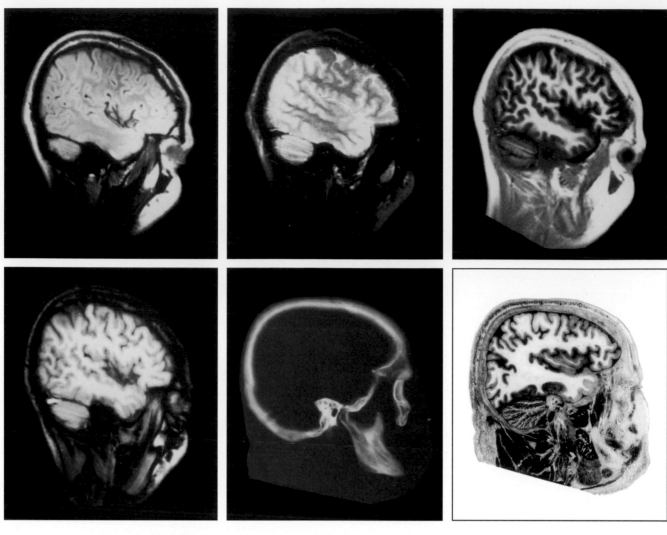

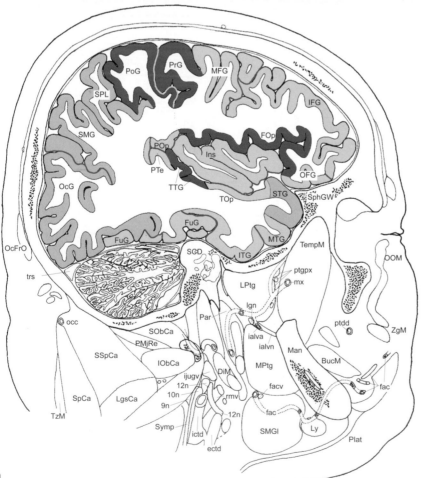

Sections 4p, 5a:

Cerebral structures:

FOp	frontal operculum
FuG	fusiform gyrus
IFG	inferior frontal gyrus
Ins	insula
ITG	inferior temporal gyrus
mcer	middle cerebral artery in lateral sulcus
MFG	middle frontal gyrus
MTG	middle temporal gyrus
OcG	occipital gyri
OFG	orbitofrontal gyri
PoG	postcentral gyrus
POp	parietal operculum
PrG	precentral gyrus
PTe	planum temporale
SMG	supramarginal gyrus
SPL	superior parietal lobule
STG	superior temporal gyrus
TOp	temporal operculum
TTG	transverse temporal gyri

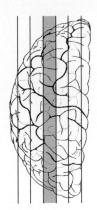

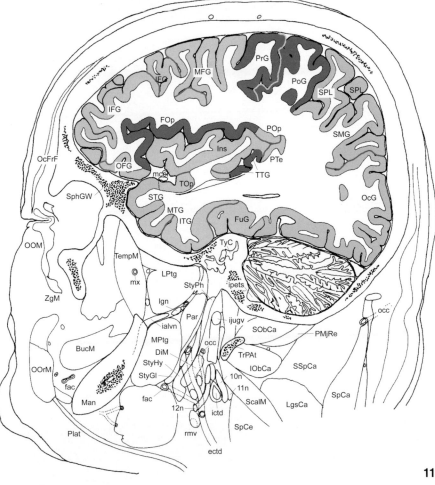

10 mm

Sections 4p, 5a:

Peripheral structures:

10n	vagus nerve
11n	accessory nerve
12n	hypoglossal nerve or its root
9n	glossopharyngeal nerve
BucM	buccinator muscle
DiM	digastric muscle
ectd	external carotid artery
fac	facial artery
facv	facial vein
ialvn	inferior alveolar nerve
ictd	internal carotid artery
ijugv	internal jugular vein
IObCa	inferior oblique capitis muscle
ipets	inferior petrosal sinus
lgn	lingual nerve
LgsCa	longissimus capitis muscle
LPtg	medial pterygoid muscle
Man	mandible
MPtg	lateral pterygoid muscle
mx	maxillary artery
Mx	maxilla
occ	occipital artery
OcFrF	occipito-frontal muscle, frontal belly
OcFrO	occipito-frontal muscle, occipital belly
OOM	orbicularis oculi muscle
OOrM	orbicularis oris muscle
Par	parotid gland
Plat	platysma
PMiRe	posterior minor rectus capitis muscle
PMjRe	posterior major rectus capitis muscle
ptdd	parotid duct
ptgpx	pterygoid plexus
rmv	retromandibular vein
ScalM	scalenus muscle
SCD	semicircular ducts
SMGl	submandibular gland
SObCa	superior oblique capitis muscle
SpCa	splenius capitis muscle
SpCe	splenius cervicis muscle
SphGW	sphenoid, greater wing
SSpCa	semispinalis capitis muscle
StyGl	styloglossus muscle
StyHy	stylohyoid muscle
StyPh	stylopharyngeus muscle
TempM	temporalis muscle
TrPAt	transverse process of atlas
trs	transverse sinus
TyC	tympanic cavity
ZgM	zygomatic muscles

111

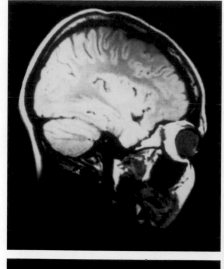
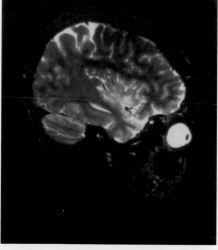
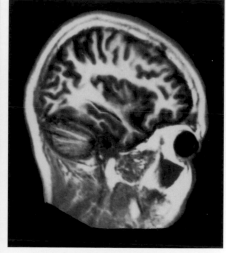

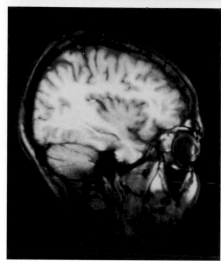
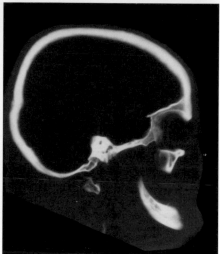
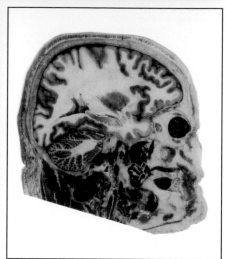

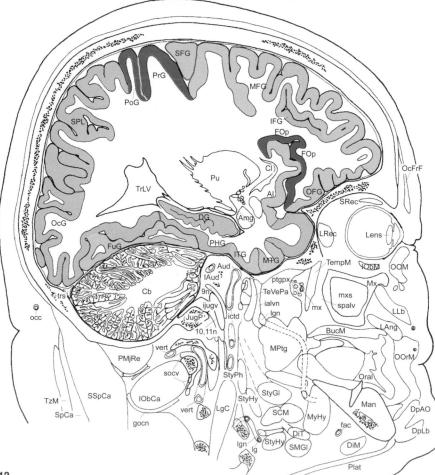

Sections 5p, 6a:

Cerebral structures:

ac	anterior commissure
AI	agranular insular cortex (claustro-cortex insularis)
Amg	amygdala
aud	auditory radiation
Cb	cerebellum
Cl	claustrum
DG	dentate gyrus
fi	fimbria of the hippocampus
FOp	frontal operculum
FuG	fusiform gyrus
GP	globus pallidus
Hi	hippocampus
IFG	inferior frontal gyrus
ITG	inferior temporal gyrus
LG	lateral geniculate nucleus
MFG	medial frontal gyrus
MTG	medial temporal gyrus
OcG	occipital gyri
OFG	orbitofrontal gyri
OLV	occipital horn of lateral ventricle
or	optic radiation
PHG	parahippocampal gyrus
PoG	postcentral gyrus
PrG	precentral gyrus
Pu	putamen
SFG	superior frontal gyrus
SMG	supramarginal gyrus
SPL	superior parietal lobule
st	stria terminalis
STG	superior temporal gyrus
TCd	tail of caudate nucleus
thr	thalamic radiation (corona radiata)
TrLV	trigone of lateral ventricle

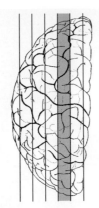

Sections 5p, 6a:

Peripheral structures:

5inf	infraorbital nerve
9n	glossopharyngeal nerve
10n	vagus nerve
11n	accessory nerve
12n	hypoglossal nerve or its root
Aud	auditory tube
AudC	auditory tube cartilage
BucM	buccinator muscle
Cb	cerebellum
DiM	digastric muscle (ant. belly, post belly)
DiT	digastric muscle, tendon
DpAO	depressor anguli oris muscle
DpLb	depressor labii inferioris muscle
fac	facial artery
facv	facial vein
gocn	greater occipital nerve
ialvn	inferior alveolar nerve
IAud	internal auditory meatus
ictd	internal carotid artery
ijugv	internal jugular vein (and sigmoid sinus)
infa	infraorbital artery
IObCa	inferior oblique capitis muscle
IObM	inferior oblique muscle
IOrbF	infraorbital foramen
ivvpx	internal vertebral venous plexus
JugF	jugular foramen
JugP	jugular process
lab	labial artery
LAng	levator anguli oris muscle
lg	lingual artery
LgC	longus capitis and colli muscles
lgn	lingual nerve
LgsCa	longissimus capitis muscle
lgv	lingual vein
LLb	levator labii superioris muscle
LPal	levator palpebrae superioris muscle
LPtg	lateral pterygoid muscle
LRec	lateral rectus muscle
LReCa	lateral rectus capitis muscle
Man	mandible
mand5	mandibular nerve
MidE	middle ear
mm	middle meningeal artery
MPtg	medial pterygoid muscle
mx	maxillary artery
Mx	maxilla
mxs	maxillary sinus
MyHy	mylohyoid muscle
occ	occipital artery and vein
OcFrF	occipito-frontal muscle, frontal belly
OOM	orbicularis oculi muscle
OOrM	orbicularis oris muscle
Oral	oral cavity
Par	parotid gland
Plat	platysma
PMjRe	posterior major rectus capitis muscle
ptgpx	pterygoid plexus
rmv	retromandibular vein
SCM	superior constrictor muscle
SMGl	submandibular gland
SObCa	superior oblique capitis muscle
socv	suboccipital venous plexus
spalv	superior posterior alveolar artery
SpCa	splenius capitis muscle
SpCe	splenius cervicis muscle
SRec	superior rectus muscle
SSpCa	semispinal capitis muscle
StyGl	styloglossus muscle
StyHy	stylohyoid muscle
StyPh	stylopharyngeus muscle
TempM	temporalis muscle
TrPAt	transverse process of atlas
trs	transverse sinus
TzM	trapezius muscle
vert	vertebral artery

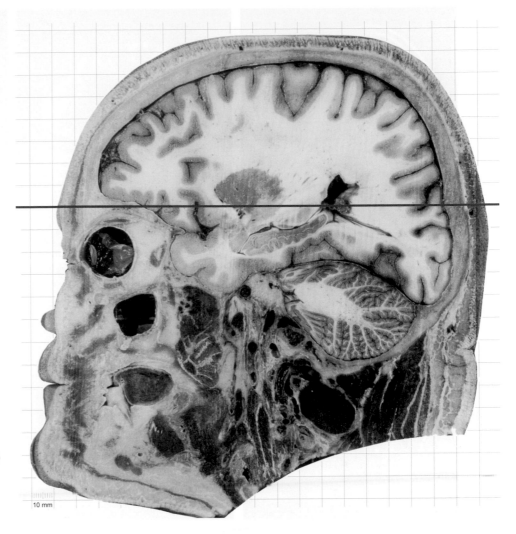

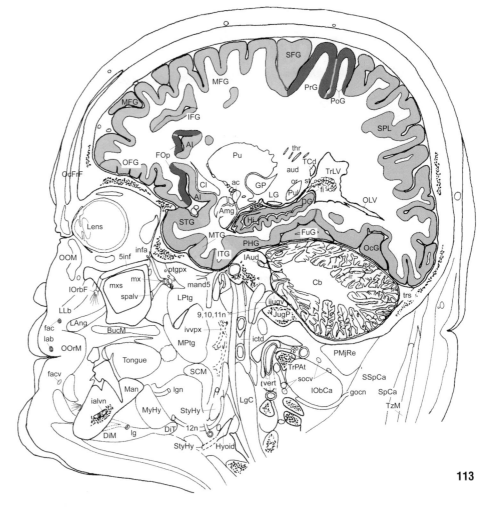

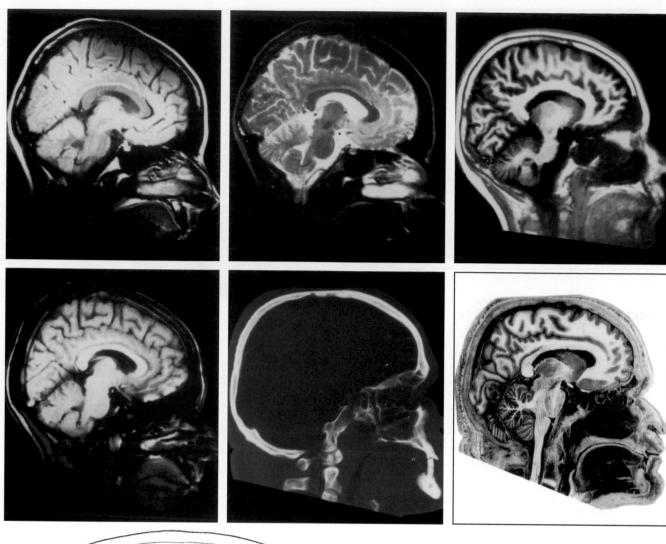

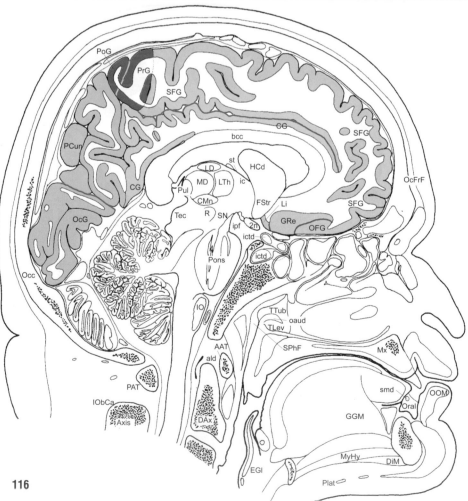

Sections 7p, 8a:

Cerebral structures:

2n	optic nerve
ac	anterior commissure
bcc	body of corpus callosum
BST	bed nucleus of the stria terminalis
CG	cingulate gyrus
CMn	centrum medianum, parafascicular nucleus
FStr	fundus striati
GP	globus pallidus
GRe	gyrus rectus
HCd	head of caudate nucleus
ic	internal capsule
IO	inferior olive
ipf	interpeduncular fossa
LC	locus coeruleus
Li	limen insulae
LTh	lateral thalamic nuclear region and reticular nucleus
MD	medial dorsal thalamic nucleus
MTec	mesencephalic tectum
OcG	occipital gyri
OFG	orbitofrontal gyri
PCun	precuneus
PoG	postcentral gyrus
Pons	pons
PrG	precentral gyrus
Pul	pulvinar
R	red nucleus
SFG	superior frontal gyrus
SN	substantia nigra
st	stria terminalis
Tec	tectum
Th	thalamus

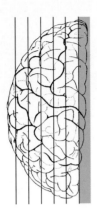

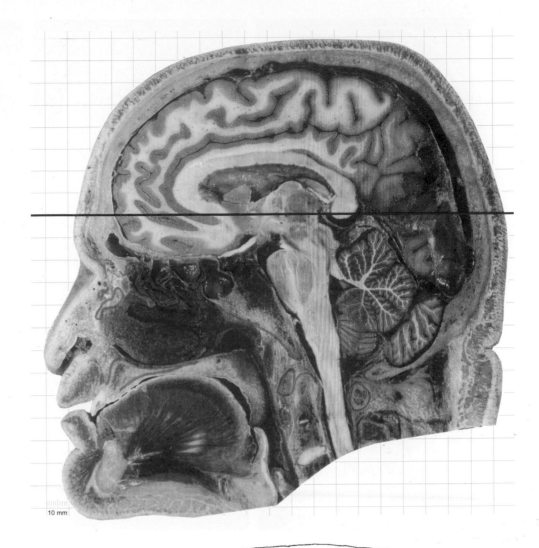

10 mm

Sections 7p, 8a:

Peripheral structures:

AAT	anterior arch of atlas
ald	apical ligament of dens
alal	alar ligament of dens
all	anterior longitudinal ligament
Atlas	atlas
AtAx	altanto-axial membrane
AtOc	atlanto-occipital membrane
Axis	axis
DAx	dens axis
DiM	digastric muscle
EGl	epiglottis
GeHy	geniohyoid muscle
GGM	genioglossus muscle
ictd	internal carotid artery
IObCa	inferior oblique capitis muscle
Man	mandible
Mx	maxilla
MyHy	mylohyoid muscle
NPhT	nasopharyngeal tonsil
oaud	opening of auditory tube
Occ	occipital bone
OcFrF	occipito-frontal muscle, frontal belly
OOM	orbicularis oculi muscle
Oral	oral cavity
PAT	posterior arch of atlas
Plat	platysma
smd	submandibular duct
SPaF	salpingopalatinal fold
SPal	soft palate
SPhF	salpingopharyngeal fold
tla	transverse ligament of atlas
TLev	torus levatorius
TTub	torus tubarius

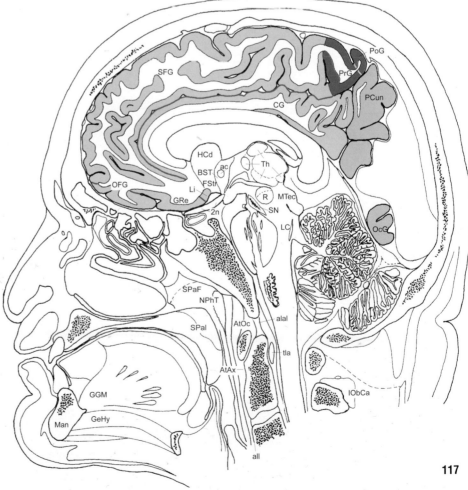

117

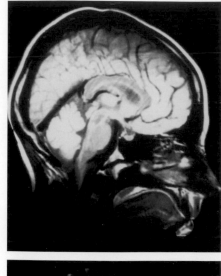
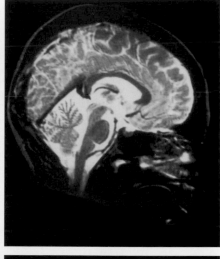
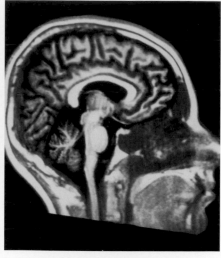
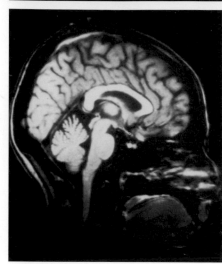
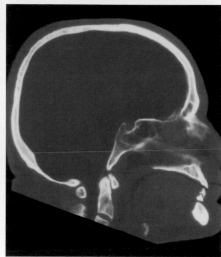
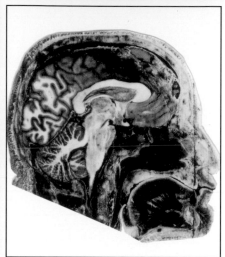

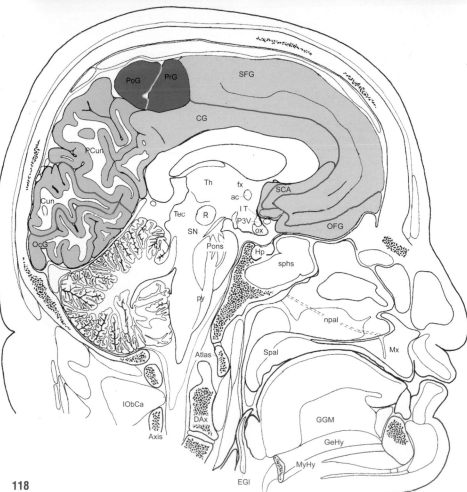

Section 8p:

Cerebral structures:

ac	anterior commissure
CG	cingulate gyrus
Cun	cuneus
fx	fornix
GRe	gyrus rectus
Hp	hypophysis
LT	lamina terminalis
npal	nasopalatine nerve
OcG	occipital gyri
OFG	orbitofrontal gyri
ox	optic chiasm
P3V	prooptic recess of the third ventricle
PCun	precuneus
PoG	postcentral gyrus
Pons	pons
PrG	precentral gyrus
py	pyramidal tract
R	red nucleus
SCA	subcallosal area
SFG	superior frontal gyrus
SN	substantia nigra
sphs	sphenoid sinus
Tec	tectum
Th	thalamus

Peripheral structures:

Atlas	atlas
Axis	axis
DAx	dens axis
EGl	epiglottis
GeHy	geniohyoid muscle
GGM	genioglossus muscle
IObCa	inferior oblique capitis muscle
Mx	maxilla
MyHy	mylohyoid muscle
Spal	soft palate

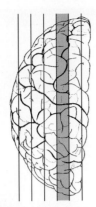

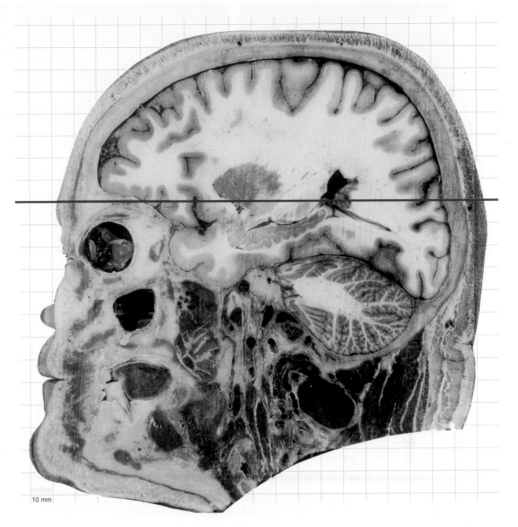

Sections 5p, 6a:

Peripheral structures:

5inf	infraorbital nerve
9n	glossopharyngeal nerve
10n	vagus nerve
11n	accessory nerve
12n	hypoglossal nerve or its root
Aud	auditory tube
AudC	auditory tube cartilage
BucM	buccinator muscle
Cb	cerebellum
DiM	digastric muscle (ant. belly, post belly)
DiT	digastric muscle, tendon
DpAO	depressor anguli oris muscle
DpLb	depressor labii inferioris muscle
fac	facial artery
facv	facial vein
gocn	greater occipital nerve
ialvn	inferior alveolar nerve
lAud	internal auditory meatus
ictd	internal carotid artery
ijugv	internal jugular vein (and sigmoid sinus)
infa	infraorbital artery
IObCa	inferior oblique capitis muscle
IObM	inferior oblique muscle
IOrbF	infraorbital foramen
ivvpx	internal vertebral venous plexus
JugF	jugular foramen
JugP	jugular process
lab	labial artery
LAng	levator anguli oris muscle
lg	lingual artery
LgC	longus capitis and colli muscles
lgn	lingual nerve
LgsCa	longissimus capitis muscle
lgv	lingual vein
LLb	levator labii superioris muscle
LPal	levator palpebrae superioris muscle
LPtg	lateral pterygoid muscle
LRec	lateral rectus muscle
LReCa	lateral rectus capitis muscle
Man	mandible
mand5	mandibular nerve
MidE	middle ear
mm	middle meningeal artery
MPtg	medial pterygoid muscle
mx	maxillary artery
Mx	maxilla
mxs	maxillary sinus
MyHy	mylohyoid muscle
occ	occipital artery and vein
OcFrF	occipito-frontal muscle, frontal belly
OOM	orbicularis oculi muscle
OOrM	orbicularis oris muscle
Oral	oral cavity
Par	parotid gland
Plat	platysma
PMjRe	posterior major rectus capitis muscle
ptgpx	pterygoid plexus
rmv	retromandibular vein
SCM	superior constrictor muscle
SMGl	submandibular gland
SObCa	superior oblique capitis muscle
socv	suboccipital venous plexus
spalv	superior posterior alveolar artery
SpCa	splenius capitis muscle
SpCe	splenius cervicis muscle
SRec	superior rectus muscle
SSpCa	semispinal capitis muscle
StyGl	styloglossus muscle
StyHy	stylohyoid muscle
StyPh	stylopharyngeus muscle
TempM	temporalis muscle
TrPAt	transverse process of atlas
trs	transverse sinus
TzM	trapezius muscle
vert	vertebral artery

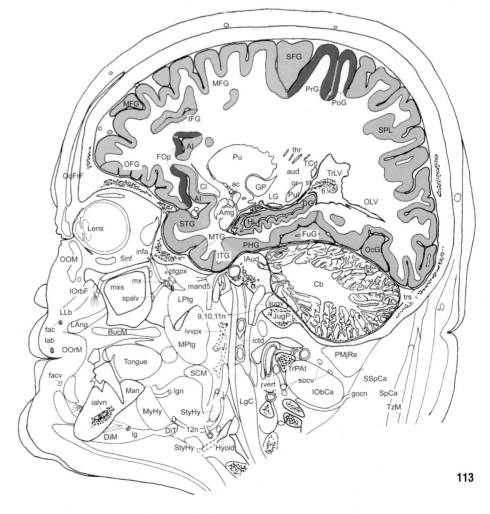

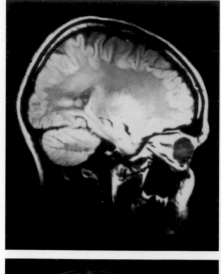
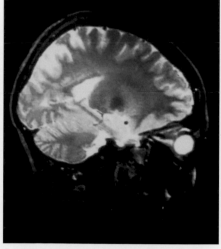
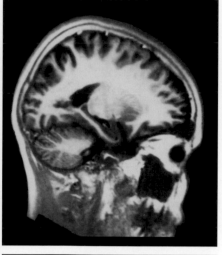
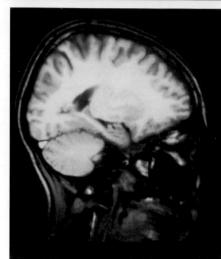
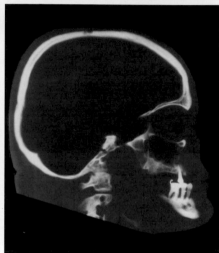
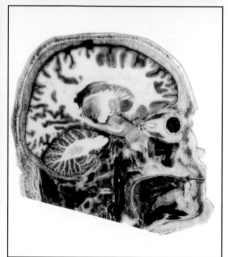

Sections 6p, 7a:

Cerebral structures:

2n	optic nerve
ac	anterior commissure
AI	claustro-cortex insularis
alv	alveus of hippocampus
Amg	amygdala
Cb	cerebellum
Cd	caudate nucleus
CG	cingulate gyrus
cp	cerebral peduncle
Cun	cuneus
DG	dentate gyrus
FG	fasciolar gyrus
FuG	fusiform gyrus
GP	globus pallidus
Hi	hippocampus
ic	internal capsule
LgG	lingual gyrus
Li	limen insulae
LTh	lateral thalamic nuclear region
mcp	middle cerebellar peduncle
MFG	medial frontal gyrus
MG	medial geniculate nucleus
OcG	occipital gyri
OFG	orbitofrontal gyri
opt	optic tract
PAC	periamygdaloid cortex
PCun	precuneus
PHG	parahippocampal gyrus
Pir	piriform cortex
PoG	postcentral gyrus
PrG	precentral gyrus
Pu	putamen
Pul	pulvinar nucleus
SB	striatal cell bridges
SFG	superior frontal gyrus
SPL	superior parietal lobule
st	stria terminalis
Th	thalamus
TLV	temporal horn of lateral ventricle

114

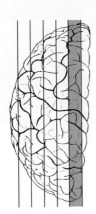

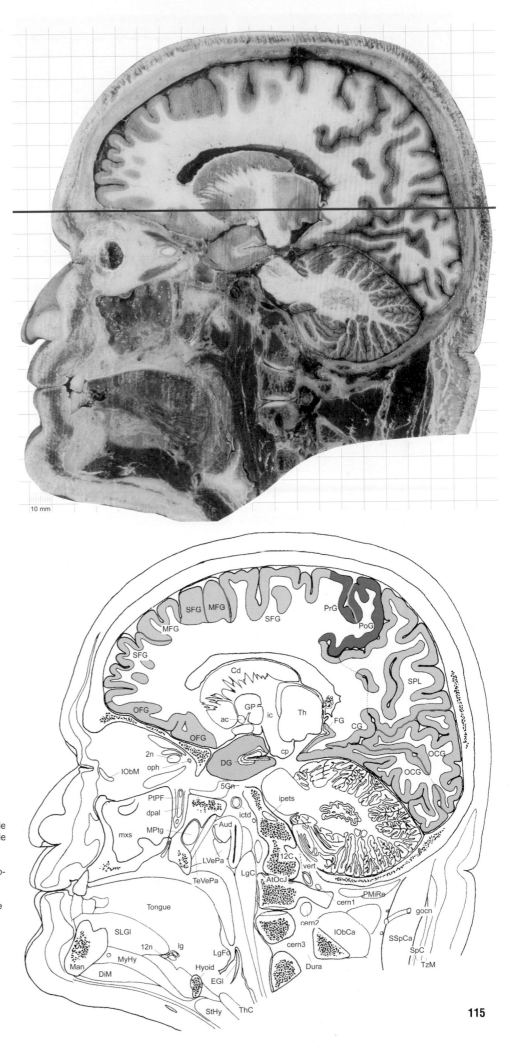

Sections 6p, 7a:

Peripheral structures:

5Gn	trigeminal ganglion
5n	trigeminal nerve
5nc	nasociliary nerve
12C	hypoglossal canal
12n	hypoglossal nerve
AReCa	anterior rectus capitis muscle
AtOcJ	atlanto-occipital joint
Aud	auditory tube
cern (1-3)	cervical nerve (1-3)
DiM	digastric muscle, ant. belly
dpal	descending palatine artery
EGl	epiglottis
gocn	greater occipital nerve
HyGl	hyoglossus muscle
Hyoid	hyoid bone
ictd	internal carotid artery
IObCa	inferior oblique capitis muscle
IObM	inferior oblique muscle
ipets	inferior petrosal sinus
lg	lingual artery
LgC	longus capitis and colli muscles
LgFo	lingual follicle
LPal	levator palpebrae muscle
LVePa	levator veli palatini muscle
Man	mandible
mand5	mandibular nerve
MPtg	medial pterygoid muscle
MRec	medial rectus muscle
Mult	multifidus muscle
mx	maxillary artery
mxs	maxillary sinus
MyHy	mylohyoid muscle
OOM	orbicularis oculi muscle
OOrM	orbicularis oris muscle
oph	ophthalmic artery
Oral	oral cavity
Plat	platysma
PlPh	palatopharyngeus muscle
PMiRe	posterior minor rectus capitis muscle
PMjRe	posterior major rectus capitis muscle
PtPF	pterygopalatine fossa
PtT	palatine tonsil
SCMPP	superior constrictor muscle, pterygo-pharyngeal part
SLGl	sublingual gland
SpC	splenius capitis and cervicis muscle
SRec	superior rectus muscle
SSpCa	semispinal capitis muscle
StHy	sternohyoid muscle
TeVePa	tensor palatini muscle
ThC	thyroid cartilage, upper horn
ThHy	thyrohyoid muscle
TzM	trapezius muscle
vert	vertebral artery

115

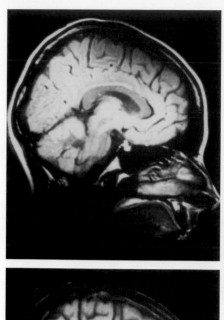
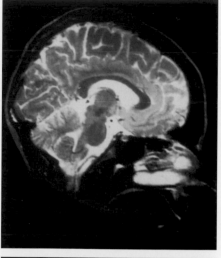
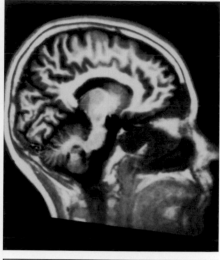

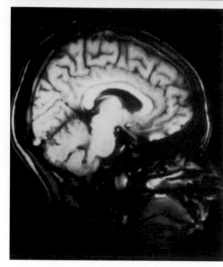
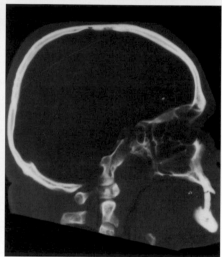
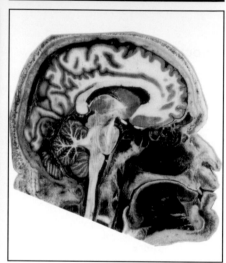

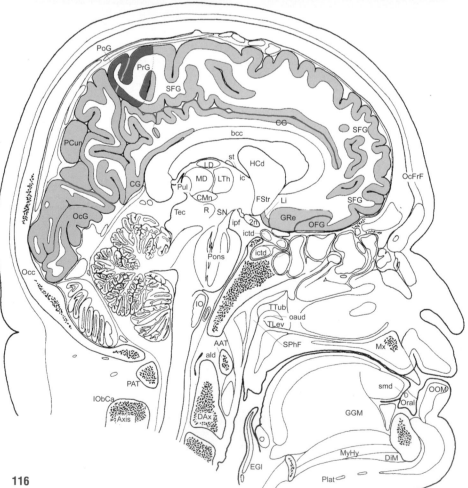

Sections 7p, 8a:

Cerebral structures:

2n	optic nerve
ac	anterior commissure
bcc	body of corpus callosum
BST	bed nucleus of the stria terminalis
CG	cingulate gyrus
CMn	centrum medianum, parafascicular nucleus
FStr	fundus striati
GP	globus pallidus
GRe	gyrus rectus
HCd	head of caudate nucleus
ic	internal capsule
IO	inferior olive
ipf	interpeduncular fossa
LC	locus coeruleus
Li	limen insulae
LTh	lateral thalamic nuclear region and reticular nucleus
MD	medial dorsal thalamic nucleus
MTec	mesencephalic tectum
OcG	occipital gyri
OFG	orbitofrontal gyri
PCun	precuneus
PoG	postcentral gyrus
Pons	pons
PrG	precentral gyrus
Pul	pulvinar
R	red nucleus
SFG	superior frontal gyrus
SN	substantia nigra
st	stria terminalis
Tec	tectum
Th	thalamus

116

4 MYELOARCHITECTONIC ATLAS

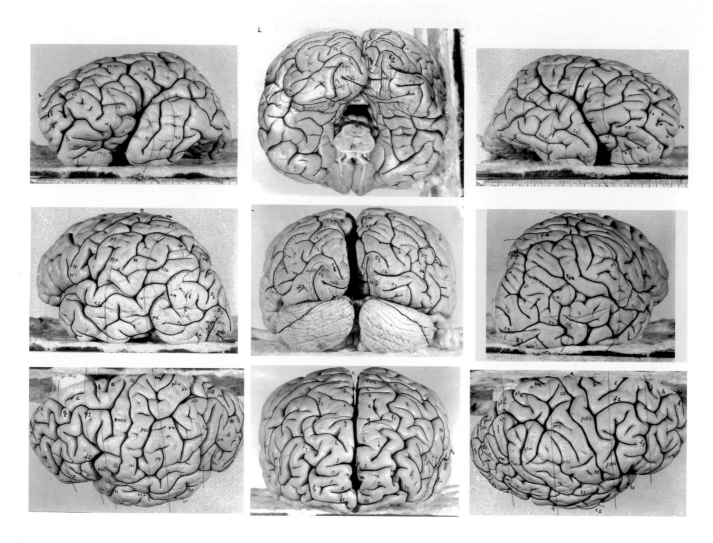

The photographs of the following myelin-stained sections were taken from sections prepared from the brain of a 24-year-old male (see Section 2.2.1). The external morphology of the formalin-fixed brain is shown below and on the diagrams on the following page (Section 4.1). Some relevant gyri are discriminated by different shadings on these diagrams. This brain was cut perpendicular to the intercommissural plane. Presentation of complete sections through the entire (right) hemisphere is provided in a set of 36 diagrams. These show each section with low-detail morphological information according to its approximate position in the topometric space, and the location of each section is found in the preceding diagram. The reader can thereby advance from the surface view of the gyral patterning to the section level. Because shading is used for discrimination between different gyri, it is not necessarily identical. The following section (4.3) shows the central region of the brain in a resolution that permits high-detail recognition of morphological structures. The photographs of myelin-stained sections are accompanied by diagrams of the same size and define the position, extent, and relationship of nuclei and pathways of the forbrain and mesencephalon. Because the brain shown in this myeloarchitectonic atlas was used by previous researchers, we have also compiled the results of their studies (Section 4.4). Delineations suggested in the previous works are not always identical to those shown in our myeloarchitectonic atlas; therefore, a set of diagrams is included integrating previous delineations. The location of these diagrams can be easily matched to those shown in the preceding sections. Finally, diagrams with suppressed details are shown, in Section 4.5 which present the brain after transformation into the mean Talairach space. The sections correspond to those shown in Section 4.1.

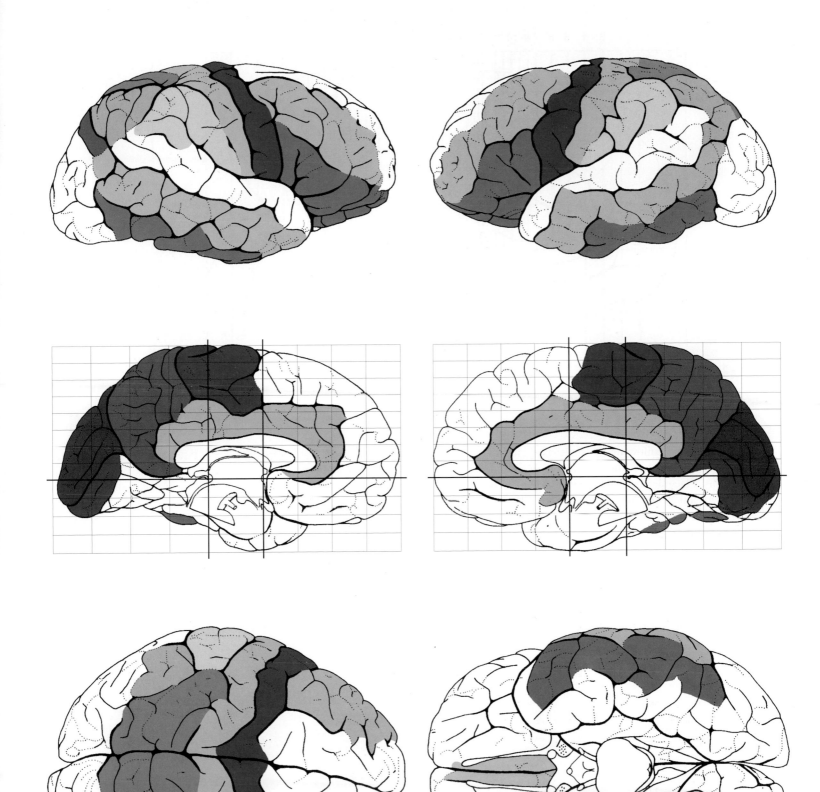

4.2 Low-Detail Diagrams

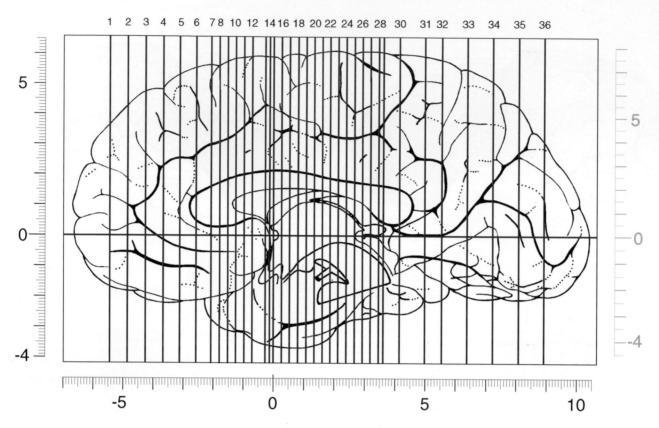

Location of the following 36 sections (pages 125–128) of the low-detail diagrams. Placement of each section is indicated along the upper line. The actual dimensions of the nonembedded, formalin-fixed brain are given on the left side and bottom line. The scale on the right side shows the dimension after transformation to the mean Talairach space. (Because the anterior–posterior extension is equivalent to the corresponding values from Talairach, no transformation was necessary for that dimension.)

Pages 125–128: Low-detail diagrams based on high-detail diagrams shown in (Section 4.3). Abbreviations used for structures in the following 36 diagrams are listed below:

17	striate area	IFGOp	inferior frontal gyrus, opercular part	MTP	medial temporopolar region	PTG	posterior temporopolar region
AG	ambiens gyrus	IFGOr	inferior frontal gyrus, orbital part	OcG	occipital gyri	ros	rostral sulcus
AnG	angular gyrus	IFGTr	inferior frontal gyrus, triangular part	olf	olfactory tract	S	subicular region
AO	anterior olfactory nucleus	ifs	inferior frontal sulcus	olfs	olfactory sulcus	sbps	subparietal sulcus
BOp	basal operculum	IG	insular gyrus	OrG	orbital gyrus (gyri)	SCA	subcallosal area
cas	callosal sulcus	imfs	intermediate frontal sulcus	PCL	paracentral lobule	SepG	separans gyrus
ccs	calcarine sulcus	IOrG	intermediate orbital gyrus	pcs	precentral sulcus	SFG	superior frontal gyrus
ce	central fissure	IPL	inferior parietal lobule	PCun	precuneus	sfs	superior frontal sulcus
CG	cingulate gyrus	ips	intraparietal sulcus	PHG	parahippocampal gyrus	SLG	semilunar gyrus
cgs	cingulate sulcus	IRoG	inferior rostral gyrus	Pir	(pre-) piriform cortex	SMG	supramarginal gyrus
cir	circular insular sulcus	ITFPG	inferior transverse frontopolar gyrus	PIR	parainsular region	SPL	superior parietal lobule
cos	collateral sulcus	ITG	inferior temporal gyrus, T3	pocs	postcentral sulcus	SRoG	superior rostral gyrus
DTP	dorsal temporopolar region	its	inferior temporal sulcus	PoG	postcentral gyrus	STFPG	superior transverse frontopolar gyrus
Ent	entorhinal cortex	lf	lateral fissure	POp	parietal operculum	STG	superior temporal gyrus, T1
FMG	frontomarginal gyrus	LOrG	lateral orbital gyrus	POrG	posterior orbital gyrus	sts	superior temporal sulcus
FOp	frontal operculum	lots	lateral occipitotemporal sulcus	pos	parietooccipital sulcus	TFPG	transverse frontopolar gyri
FPG	frontopolar gyrus	LTP	lateral temporopolar region	PPo	planum polare	TFPG	transverse frontopolar gyrus
FuG	fusiform gyrus, T4	MFG	medial frontal gyrus	pps	posterior parolfactory sulcus	TmP	temporal pole
GR	gyrus rectus	MOrG	medial orbital gyrus	PRC	perirhinal cortex	TrG1	anterior transverse temporal gyrus
Hi	hippocampus	MTFPG	medial transverse frontopolar gyrus	PrG	precentral gyrus	TrG2	posterior transverse temporal gyrus
ICG	isthmus cinguli	MTG	medial temporal gyrus, T2	PTe	planum temporale	Un	uncus

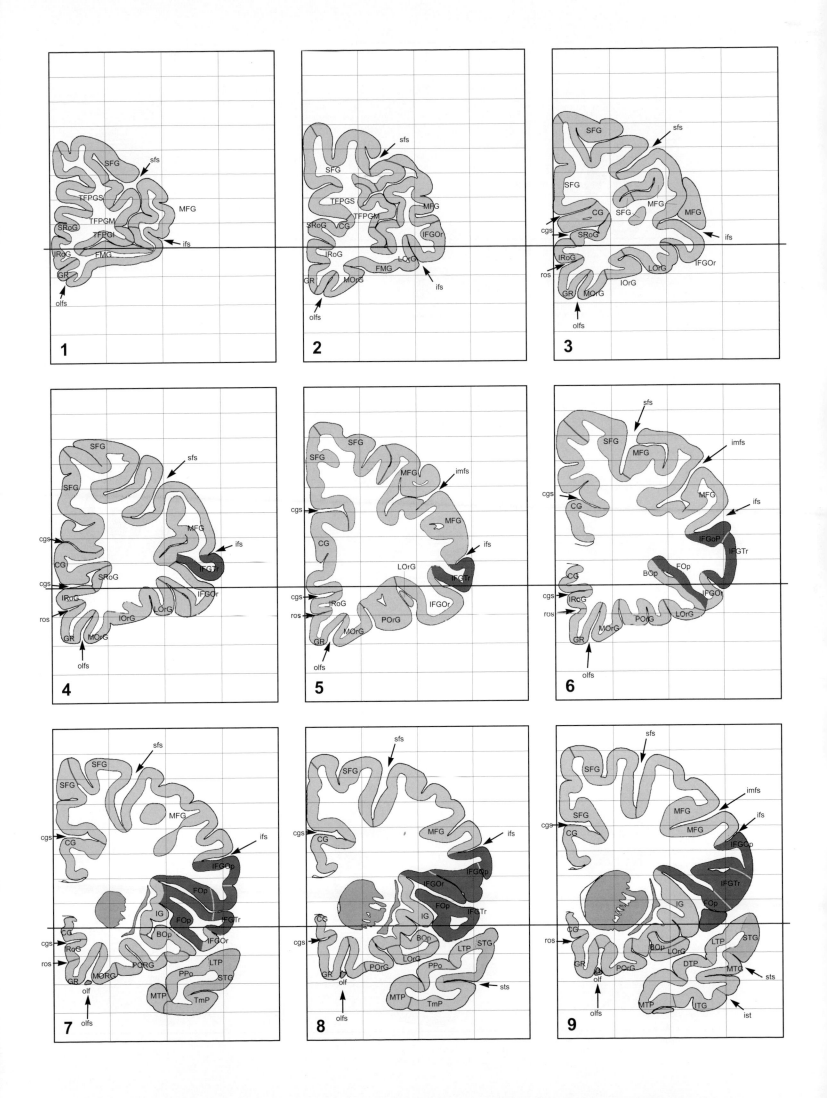

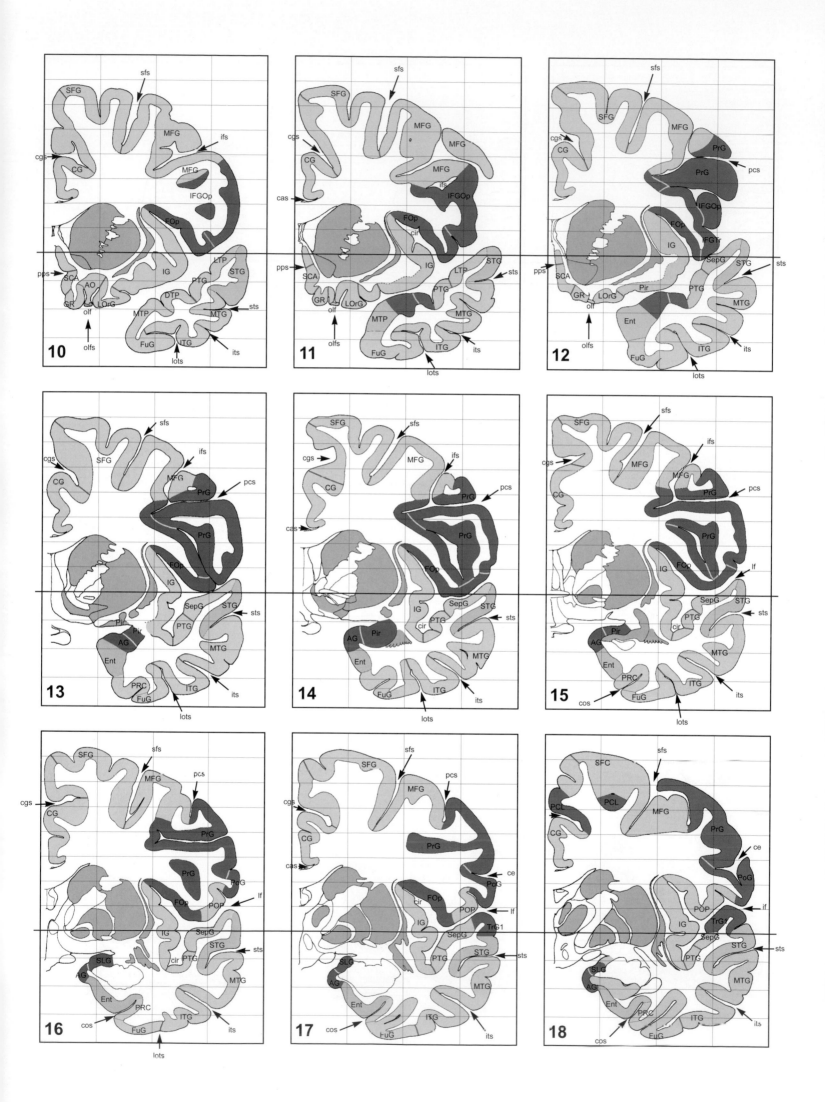

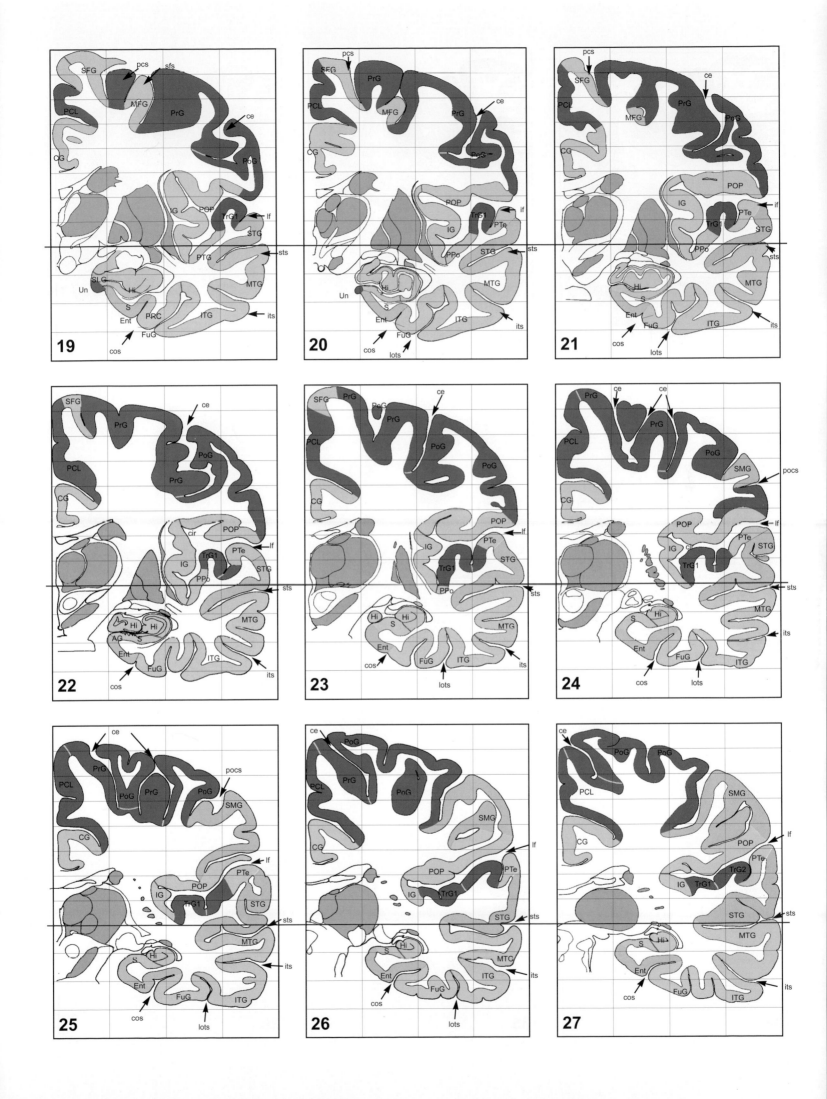

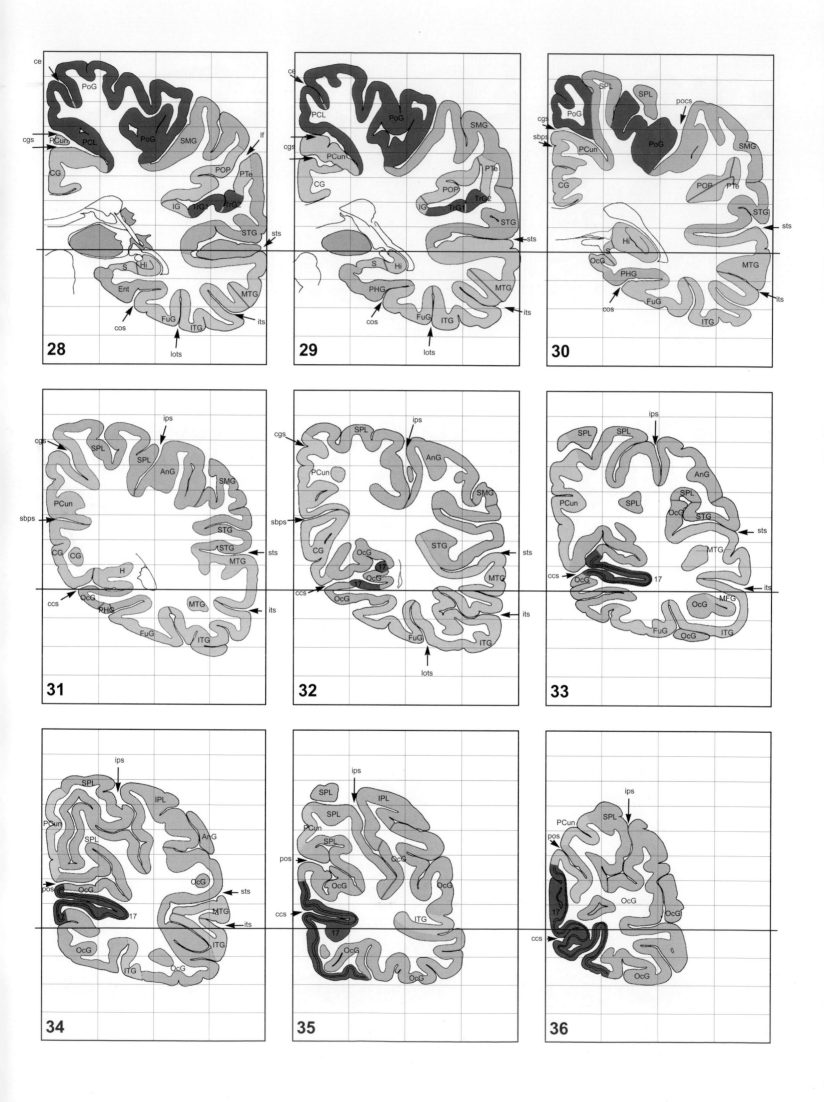

4.3 High-Detail Diagrams

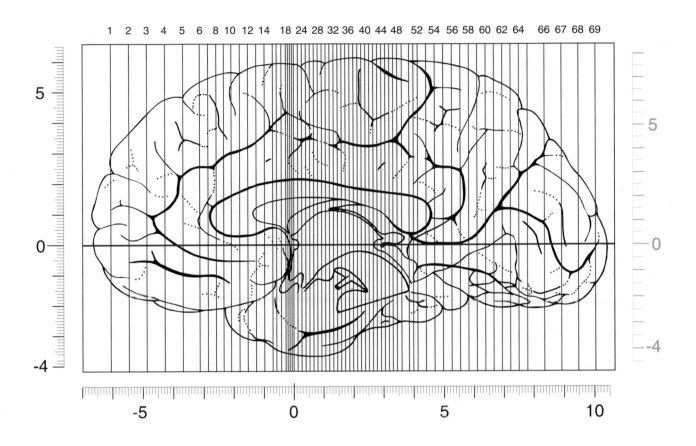

Location of the following 69 brain sections and accompanying high-detail diagrams. The metric scales at the left and lower side show the dimensions of the formalin-fixed brain. The scale on the right side shows the dimension calculated for the *in vivo* brain. Shrinkage was corrected separately for the volumes above and below the intercommissural line. (Shrinkage in the anterior–posterior dimension was neglegible and therefore the scale at the bottom represents both *in vivo* and *in vitro* dimensions.) The intersection of the intercommissural plane with the vertical through the center of the anterior commissure shows the source of both scalings (see Section 2.2.5) .

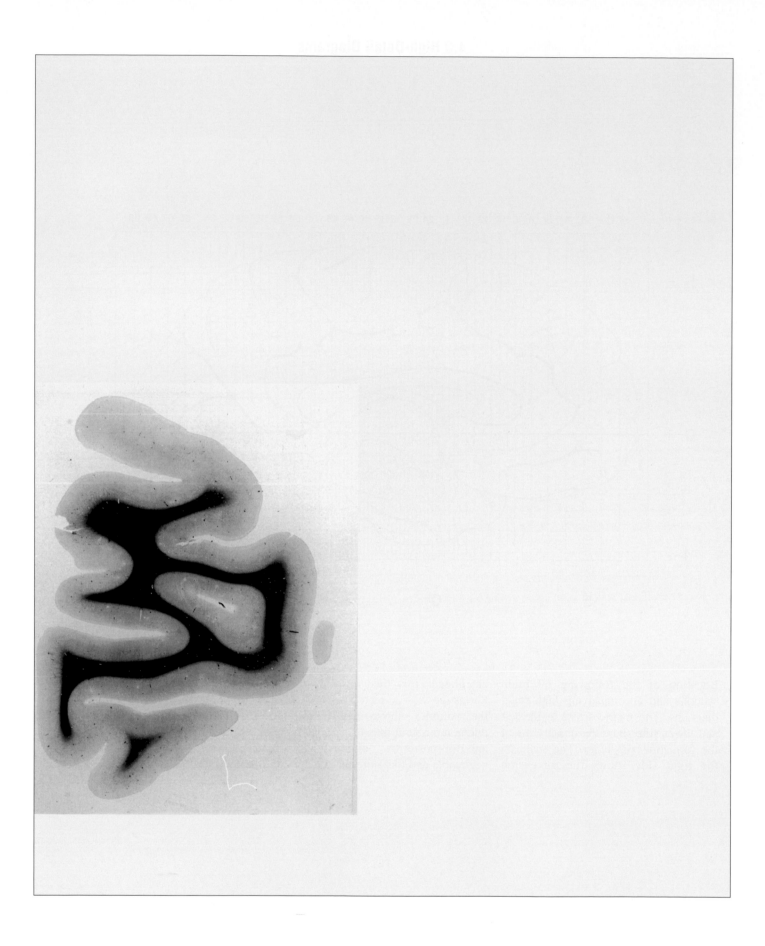

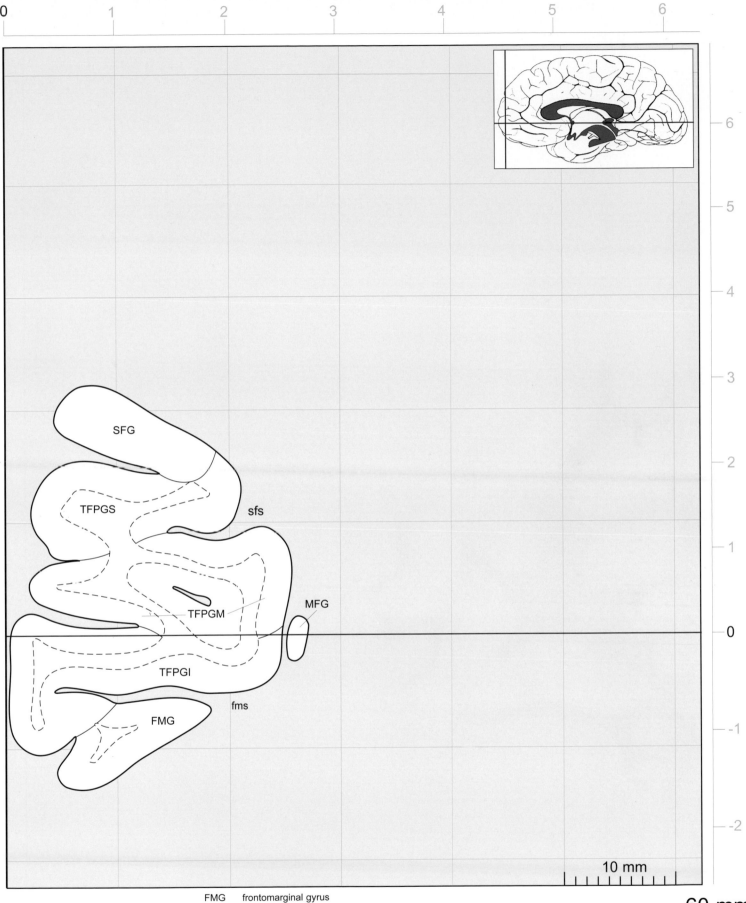

FMG frontomarginal gyrus
fms frontomarginal sulcus
MFG medial frontal gyrus
SFG superior frontal gyrus
sfs superior frontal sulcus
TFPGI inferior transverse frontopolar gyrus
TFPGM medial transverse frontopolar gyrus
TFPGS superior transverse frontopolar gyrus

10 mm

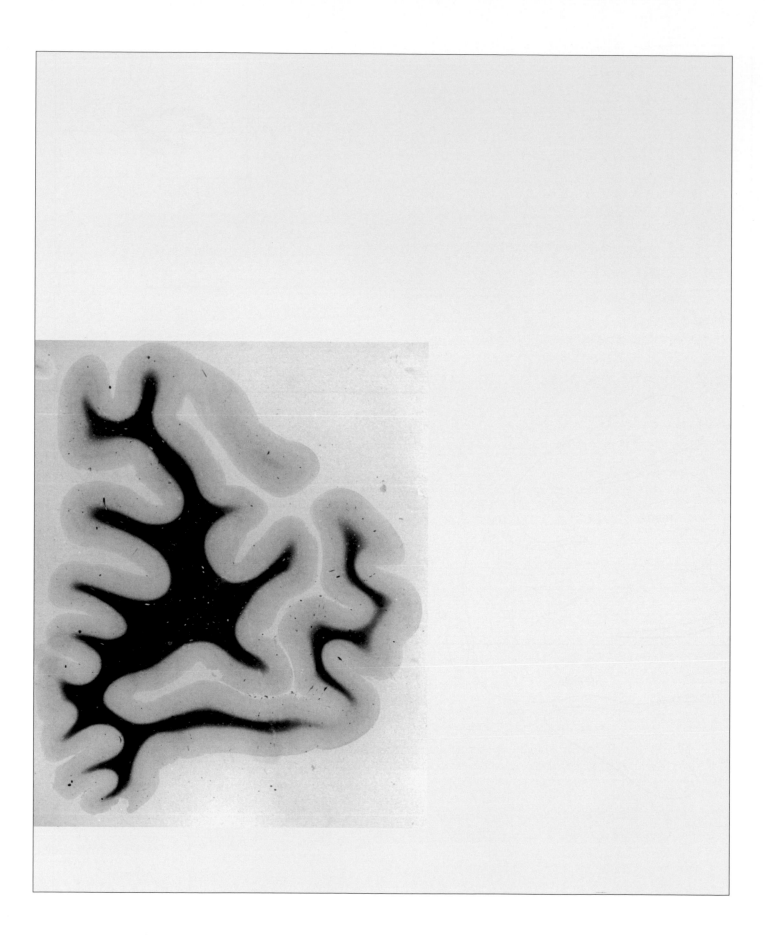

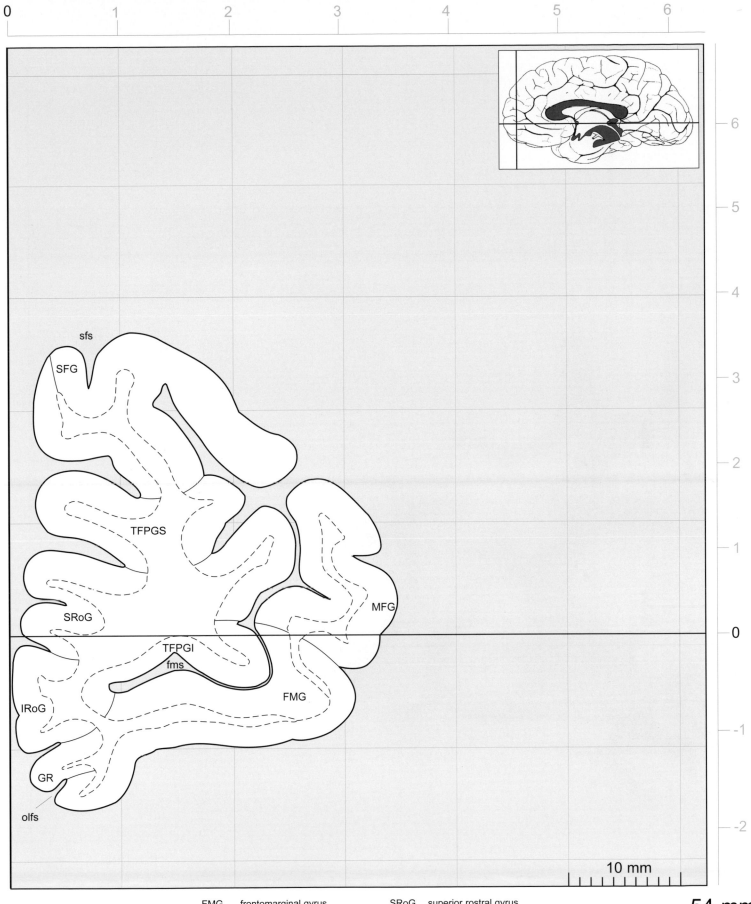

0   1   2   3   4   5   6

sfs

SFG

TFPGS

SRoG

MFG

TFPGI
fms

IRoG

FMG

GR

olfs

10 mm

-54 mm

FMG	frontomarginal gyrus		SRoG	superior rostral gyrus
fms	frontomarginal sulcus		TFPGI	inferior transverse frontopolar
GR	gyrus rectus			gyrus
ifs	inferior frontal sulcus		TFPGM	medial transverse frontopolar
IRoG	inferior rostral gyrus			gyrus
MFG	medial frontal gyrus		TFPGS	superior transverse frontopolar
olfs	olfactory sulcus			gyrus
SFG	superior frontal gyrus			
sfs	superior frontal sulcus			

02

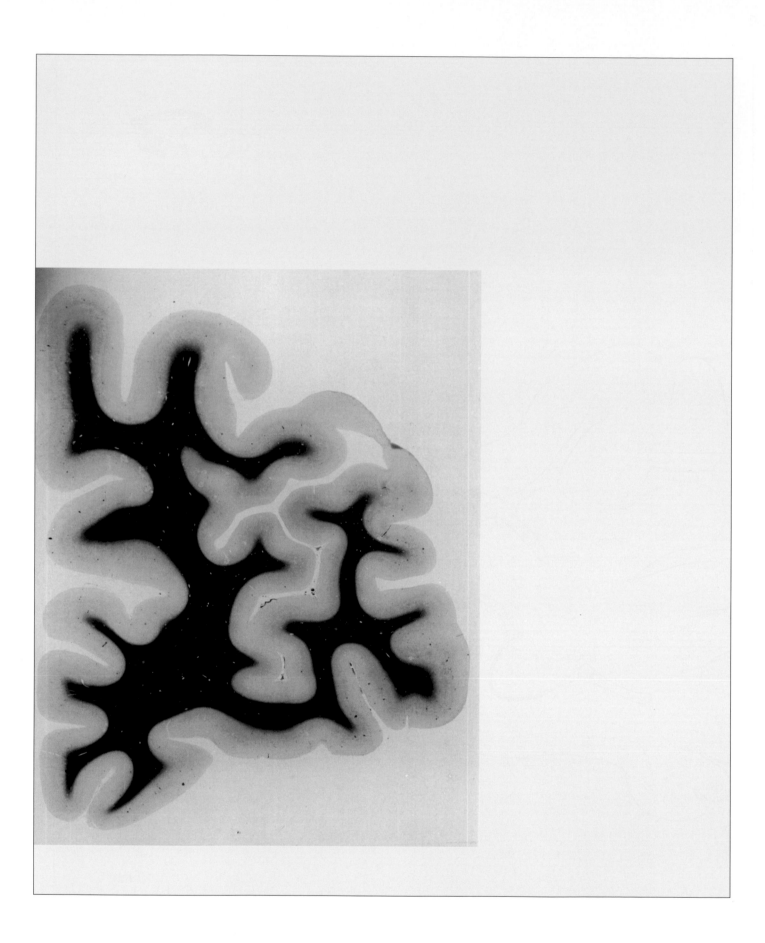

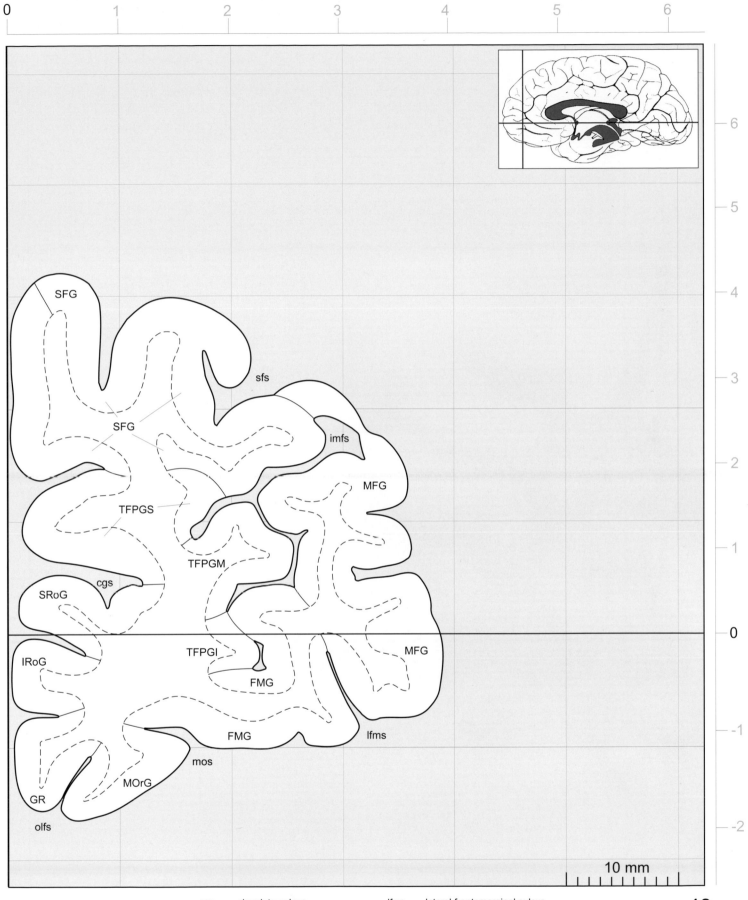

cgs	cingulate sulcus	lfms	lateral frontomarginal sulcus
FMG	frontomarginal gyrus	mos	medial orbital sulcus
fms	frontomarginal sulcus	sfs	superior frontal sulcus
GR	gyrus rectus	SRoG	superior rostral gyrus
IRoG	inferior rostral gyrus	TFPGI	inferior transverse frontopolar gyrus
MFG	medial frontal gyrus		
MOrG	medial orbital gyrus	TFPGM	medial transverse frontopolar gyrus
olfs	olfactory sulcus		
SFG	superior frontal gyrus	TFPGS	superior transverse frontopolar gyrus
imfs	intermediate frontal sulcus		

-48 mm

03

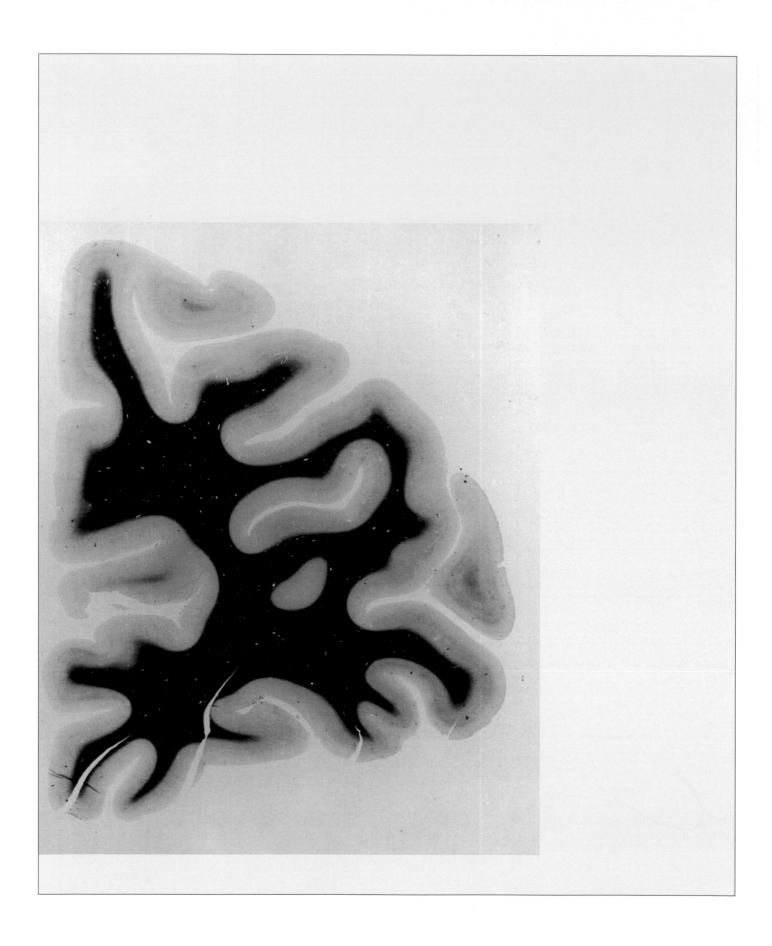

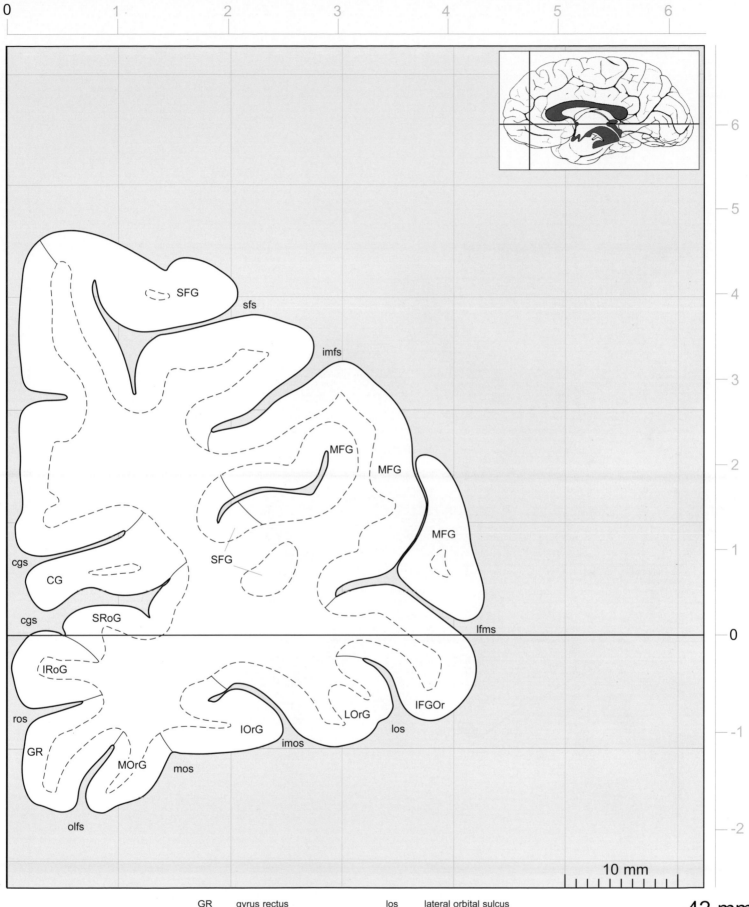

0 1 2 3 4 5 6

6

5

4

3

2

1

0

-1

-2

SFG
sfs
imfs
MFG
MFG
MFG
cgs
CG
SFG
cgs
SRoG
lfms
IRoG
IFGOr
ros
LOrG
los
IOrG
imos
GR
MOrG
mos
olfs

10 mm

-42 mm

GR	gyrus rectus	los	lateral orbital sulcus
IFGOr	inferior frontal gyrus, orbital part	MFG	medial frontal gyrus
ifs	inferior frontal sulcus	MOrG	medial orbital gyrus
imfs	intermediate frontal sulcus	mos	medial orbital sulcus
imos	intermediate orbital sulcus	olfs	olfactory sulcus
IOrG	intermediate orbital gyrus	ros	rostral sulcus
IRoG	inferior rostral gyrus	SFG	superior frontal gyrus
CG	cingulate gyrus	lfms	lateral frontomarginal sulcus	sfs	superior frontal sulcus
cgs	cingulate sulcus	LOrG	lateral orbital gyrus	SRoG	superior rostral gyrus

04

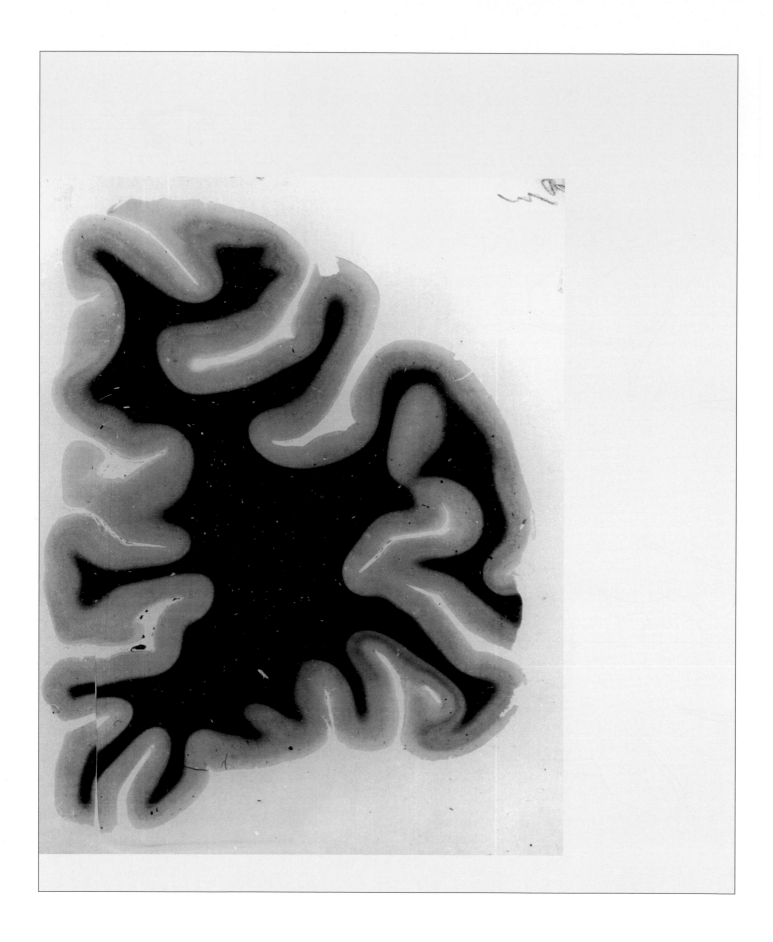

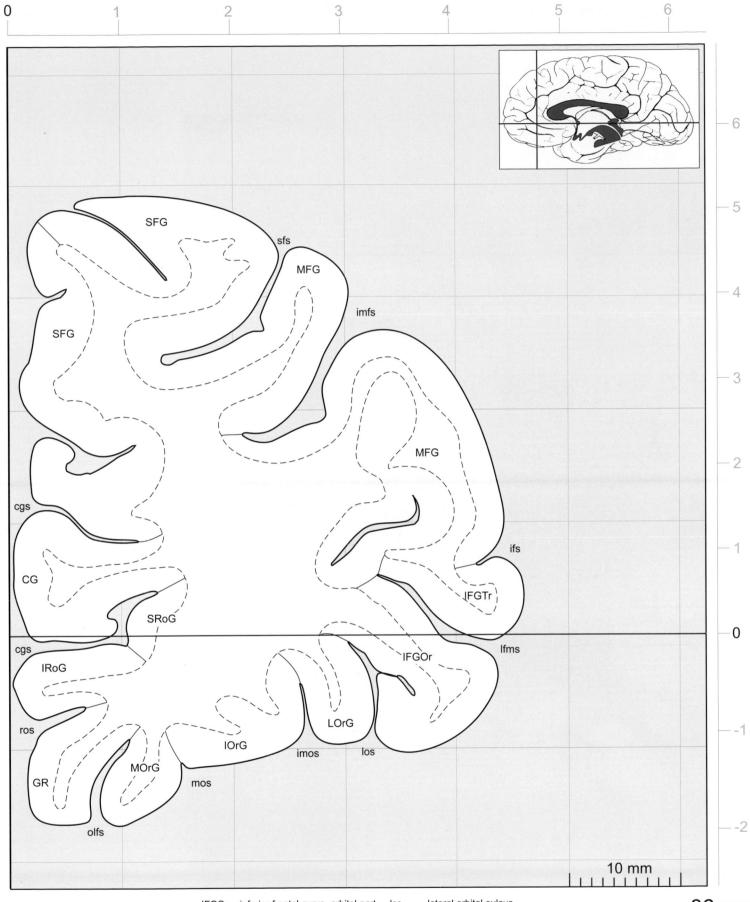

		IFGOr	inferior frontal gyrus, orbital part	los	lateral orbital sulcus
		IFGTr	IFG triangular part	MFG	medial frontal gyrus
		ifs	inferior frontal sulcus	MOrG	medial orbital gyrus
		imfs	intermediate frontal sulcus	mos	medial orbital sulcus
		imos	intermediate orbital sulcus	olfs	olfactory sulcus
		IOrG	intermediate orbital gyrus	ros	rostral sulcus
CG	cingulate gyrus	IRoG	inferior rostral gyrus	SFG	superior frontal gyrus
cgs	cingulate sulcus	lfms	lateral frontomarginal sulcus	sfs	superior frontal sulcus
GR	gyrus rectus	LOrG	lateral orbital gyrus	SRoG	superior rostral gyrus

-36 mm

05

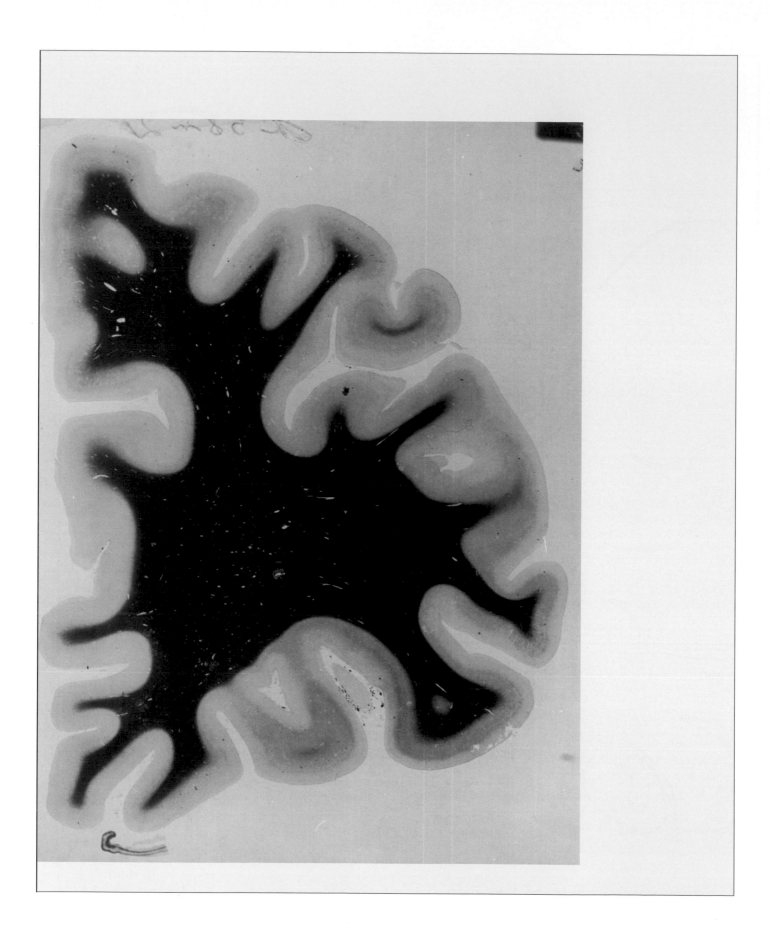

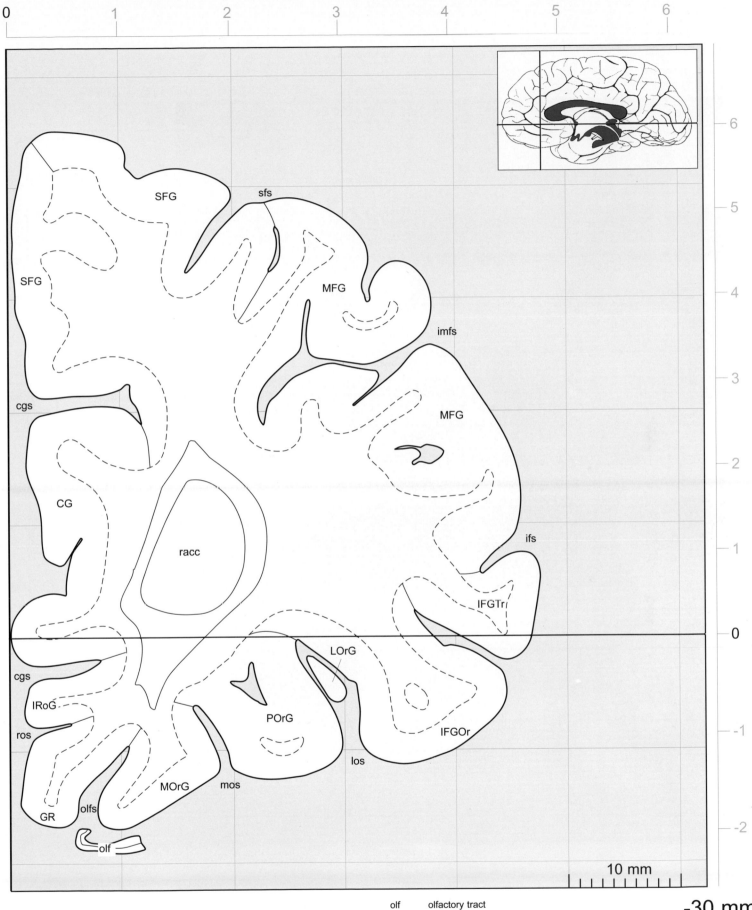

		imfs	intermediate frontal sulcus	olf	olfactory tract	
		ifs	inferior frontal sulcus	olfs	olfactory sulcus	
CG	cingulate gyrus	IRoG	inferior rostral gyrus	POrG	posterior orbital gyrus	
cgs	cingulate sulcus	LOrG	lateral orbital gyrus	racc	radiation of corpus callosum	
GR	gyrus rectus	los	lateral orbital sulcus	ros	rostral sulcus	
IFGOr	inferior frontal gyrus, orbital part	MFG	medial frontal gyrus	SCS	subcallosal stratum	
IFGTr	inferior frontal gyrus, triangular	MOrG	medial orbital gyrus	SFG	superior frontal gyrus	
	part	mos	medial orbital sulcus	sfs	superior frontal sulcus	
				SRoG	superior rostral gyrus	

-30 mm

06

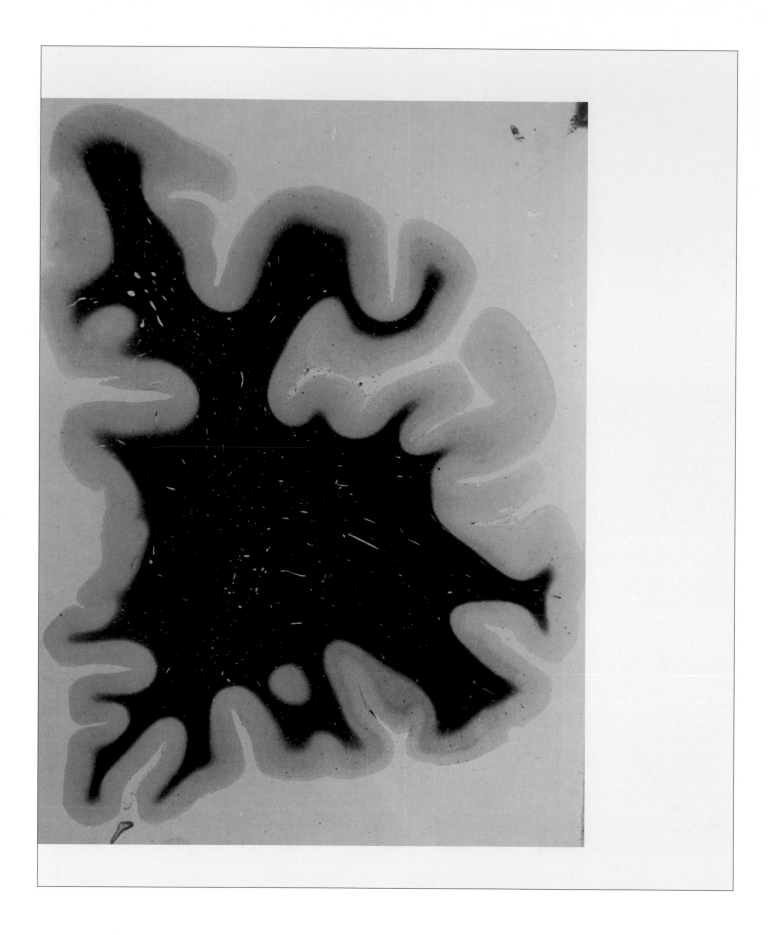

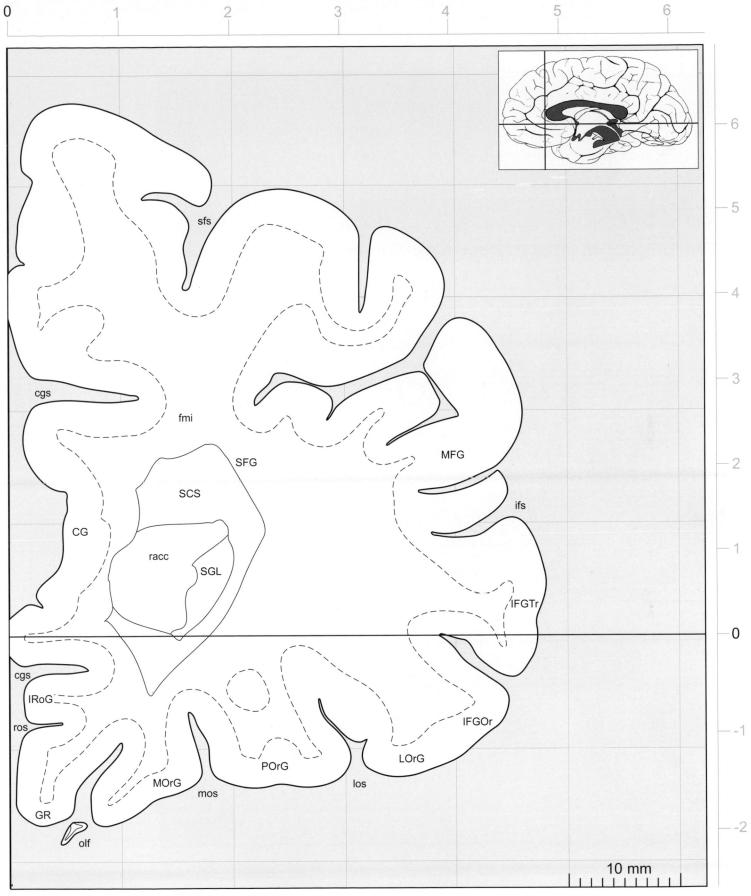

CG	cingulate gyrus	ifs	inferior frontal sulcus	ors	orbital sulcus
cgs	cingulate sulcus	imfs	intermediate frontal sulcus	POrG	posterior orbital gyrus
fmi	forceps minor of the corpus	IRoG	inferior rostral gyrus	racc	radiation of corpus callosum
	callosum	LOrG	lateral orbital gyrus	ros	rostral sulcus
GR	gyrus rectus	los	lateral orbital sulcus	SCS	subcallosal stratum
IFGOr	inferior frontal gyrus, orbital part	MFG	medial frontal gyrus	SFG	superior frontal gyrus
IFGTr	inferior frontal gyrus, triangular	MOrG	medial orbital gyrus	sfs	superior frontal sulcus
	part	mos	medial orbital sulcus	SGL	substantia gliosa
		olf	olfactory tract		(subependymal gray)

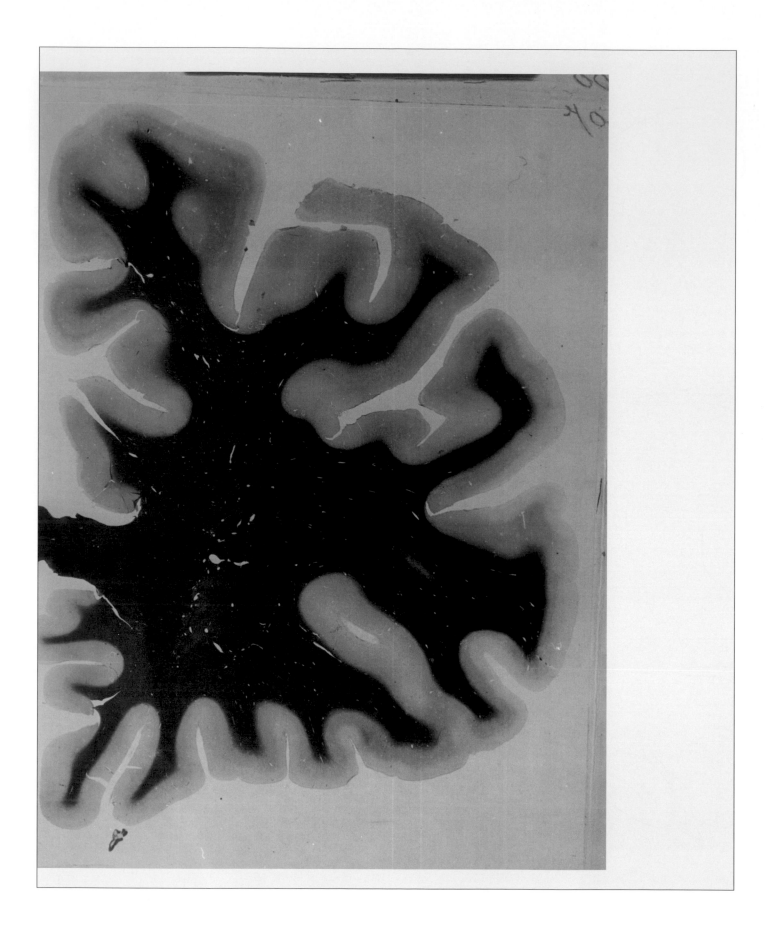

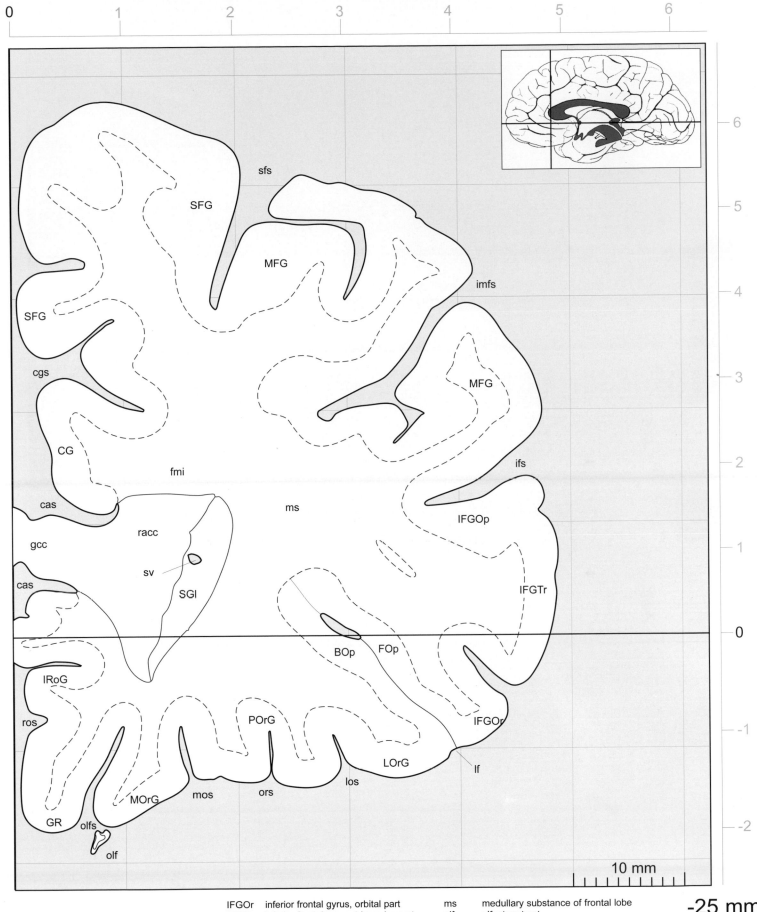

-25 mm

08

BOp	basal operculum	IFGOr	inferior frontal gyrus, orbital part	ms	medullary substance of frontal lobe
cas	callosal sulcus	IFGTr	inferior frontal gyrus, triangular part	olf	olfactory tract
CG	cingulate gyrus	ifs	inferior frontal sulcus	olfs	olfactory sulcus
cgs	cingulate sulcus	imfs	intermediate frontal sulcus	ors	orbital sulcus
fmi	forceps minor of the corpus callosum	IRoG	inferior rostral gyrus	POrg	posterior orbital gyrus
FOp	frontal operculum	lf	lateral fissure, horizontal ramus	racc	radiation of corpus callosum
gcc	genu of the corpus callosum	LOrG	lateral orbital gyrus	ros	rostral sulcus
GR	gyrus rectus	los	lateral orbital sulcus	SFG	superior frontal gyrus
IFGOp	inferior frontal gyrus, opercular part	MFG	medial frontal gyrus	sfs	superior frontal sulcus
		MOrG	medial orbital gyrus	SGl	substantia gliosa
		mos	medial orbital sulcus	sv	septal vein

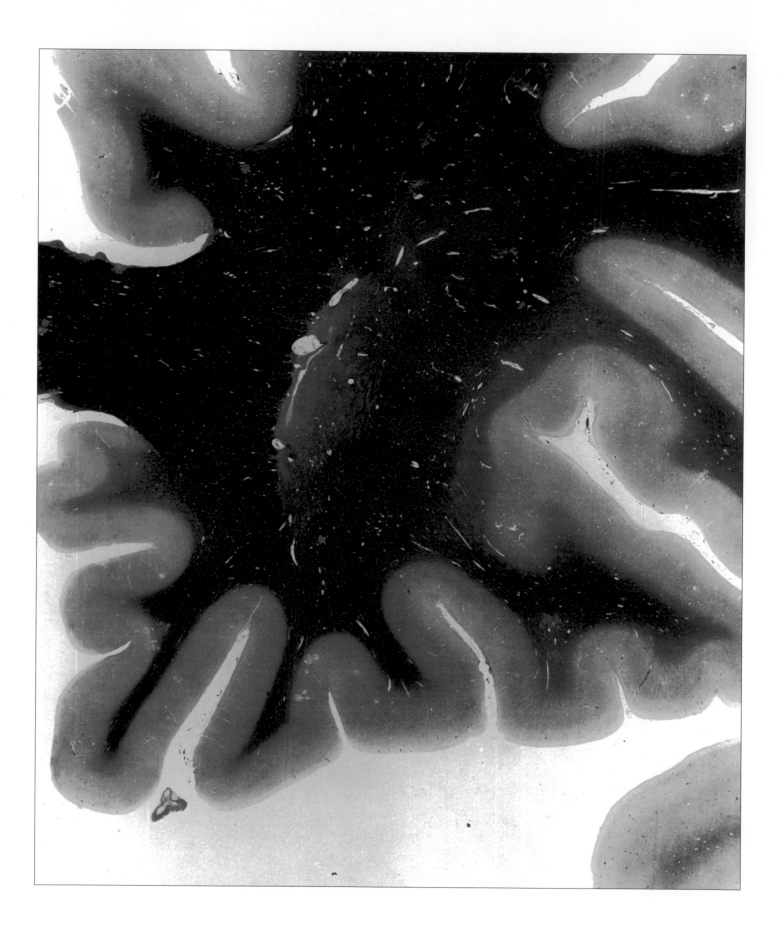

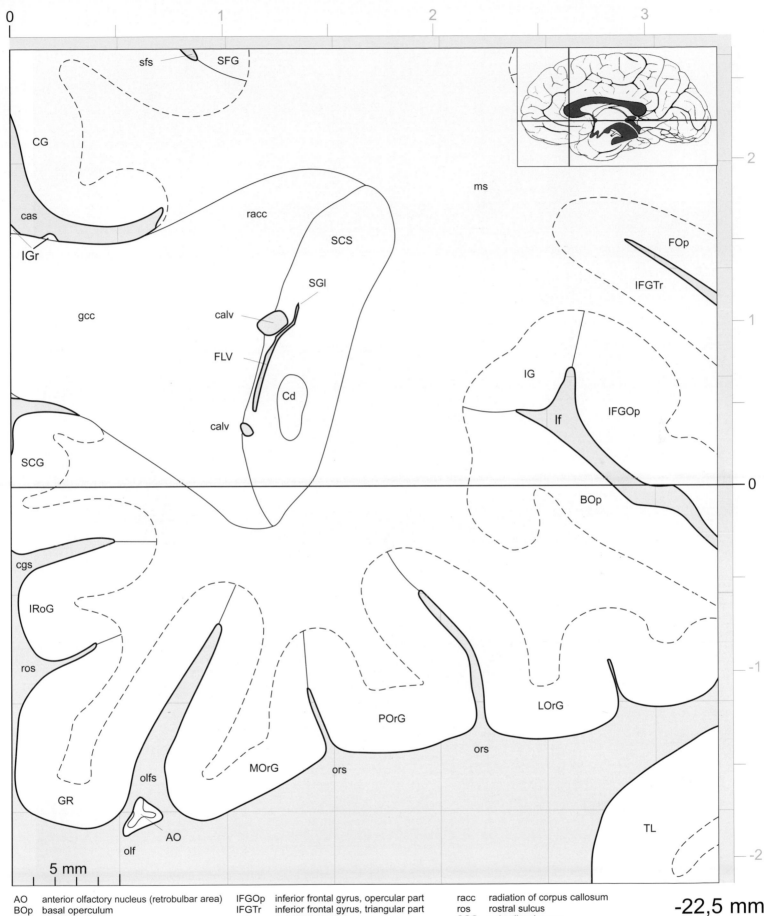

AO	anterior olfactory nucleus (retrobulbar area)	
BOp	basal operculum	
calv	callosal vein	
cas	callosal sulcus	
Cd	caudate nucleus	
CG	cingulate gyrus	
cgs	cingulate sulcus	
FLV	frontal horn of lateral ventricle	
FOp	frontal operculum	
gcc	genu of the corpus callosum	
GR	gyrus rectus	
IFGOp	inferior frontal gyrus, opercular part	
IFGTr	inferior frontal gyrus, triangular part	
IGr	indusium griseum	
IRoG	inferior rostral gyrus	
LOrG	lateral orbital gyrus	
MOrG	medial orbital gyrus	
ms	medullary substance of frontal lobe	
olf	olfactory tract	
olfs	olfactory sulcus	
ors	orbital sulcus	
POrG	posterior orbital gyrus	
racc	radiation of corpus callosum	
ros	rostral sulcus	
SCG	subcallosal gyrus	
SCS	subcallosal stratum	
SFG	superior frontal gyrus	
sfs	superior frontal sulcus	
SGl	substantia gliosa	
TL	temporal lobe	
lf	lateral fissure	

-22,5 mm

09

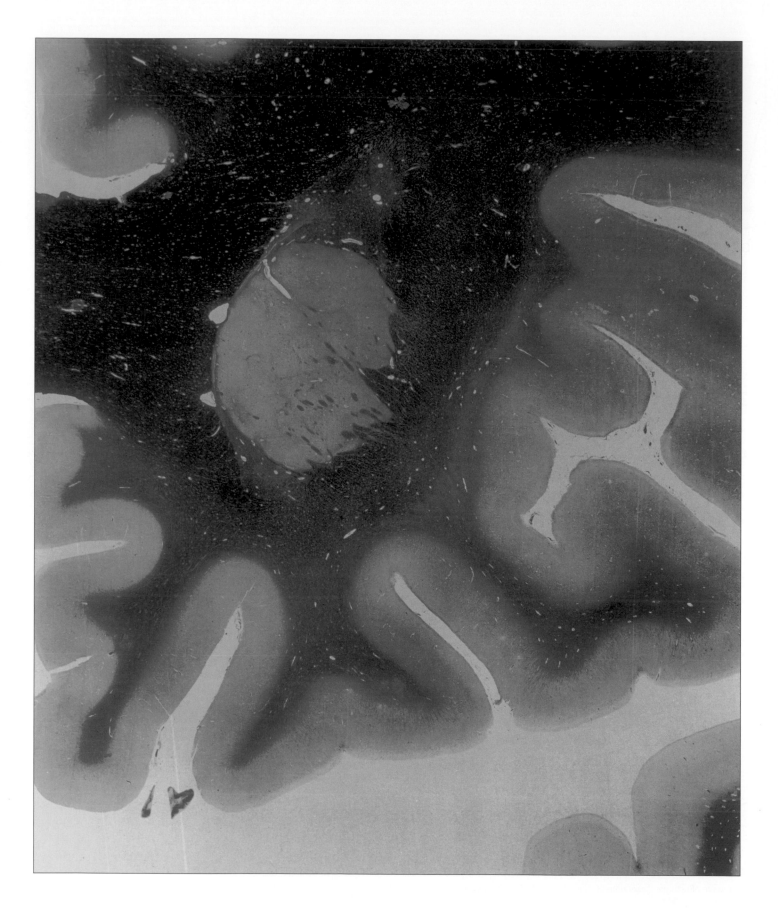

BOp   basal operculum
calv   callosal vein
cas   callosal sulcus
CdL   lateral caudate nucleus
CdM   medial caudate nucleus
CG   cingulate gyrus
cgs   cingulate sulcus

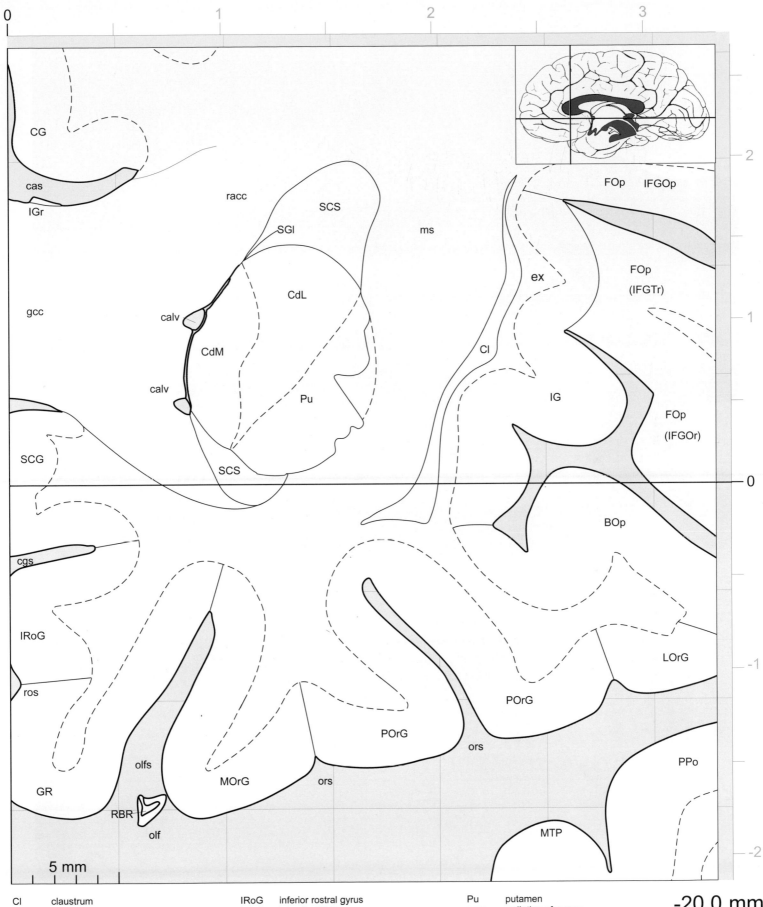

CG

cas

IGr

racc

SCS

SGI

ms

gcc

calv

CdL

ex

CdM

calv

Cl

Pu

IG

SCG

SCS

cgs

BOp

IRoG

ros

LOrG

POrG

olfs

POrG

ors

GR

MOrG

ors

PPo

RBR

olf

MTP

FOp   IFGOp

FOp
(IFGTr)

FOp
(IFGOr)

5 mm

-20,0 mm

Cl	claustrum	IRoG	inferior rostral gyrus	Pu	putamen	
ex	extreme capsule	LOrG	lateral orbital gyrus	racc	radiation of corpus	
FOp	frontal operculum	MOrG	medial orbital gyrus		callosum	
gcc	genu of the corpus callosum	ms	medullary substance of frontal lobe	RBR	retrobulbar region	
GR	gyrus rectus	MTP	medial temporopolar region	ros	rostral sulcus	
IFGOp	inferior frontal gyrus, opercular part	olf	olfactory tract	SCG	subcallosal gyrus	
IFGOr	inferior frontal gyrus, orbital part	olfs	olfactory sulcus	SCS	subcallosal stratum	
IFGTr	inferior frontal gyrus, triangular part	ors	orbital sulcus	SGI	substantia gliosa	
IG	insular gyrus	POrG	posterior orbital gyrus			
IGr	indusium griseum	PPo	planum polare			

10

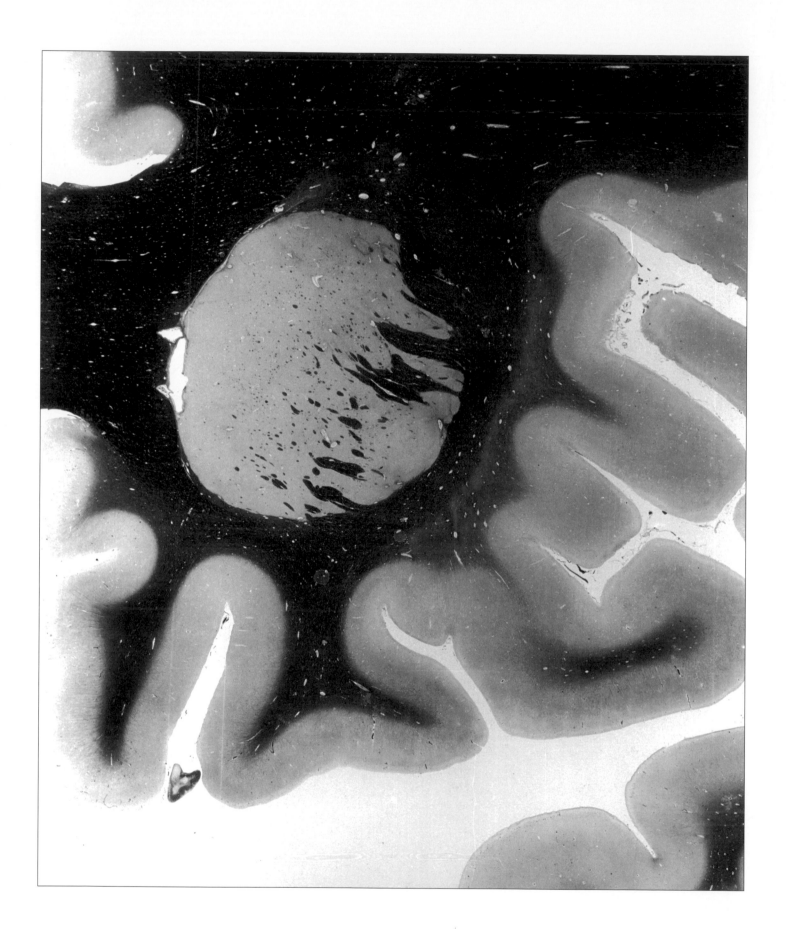

AcSV   accumbens nucl.,
       subventricular region
BOp   basal operculum
calv   callosal vein

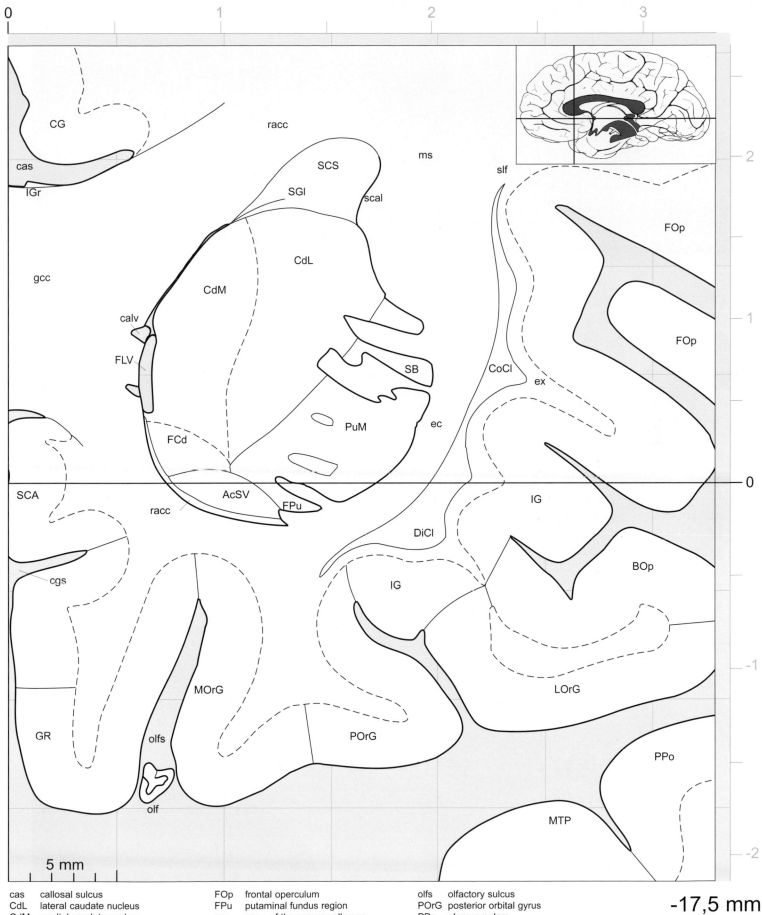

cas	callosal sulcus	FOp	frontal operculum	olfs	olfactory sulcus
CdL	lateral caudate nucleus	FPu	putaminal fundus region	POrG	posterior orbital gyrus
CdM	medial caudate nucleus	gcc	genu of the corpus callosum	PPo	planum polare
CG	cingulate gyrus	GR	gyrus rectus	PuM	medial putamen
cgs	cingulate sulcus	IG	insular gyrus	racc	radiation of corpus callosum
CoCl	compact insular claustrum	IGr	indusium griseum	SB	striatal cell bridges
DiCl	diffuse insular claustrum	LOrG	lateral orbital gyrus	SCA	subcallosal area
ec	external capsule	MOrG	medial orbital gyrus	scal	subcallosal fasciculus
ex	extreme capsule	ms	medullary substance of frontal lobe	SCS	subcallosal stratum
FCd	caudate fundus region	MTP	medial temporopolar gyrus	SGl	substantia gliosa
FLV	frontal horn of lateral ventricle	olf	olfactory tract	slf	superior fronto-occipital fasciculus

-17,5 mm

11

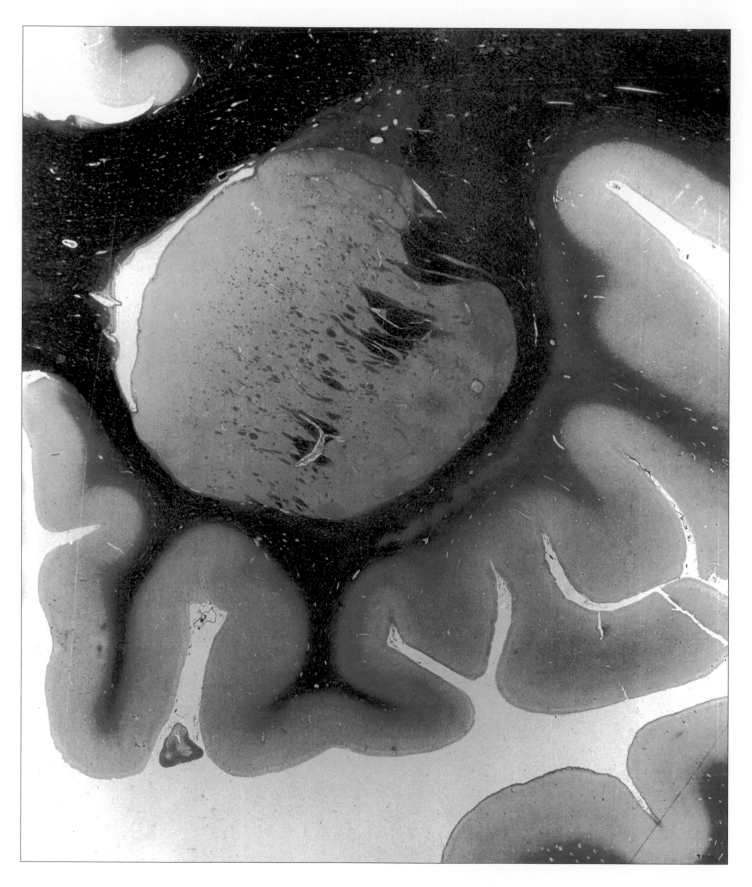

AcSV	accumbens n., subventricular region	cas	callosal sulcus
		CdL	lateral caudate nucleus
aic	anterior limb of internal capsule	CdM	medial caudate nucleus
		CG	cingulate gyrus
AO	anterior olfactory nucleus (retrobulbar region)	cgs	cingulate sulcus
		Cl	claustrum
BOp	basal operculum	ec	external capsule
calv	callosal vein	ex	extreme capsule

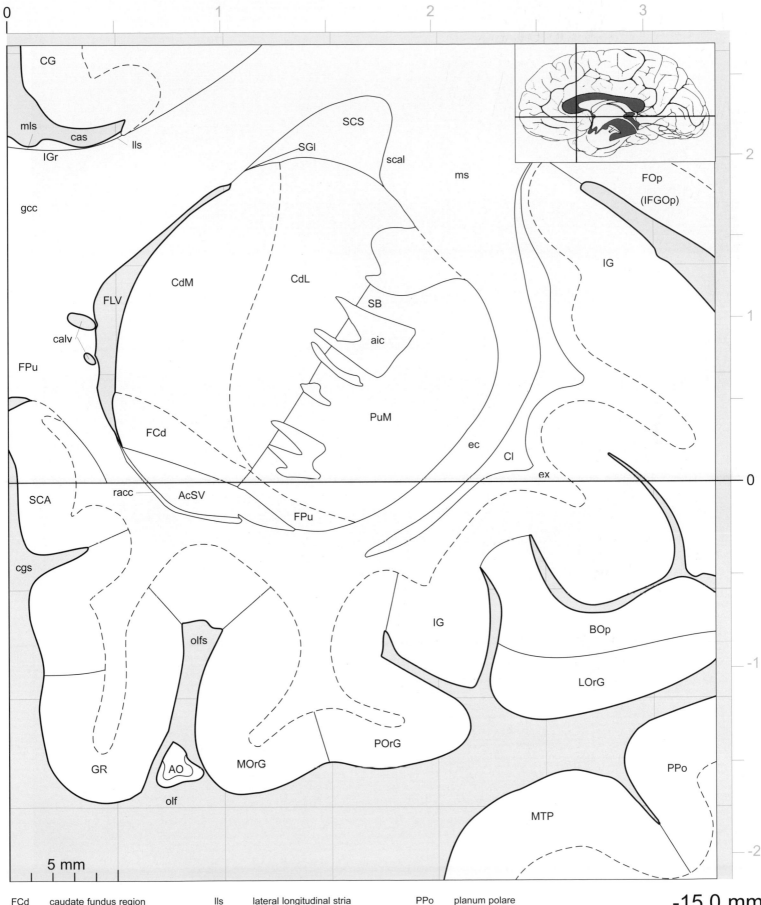

CG

mls
cas
lGr   lls

gcc

SCS
SGl
scal

ms

FOp
(IFGOp)

IG

CdM   CdL

FLV   SB

aic

calv

FPu

PuM

FCd   ec   Cl

ex

0

SCA   racc   AcSV   FPu

cgs

IG   BOp

olfs   LOrG

GR   AO   MOrG   POrG   PPo

olf   MTP

5 mm

-15,0 mm

12

FCd	caudate fundus region	lls	lateral longitudinal stria	PPo	planum polare
FLV	frontal horn of lateral ventricle	LOrG	lateral orbital gyrus	PuM	medial putamen
FOp	frontal operculum	mls	medial longitudinal stria	racc	radiation of corpus callosum
FPu	putaminal fundus region	MOrG	medial orbital gyrus	RBR	retrobulbar region
gcc	genu of the corpus callosum	ms	medullary substance of frontal lobe	SB	striatal cell bridges
GR	gyrus rectus	MTP	medial temporopolar gyrus	SCA	subcallosal area
IFGOp	inferior frontal gyrus, opercular part	olf	olfactory tract	scal	subcallosal fasciculus
IG	insular gyrus	olfs	olfactory sulcus	SCS	subcallosal stratum
IGr	indusium griseum	POrG	posterior orbital gyrus	SGl	substantia gliosa

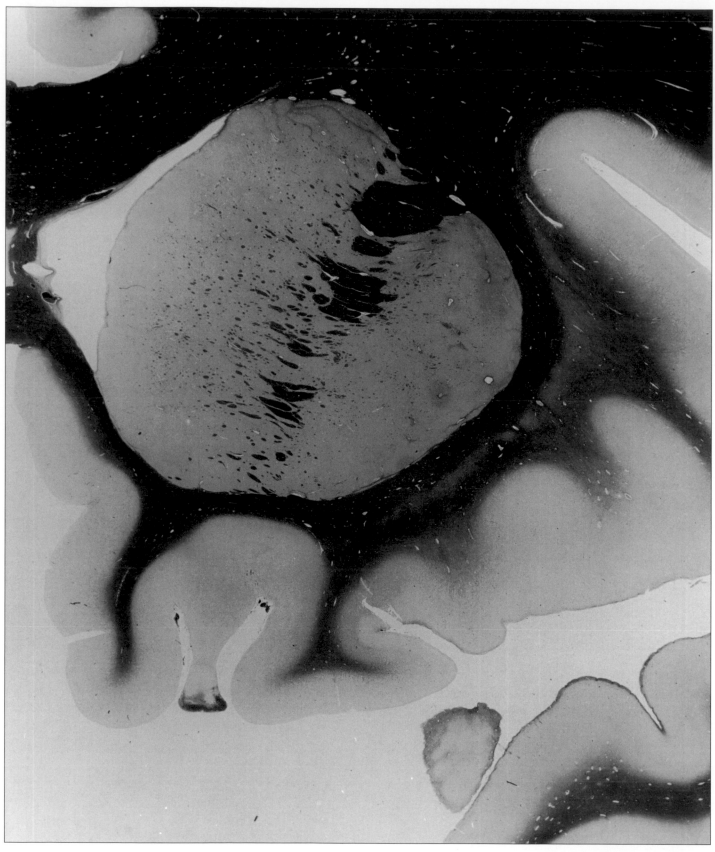

AcSV   accumbens n., subventricular
        region
aic   anterior limb of internal
        capsule
AO   anterior olfactory nucleus
        (retrobulbar
        region)
aps   anterior parolfactory sulcus
cas   callosal sulcus

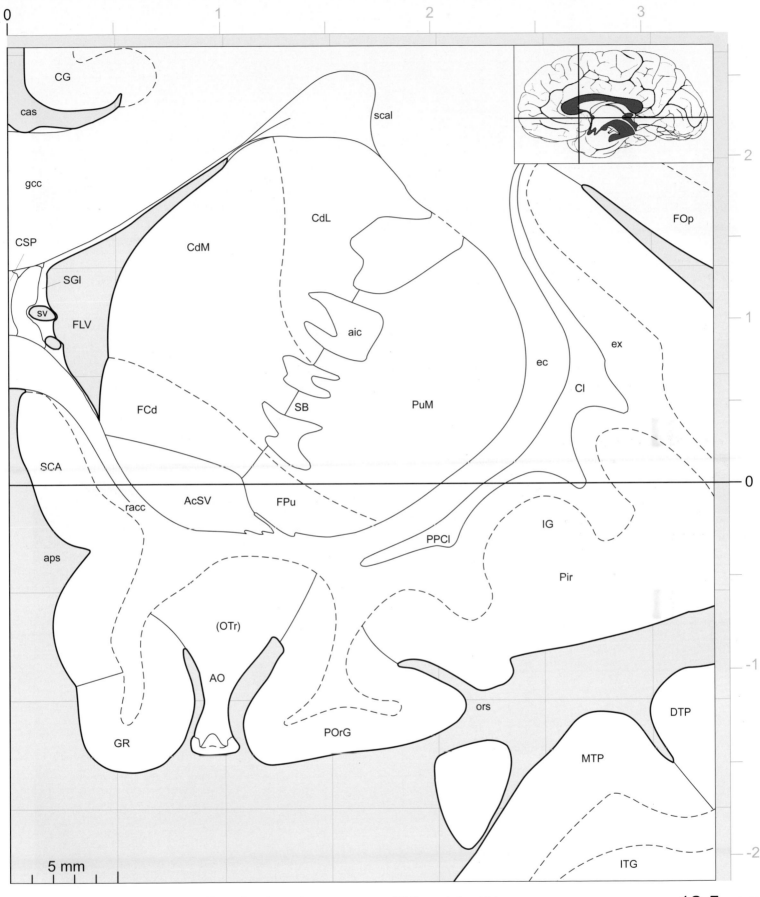

CdL	lateral caudate nucleus	FOp	frontal operculum	POrG	posterior orbital gyrus
CdM	medial caudate nucleus	FPu	putaminal fundus region	PPCl	prepiriform claustrum
CG	cingulate gyrus	gcc	genu of the corpus callosum	PuM	medial putamen
Cl	claustrum	GR	gyrus rectus	racc	radiation of corpus callosum
DTP	dorsal temporopolar gyrus	IG	insular gyrus	SB	striatal cell bridges
ec	external capsule	MTP	medial temporopolar region	SCA	subcallosal area
ex	extreme capsule	ors	orbital sulcus	scal	aubcallosal fasciculus
FCd	caudate fundus region	OTr	olfactory trigone	SGl	substantia gliosa
FLV	frontal horn of lateral ventricle	Pir	cortex (pre-)piriformis	sv	septal vein

-12,5 mm

13

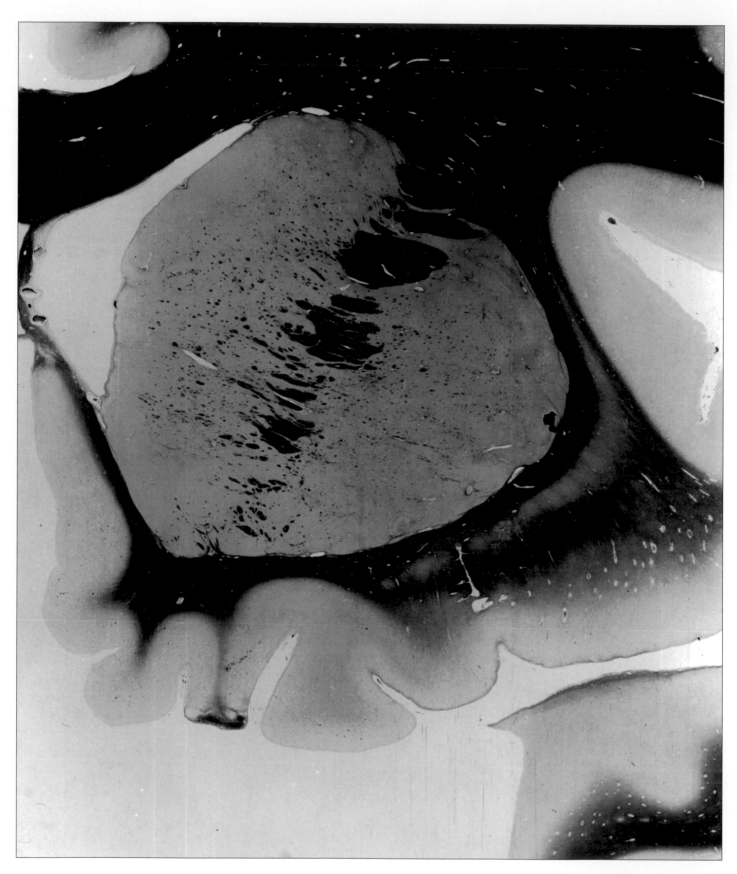

AcCL	accumbens n., centrolateral part	apsi	anterior parolfactory sulcus, inf.branch	CG	cingulate gyrus
AcM	accumbens n., medial part	apss	anterior parolfactory sulcus, sup. branch	cir	circular insular sulcus
AcSV	accumbens n., subventricular part			CoCl	compact insular claustrum
		bcc	body of the corpus callosum	CSP	cavity of septum pellucidum
aic	anterior limb of internal capsule	cas	callosal sulcus	DTP	dorsal temporopolar region
		CdL	lateral caudate nucleus	ec	external capsule
AO	anterior olfactory nucleus	CdM	medial caudate nucleus	ex	extreme capsule
				FCd	caudate fundus region

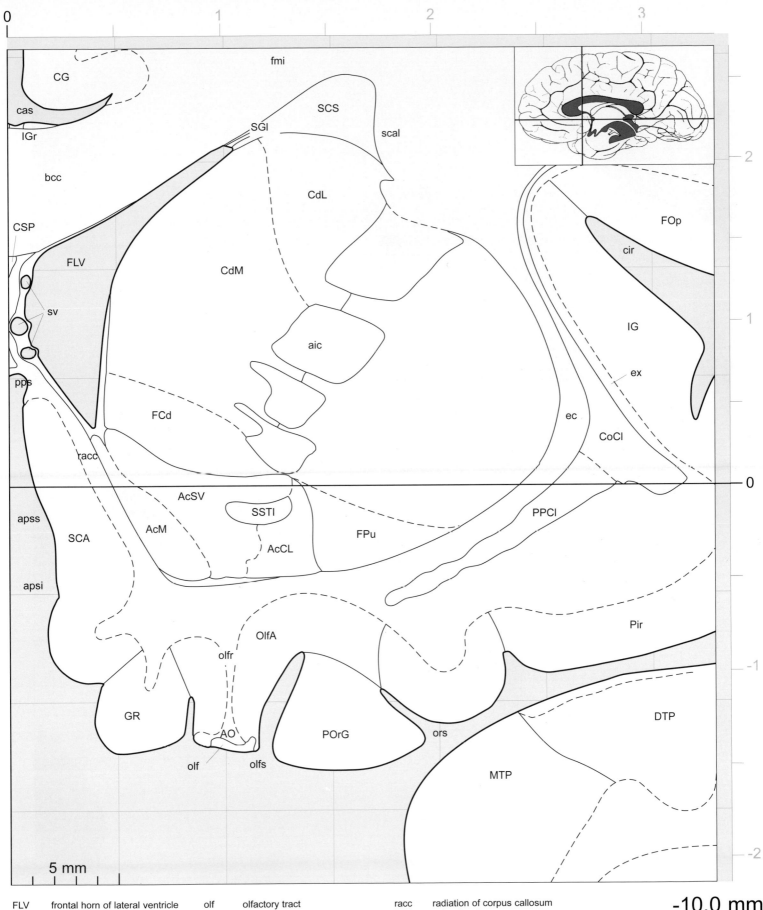

0   1   2   3

5 mm

-10,0 mm

14

FLV	frontal horn of lateral ventricle	olf	olfactory tract	racc	radiation of corpus callosum
fmi	forceps minor of the corpus callosum	OlfA	olfactory area	SCA	subcallosal area
		olfr	olfactory radiation	scal	aubcallosal fasciculus
FOp	frontal operculum	olfs	olfactory sulcus	SCS	subcallosal stratum
FPu	putaminal fundus region	ors	orbital sulcus	SGl	substantia gliosa
GR	gyrus rectus	Pir	cortex (pre-)piriformis	SSTI	substriatal terminal island
IG	insular gyrus	POrG	posterior orbital gyrus	sv	septal vein
IGr	indusium griseum	PPCl	prepiriform claustrum		
MTP	medial temporopolar region	pps	posterior parolfactory sulcus		

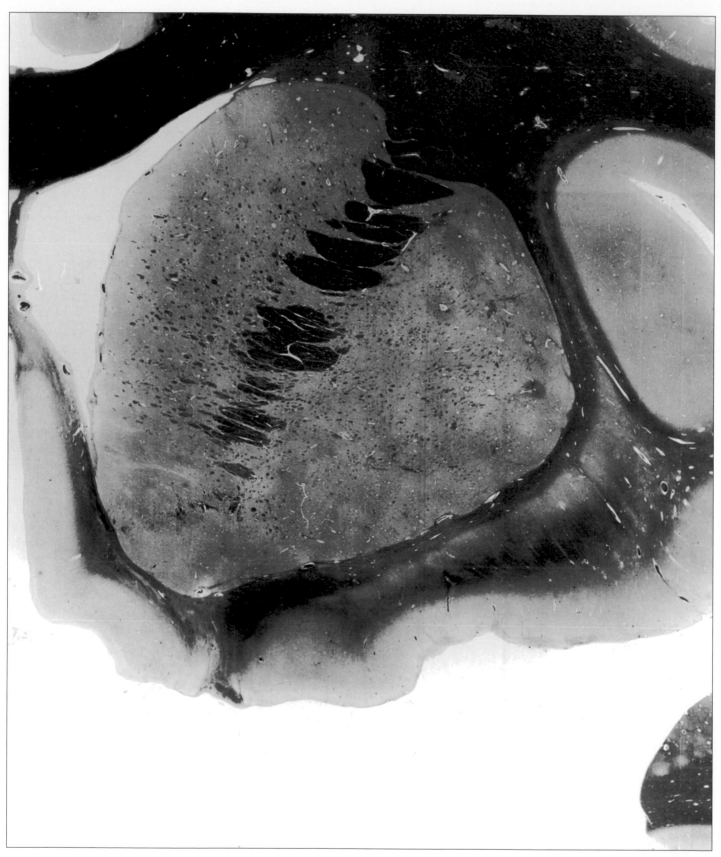

AcCL	centrolateral part of accumbens nucl.	CdM	medial caudate nucleus
AcCM	centromedial part of accumbens nucl.	CG	cingulate gyrus
AcL	lateral accumbens nucleus	cgs	cingulate sulcus
AcM	medial accumbens nucleus	cir	circular insular sulcus
aic	anterior limb of internal capsule	CoCl	compact insular claustrum
AOP	anterior olfactory nucleus, posterior part	ec	external capsule
apss	anterior parolfactory sulcus, sup. branch	ex	extreme capsule
bcc	body of the corpus callosum	FCd	caudate fundus region
CdL	lateral caudate nucleus	FPu	putaminal fundus region

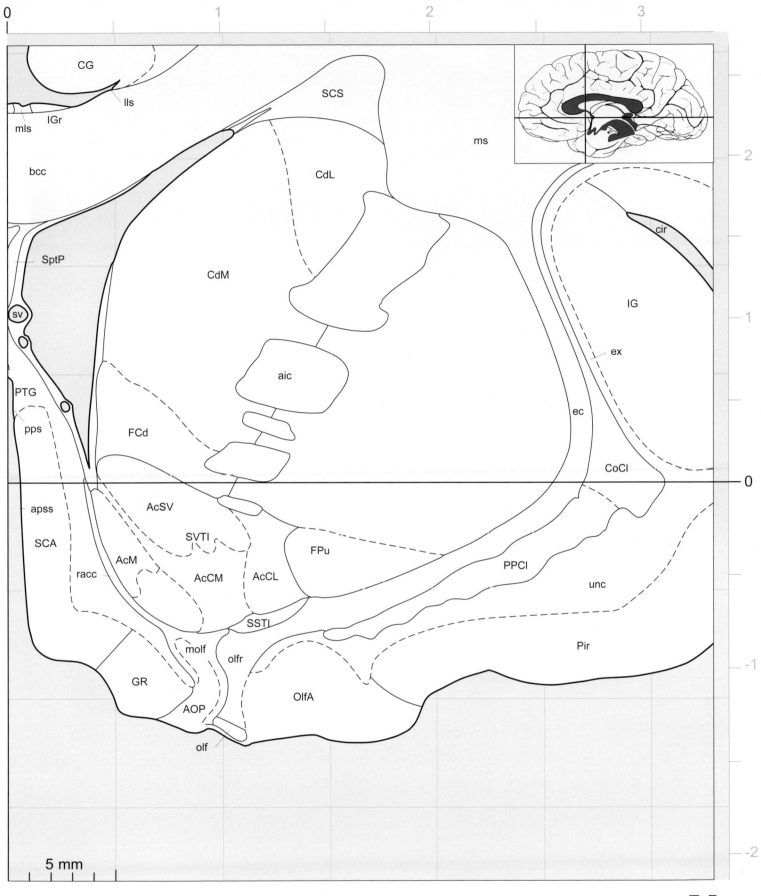

-7,5 mm

15

GR	gyrus rectus
IG	insular gyrus
IGr	indusium griseum
lls	lateral longitudinal stria
mls	medial longitudinal stria
molf	medial olfactory radiation
ms	medullary substance of frontal lobe
olf	olfactory tract

OlfA	olfactory area
olfr	olfactory radiation
Pir	cortex (pre-)piriformis
PPCl	prepiriform claustrum
pps	posterior parolfactory sulcus
PTG	paraterminal gyrus
racc	radiation of corpus callosum
SCA	subcallosal area
SCS	subcallosal stratum

SptP	septum pellucidum
SSTI	substriatal terminal island
SVTI	subventricular terminal island
sv	septal vein
unc	uncinate fasciculus

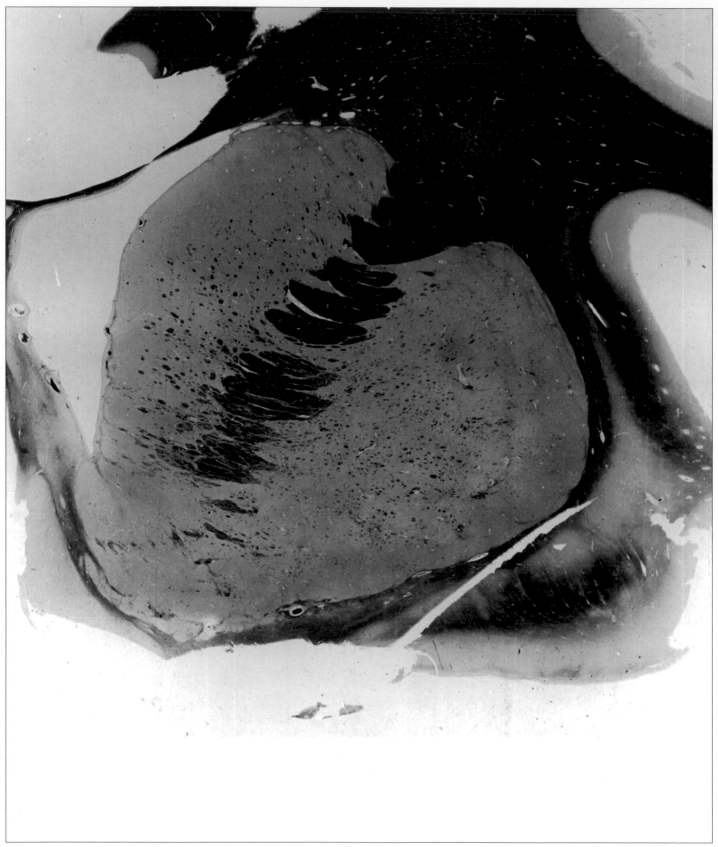

AcCL	accumbens n., centrolateral part	AOP	anterior olfactory nucleus, posterior part
AcCM	accumbens n., centromedial part	bcc	body of the corpus callosum
		CdL	lateral caudate nucleus
AcM	accumbens n., medial part	CdM	medial caudate nucleus
AcSV	accumbens n., subventricular part	CG	cingulate gyrus
		cir	circular insular sulcus
aic	anterior limb of internal capsule	CoCl	(compact) insular claustrum
		db	diagonal band

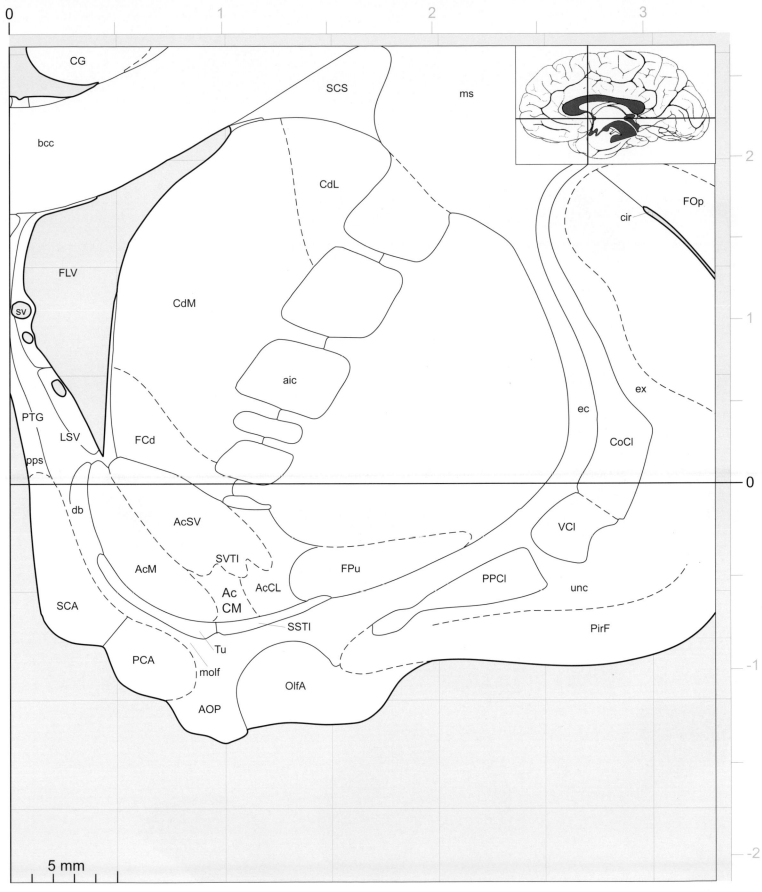

ec	external capsule	molf	medial olfactory radiation	SCA	subcallosal area
ex	extreme capsule	ms	medullary substance of frontal	SCS	subcallosal stratum
FCd	accumbens n., caudate fundus		lobe	SSTI	substriatal terminal island
	region	OlfA	olfactory area	sv	septal vein
FLV	frontal horn of lateral ventricle	PCA	precommissural archicortex	SVTI	subventricular terminal island
FOp	frontal operculum	PirF	(pre-)piriform cortex, frontal area	Tu	olfactory tubercle
FPu	accumbens n., putaminal fundus	PPCl	prepiriform claustrum	unc	uncinate fasciculus
	region	pps	posterior parolfactory sulcus	VCl	ventral claustrum
LSV	ventrolateral septal nucleus	PTG	paraterminal gyrus		

-5,8 mm

16

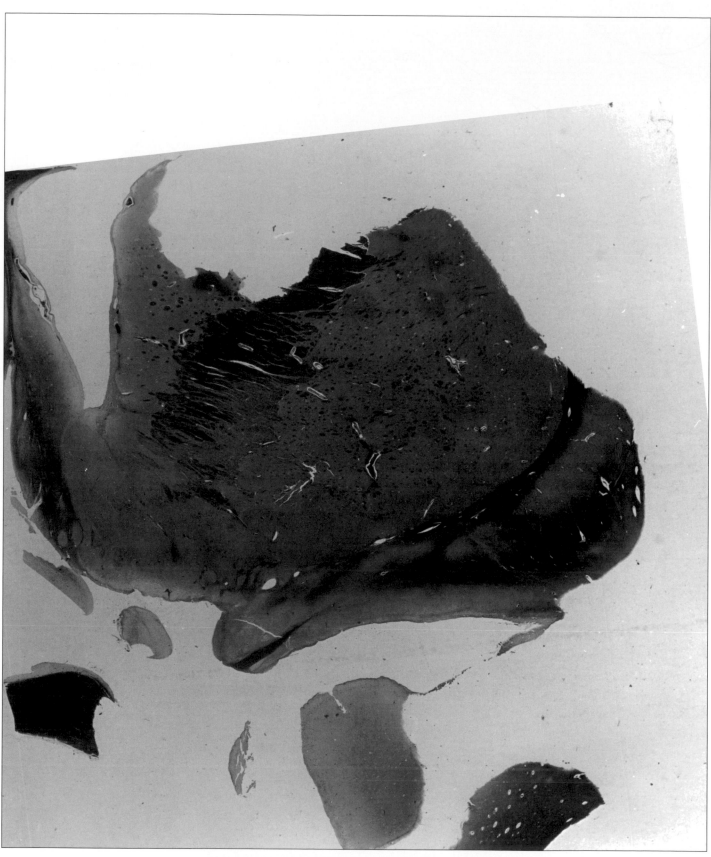

AcCL	accumbens n., centrolateral part	cir	circular insular sulcus	FOp	frontal operculum
AcCM	accumbens n., centromedial part	CoCl	(compact) insular claustrum	FPu	accumbens n., putaminal
AcM	accumbens n., medial part	DiCl	diffuse insular claustrum		fundus region
AcSV	accumbens n., subventricular part	ec	external capsule	GTI	great terminal island
aic	anterior limb of internal capsule	EGP	external globus pallidus	IG	insular gyrus
bcc	body of the corpus callosum	Ent	entorhinal cortex	ilf	inferior longitudinal fasciculus
CdL	lateral caudate nucleus	ex	extreme capsule	Li	limen insulae
CdM	medial caudate nucleus	FCd	accumbens n., caudate	lml	lateral medullary lamina of
CG	cingulate gyrus		fundus region		the globus pallidus

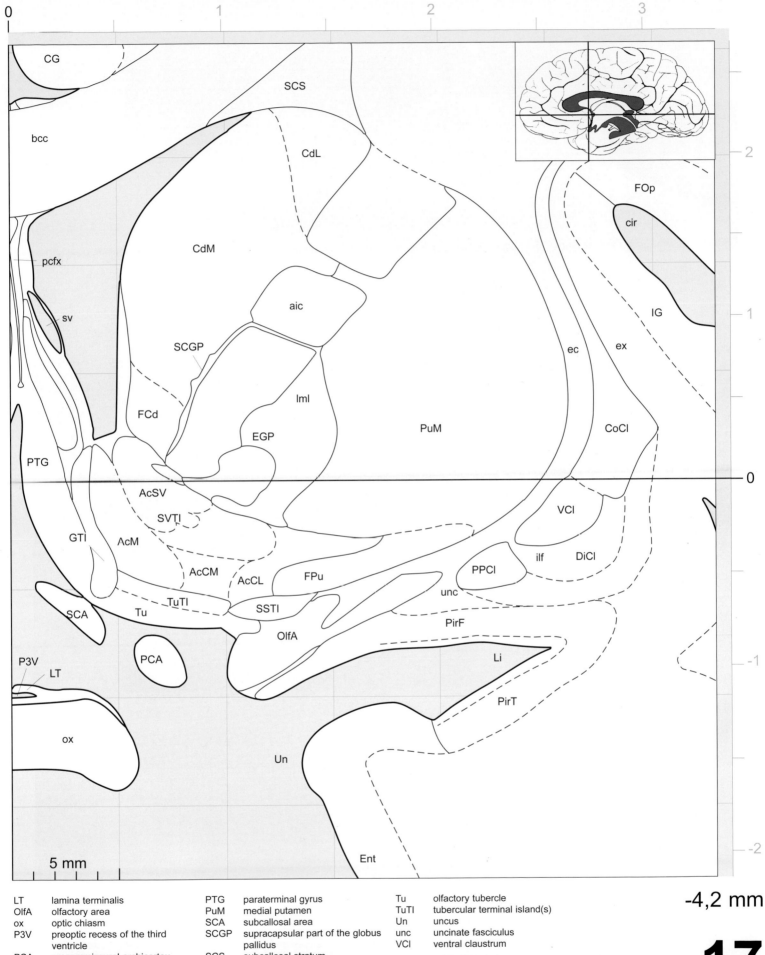

LT	lamina terminalis	PTG	paraterminal gyrus
OlfA	olfactory area	PuM	medial putamen
ox	optic chiasm	SCA	subcallosal area
P3V	preoptic recess of the third ventricle	SCGP	supracapsular part of the globus pallidus
PCA	precommissural archicortex	SCS	subcallosal stratum
pcfx	precommissural fornix	SSTI	substriatal terminal island
Pir	(pre-)piriform cortex	sv	septal vein
PPCl	prepiriform claustrum	SVTI	subventricular terminal island

Tu	olfactory tubercle
TuTI	tubercular terminal island(s)
Un	uncus
unc	uncinate fasciculus
VCl	ventral claustrum

5 mm

-4,2 mm

17

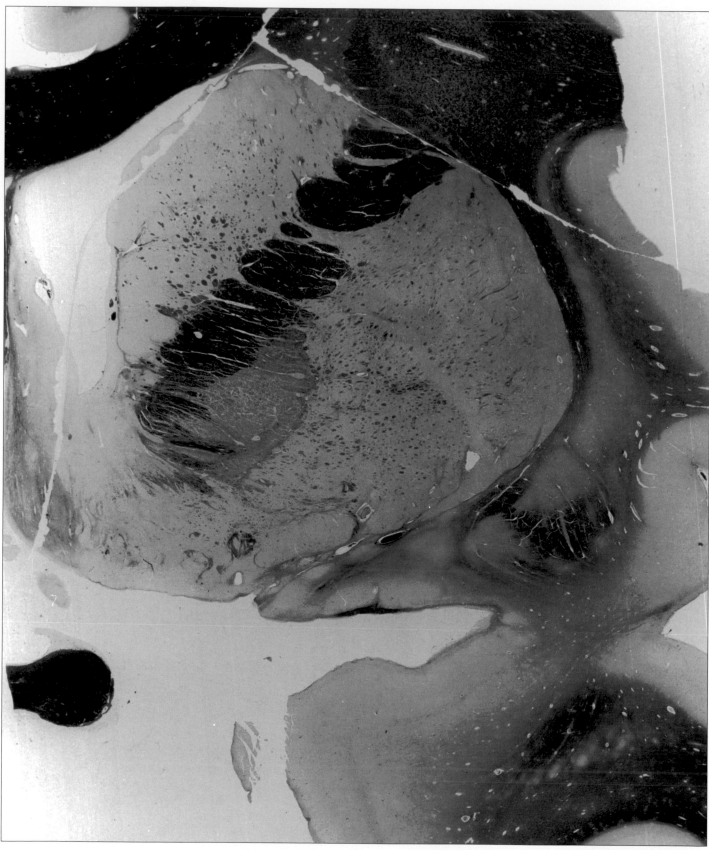

ac	anterior commissure		terminalis, lateral division	EGP	external globus pallidus	ilf	inferior longitudinal fasciculus
AcCL	accumbens n., centrolateral part	CdL	lateral caudate nucleus	Ent	entorhinal cortex	Li	limen insulae
AcCM	accumbens n., centromedial part	CdM	medial caudate nucleus	ex	extreme capsule	lml	lateral medullary lamina of the
AcM	accumbens n., medial part	CdV	ventral caudate nucleus	FCd	caudate fundus region		globus pallidus
aic	anterior limb of internal capsule	CG	cingulate gyrus	FOp	frontal operculum	LSV	ventrolateral septal nucleus
bcc	body of the corpus callosum	cir	circular insular sulcus	FPu	putaminal fundus region	LT	lamina terminalis
BSTC	bed nucleus of the stria	CoCl	(compact) insular claustrum	GTI	great terminal island	mfb	medial forebrain bundle
	terminalis, central division	DiCl	diffuse insular claustrum	IG	insular gyrus	mls	medial longitudinal stria
BSTL	bed nucleus of the stria	ec	external capsule	IGr	indusium griseum	ox	optic chiasm

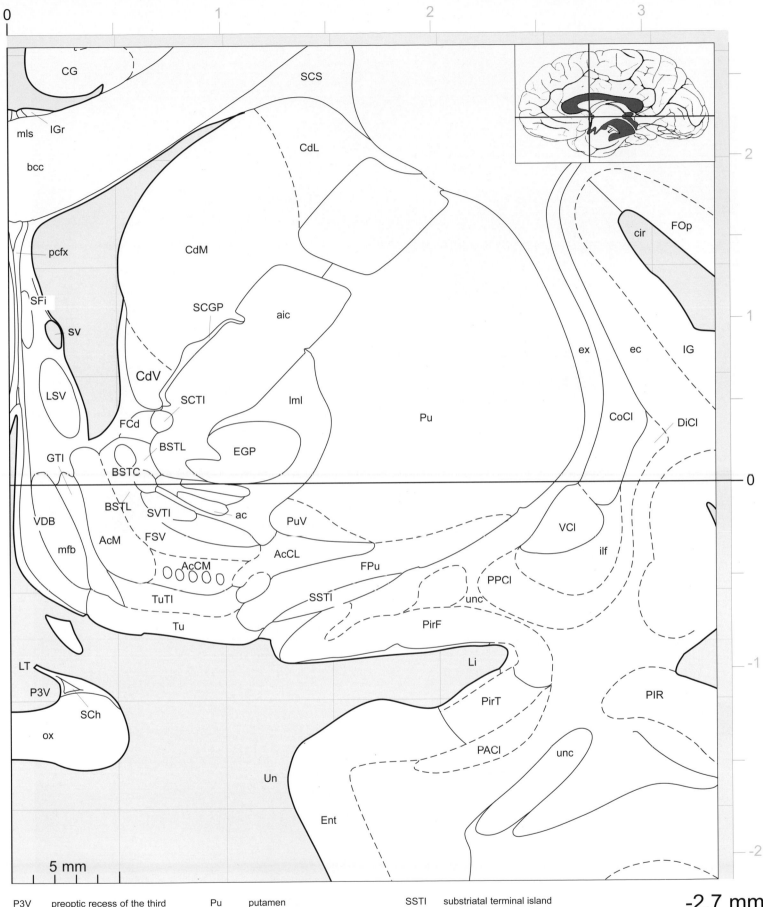

0   1   2   3

CG

SCS

mls   IGr

bcc

CdL

pcfx

CdM

SFi

SCGP   aic

sv

CdV

LSV

SCTI   lml

FCd

GTI   BSTL

BSTC   EGP

Pu

CoCl

DiCl

VCl

ex   ec   IG

cir   FOp

BSTL   SVTI   ac

VDB   AcM   FSV   PuV

mfb   AcCL

AcCM   FPu

TuTI   SSTI   PPCl   unc

ilf

Tu   PirF

LT   Li

P3V   PirT   PIR

SCh   PACl   unc

ox

Un

Ent

5 mm

-2,7 mm

18

P3V	preoptic recess of the third ventricle	Pu	putamen	
PACl	preamygdalar claustrum	PuV	ventral putamen	
pcfx	precommissural fornix	SCGP	supracapsular part of the globus pallidus	
PIR	parainsular region			
PirF	(pre-)piriform cortex, frontal area	SCh	suprachiasmatic nucleus	
PirT	(pre-)piriform cortex, temporal area	SCS	subcallosal stratum	
		SCTI	subcaudate terminal island	
PPCl	prepiriform claustrum	SFi	septofimbrial nucleus	
		SLG	semilunar gyrus	

SSTI	substriatal terminal island
sv	septal vein
SVTI	subventricular terminal island
Tu	olfactory tubercle
TuTI	tubercular terminal island(s)
Un	uncus
unc	uncinate fasciculus
VCl	ventral claustrum
VDB	vertical limb of the diagonal band

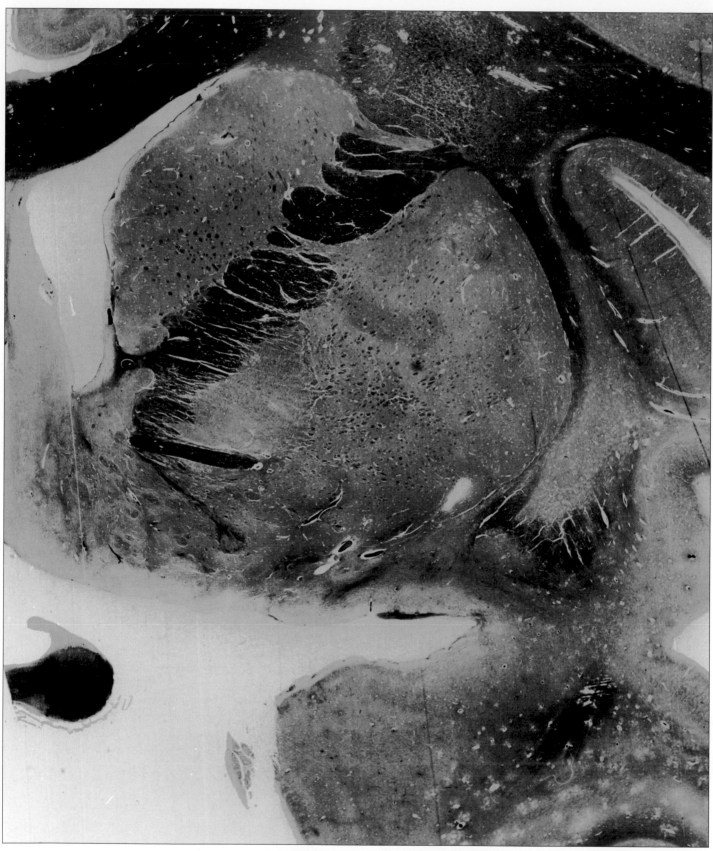

ac	anterior commisure	BSTLJ	bed nucleus of the stria terminalis, lateral division, juxtacapsular part	DiCl	diffuse insular claustrum	IGr	indusium griseum
AcCL	accumbens n., centrolateral part			ec	external capsule	ilf	inferior longitudinal fasciculus
AcCM	accumbens n., centromedial part	BSTM	bed nucleus of the stria terminalis, medial division	EGP	external globus pallidus	Li	limen insulae
AcM	accumbens n., medial part			Ent	entorhinal cortex	lml	external medullary lamina of the globus pallidus
aco	anterior commissure, olfactory limb	CdL	lateral caudate nucleus	ex	extreme capsule		
AcSV	accumbens n., subventricular part	CdM	medial caudate nucleus	FLV	frontal horn of lateral ventricle	lo	lateral olfactory tract
aic	anterior limb of internal capsule	CdV	ventral caudate nucleus	FOp	frontal operculum	LSD	dorsolateral septal nucleus
bcc	body of the corpus callosum	CG	cingulate gyrus	FPu	putaminal fundus region	LSI	intermediolateral septal nucleus
BSTC	bed nucleus of the stria terminalis, central division	cir	circular insular sulcus	GTI	great terminal island	LSV	ventrolateral septal nucleus
		CoCl	(compact) insular claustrum	IG	insular gyrus	LT	lamina terminalis

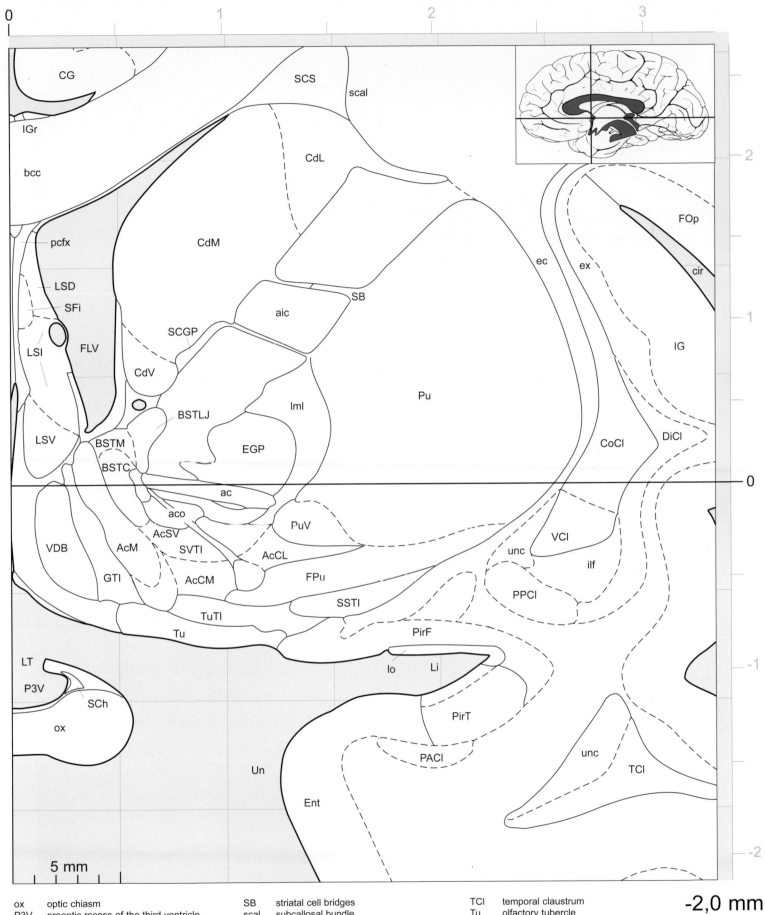

0   1   2   3

CG

SCS

scal

IGr

CdL

bcc

CdM

pcfx

SB

LSD

SFi

aic

SCGP

LSI

FLV

CdV

IG

Pu

BSTLJ

lml

LSV

EGP

CoCl

DiCl

BSTM

BSTC

ac

0

aco

PuV

AcSV

VCl

VDB

AcM

SVTI

unc

ilf

AcCL

GTI

AcCM

FPu

PPCl

SSTI

TuTI

PirF

Tu

LT

lo

Li

P3V

SCh

PirT

ox

PACl

unc

TCl

Un

Ent

FOp

ec

ex

cir

5 mm

-2,0 mm

ox	optic chiasm	SB	striatal cell bridges
P3V	preoptic recess of the third ventricle	scal	subcallosal bundle
PACl	preamygdalar claustrum	SCGP	supracapsular part of the globus pallidus
pcfx	precommissural fornix	SCh	suprachiasmatic nucleus
PirF	(pre-)piriform cortex, frontal area	SCS	subcallosal stratum
PirT	(pre-)piriform cortex, temporal area	SFi	septofimbrial nucleus
PPCl	(pre-)piriform claustrum	SLG	semilunar gyrus
Pu	putamen	SSTI	substriatal terminal island
PuV	ventral putamen	SVTI	subventricular terminal island

TCl	temporal claustrum
Tu	olfactory tubercle
TuTI	tubercular terminal island(s)
Un	uncus
unc	uncinate fasciculus
VCl	ventral claustrum
VDB	vertical limb of the diagonal band

19

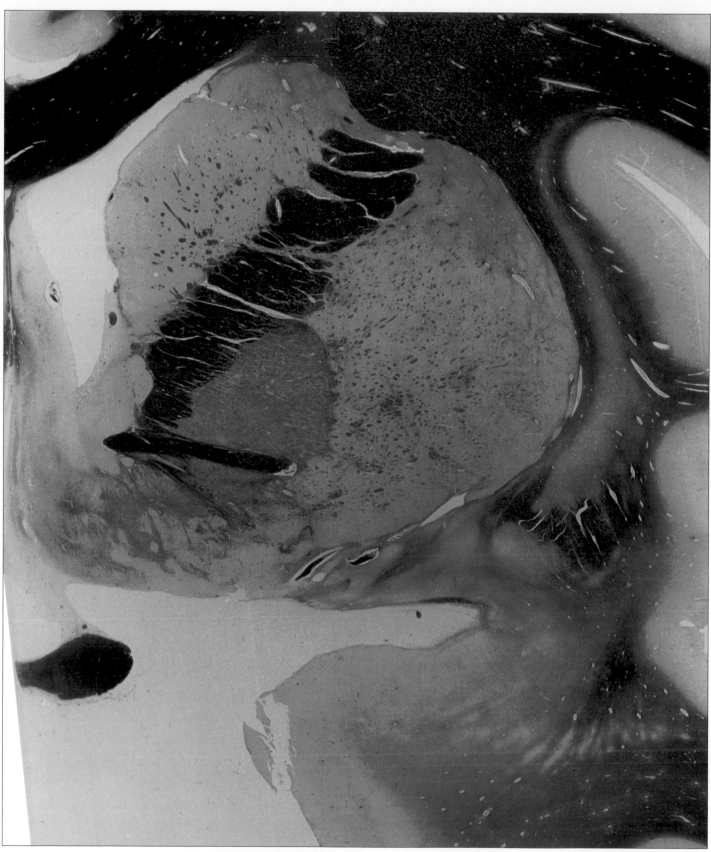

ac	anterior commissure	BSTL	bed nucleus of the stria	DB	nucleus of the diagonal band	FPu	putaminal fundus region
AcCL	accumbens n., centrolateral part		terminalis, lateral division	DiCl	diffuse insular claustrum	GTI	great terminal island
AcCM	accumbens n., centromedial part	BSTM	bed nucleus of the stria	DPe	dorsal periventricular	HDB	horizontal limb of the diagonal band
AcM	accumbens n., medial part		terminalis, medial division		hypothalamic nucleus	IG	insular gyrus
aco	anterior commissure, olfactory limb	CdL	lateral caudate nucleus	ec	external capsule	ilf	inferior longitudinal fasciculus
aic	anterior limb of internal capsule	CdM	medial caudate nucleus	EGP	external globus pallidus	Li	limen insulae
AMPO	anterior medial preoptic nucleus	CdV	ventral caudate nucleus	Ent	entorhinal cortex	lml	external medullary lamina of the
bcc	body of the corpus callosum	CG	cingulate gyrus	ex	extreme capsule		globus pallidus
BSTC	bed nucleus of the stria terminalis,	cir	circular insular sulcus	FLV	frontal horn of lateral ventricle	lo	laterao olfactory tract
	central division	CoCl	compact insular claustrum	FOp	frontal operculum	LSD	dorsolateral septal nucleus

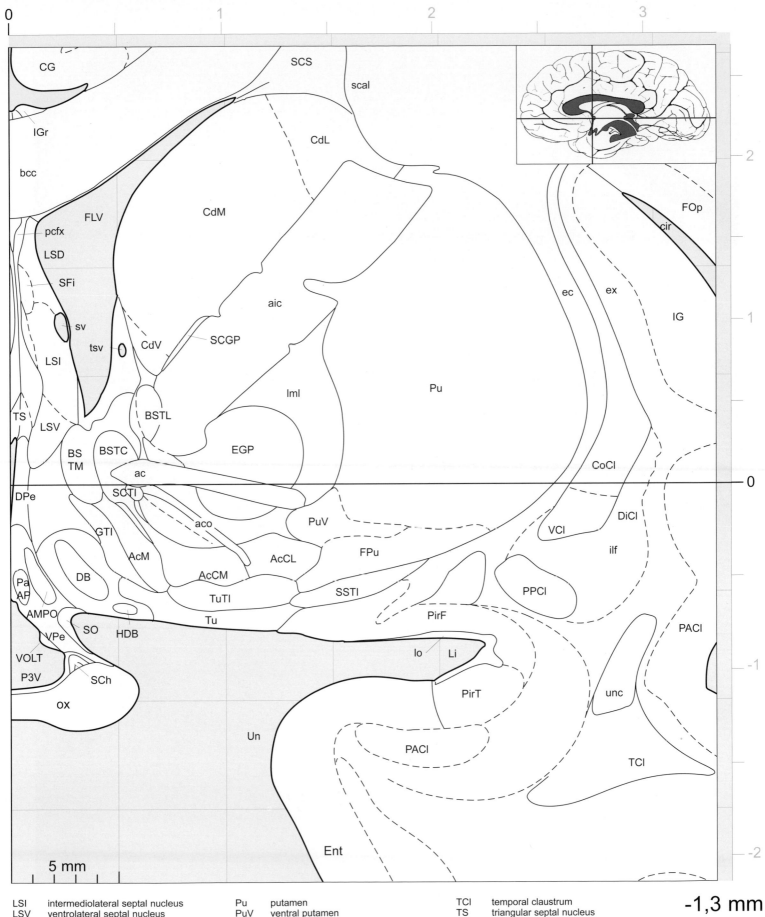

LSI	intermediolateral septal nucleus		Pu	putamen		TCl	temporal claustrum
LSV	ventrolateral septal nucleus		PuV	ventral putamen		TS	triangular septal nucleus
ox	optic chiasm		SCGP	supracapsular part of the globus pallidus		tsv	thalamostriate vein
P3V	preoptic recess of the third ventricle		SCh	suprachiasmatic nucleus		Tu	olfactory tubercle
PaAP	paraventricular hypothalamic nucleus, anterior parvocellular part		SCS	subcallosal stratum		TuTl	tubercular terminal island(s)
			SCTI	subcaudate terminal island		Un	uncus
PACl	preamygdalar claustrum		SFi	septofimbrial nucleus		unc	uncinate fasciculus
pcfx	precommissural fornix		SLG	semilunar gyrus		VCl	ventral claustrum
PirF	(pre-)piriform cortex, frontal area		SO	supraoptic nucleus		VOLT	vascular organ of the lamina terminalis
PirT	(pre-)piriform cortex, temporal area		SSTI	substriatal terminal island		VPe	ventral periventricular hypothalamic
PPCl	prepiriform claustrum		sv	septal vein			nucleus

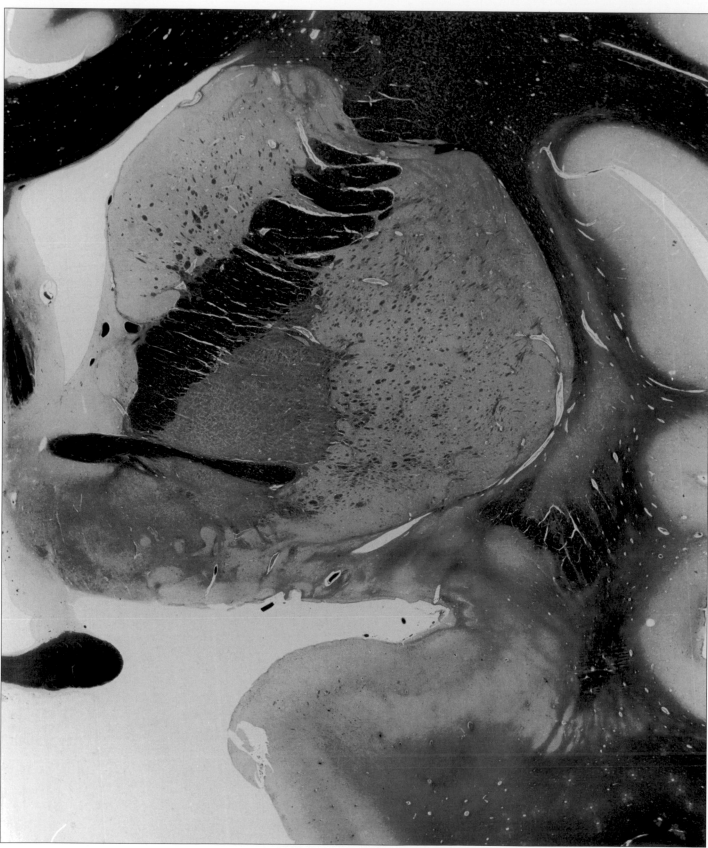

ac	anterior commissure	AMPO	anterior medial preoptic nucleus	CdL	lateral caudate nucleus	EGP	external globus pallidus
AcC	accumbens n., central part			CdM	medial caudate nucleus	Ent	entorhinal cortex
AcM	accumbens n., medial part	bcc	body of the corpus callosum	CdV	ventral caudate nucleus	ex	extreme capsule
aco	anterior commissure, olfactory limb	BM	basomedial amygdaloid nucleus	CG	cingulate gyrus	FLV	frontal horn of lateral ventricle
				cir	circular insular sulcus	FOp	frontal operculum
AcSV	accumbens n., subventricular part	BSTC	bed nucleus of the stria terminalis, central division	CoCl	compact insular claustrum	FPu	putaminal fundus region
ADB	nucleus of the diagonal band, angular part			CxA	cortico-amygdaloid transition area	fx	fornix longus
		BSTL	bed nucleus of the stria terminalis, lateral division	DiCl	diffuse insular claustrum	GTI	great terminal island
AG	ambiens gyrus			DPe	dorsal periventricular hypothalamic nucleus	HDB	horizontal limb of the diagonal band
aic	anterior limb of internal capsule	BSTM	bed nucleus of the stria terminalis, medial division			IG	insular gyrus
ALPO	anterior lateral preoptic nucleus			ec	external capsule	ilf	inferior longitudinal fasciculus

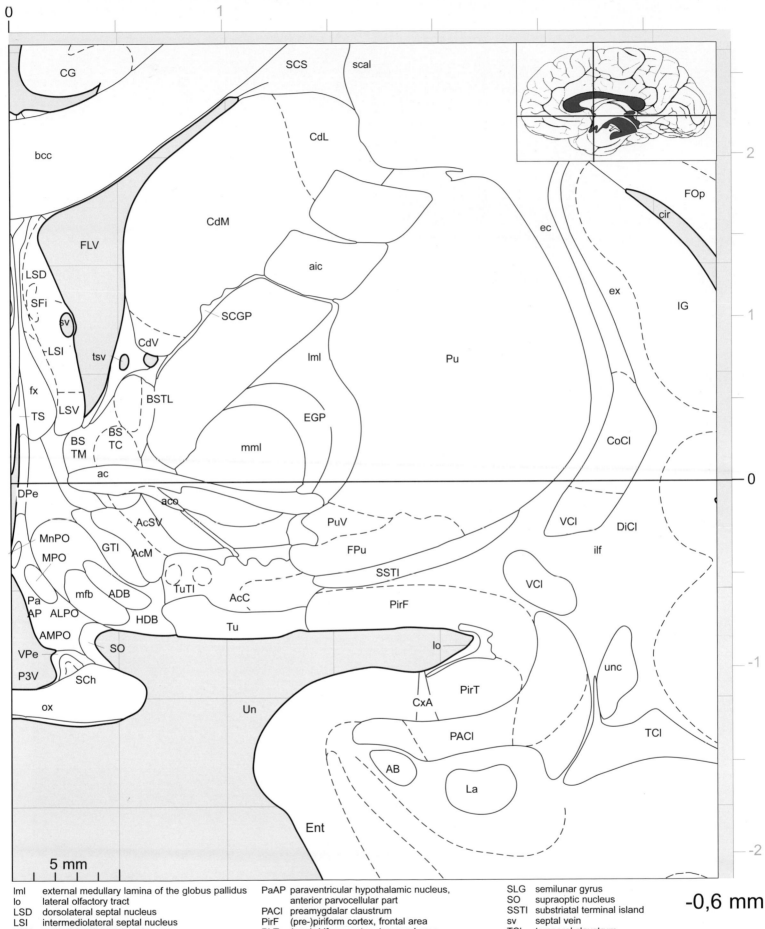

0   1

5 mm

-0,6 mm

21

lml	external medullary lamina of the globus pallidus
lo	lateral olfactory tract
LSD	dorsolateral septal nucleus
LSI	intermediolateral septal nucleus
LSV	ventrolateral septal nucleus
mfb	medial forebrain bundle
mml	medial medullary lamina
MnPO	median preoptic nucleus
MPO	medial preoptic nucleus
ox	optic chiasm
P3V	preoptic recess of the third ventricle
PaAP	paraventricular hypothalamic nucleus, anterior parvocellular part
PACl	preamygdalar claustrum
PirF	(pre-)piriform cortex, frontal area
PirT	(pre-)piriform cortex, temporal area
Pu	putamen
PuV	ventral putamen
scal	subcallosal bundle
SCGP	supracapsular part of the globus pallidus
SCh	suprachiasmatic nucleus
SCS	subcallosal stratum
SFi	septofimbrial nucleus
SLG	semilunar gyrus
SO	supraoptic nucleus
SSTI	substriatal terminal island
sv	septal vein
TCl	temporal claustrum
TS	triangular septal nucleus
tsv	thalamostriate vein
Tu	olfactory tubercle
TuTI	tubercular terminal islands
Un	uncus
unc	uncinate fasciculus
VCl	ventral claustrum

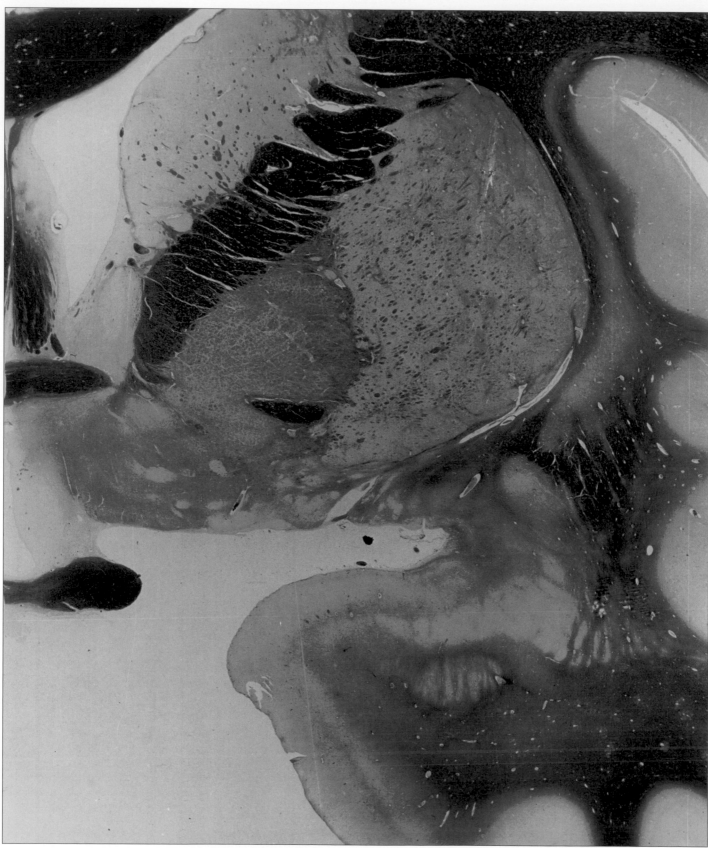

3V	third ventricle	BSTL	bed nucleus of the stria terminalis, lateral division	CoCl	compact insular claustrum	FPu	putaminal fundus region
ac	anterior commissure			CxA	cortico-amygdaloid transition area	fx	fornix
AcC	accumbens n., central part	BSTM	bed nucleus of the stria terminalis, medial division	db	diagonal band	GTI	great terminal island
AcM	accumbens n., medial part			DiCl	diffuse insular claustrum	ic	internal capsule
aic	anterior limb of internal capsule	BSTV	bed nucleus of the stria terminalis, ventral division	DPe	dorsal periventricular hypothalamic nucleus	IG	insular gyrus
BLVM	basolateral amygdaloid nucleus, ventromedial part	CdL	lateral caudate nucleus			ilf	inferior longitudinal fasciculus
		CdM	medial caudate nucleus	EGP	external globus pallidus	InfS	infundibular stalk
BM	basomedial amygdaloid nucleus	CdV	ventral caudate nucleus	Ent	entorhinal cortex	La	lateral amygdaloid nucleus
BSTC	bed nucleus of the stria terminalis, central division	CG	cingulate gyrus	FLV	frontal horn of lateral ventricle	lml	external medullary lamina of the obus pallidus
				FOp	frontal operculum		

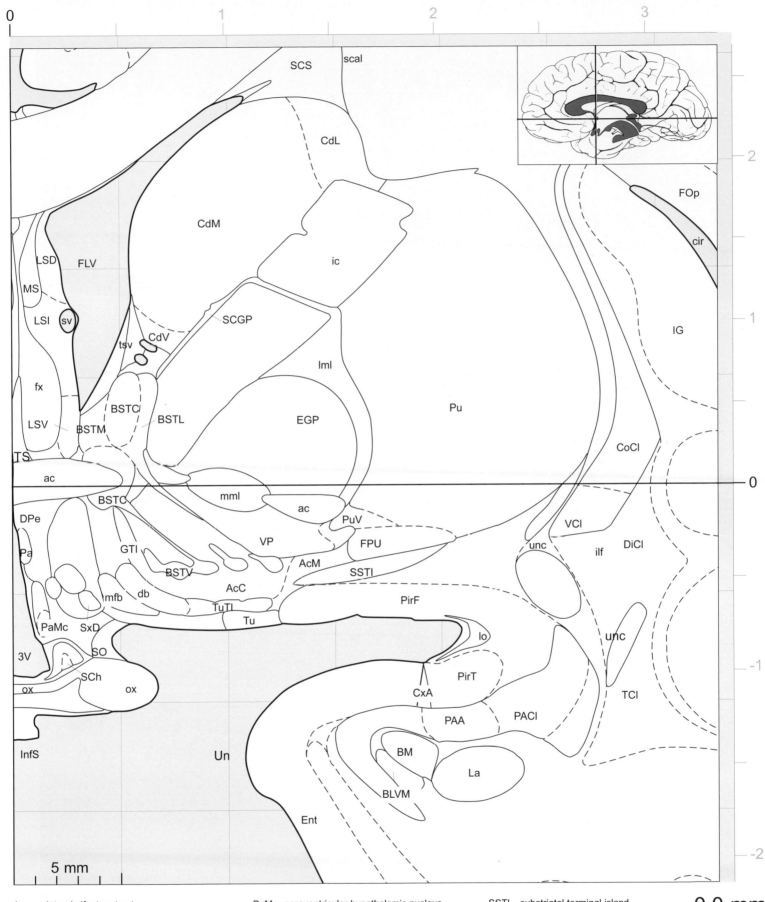

0,0 mm

22

lo — lateral olfactory tract
LSD — dorsolateral septal nucleus
LSI — intermediolateral septal nucleus
LSV — ventrolateral septal nucleus
mfb — medial forebrain bundle
mml — medial medullary lamina of the globus pallidus
MS — medial septal nucleus
ox — optic chiasm
Pa — paraventricular hypothalamic nucleus
PAA — periamygdalar area
PACl — preamygdalar claustrum

PaMc — paraventricular hypothalamic nucleus, magnocellular part
PirF — (pre-)piriform cortex, frontal area
PiT — (pre-)piriform cortex, temporal area
Pu — putamen
PuV — ventral putamen
scal — subcallosal bundle
SCGP — supracapsular part of the globus pallidus
SCh — suprachiasmatic nucleus
SCS — subcallosal stratum
SO — supraoptic nucleus

SSTI — substriatal terminal island
sv — septal vein
SxD — sexual dimorphic ncl.
TCl — temporal claustrum
TS — triangular septal nucleus
tsv — thalamostriate vein
Tu — olfactory tubercle
TuTI — tubercular terminal island(s)
Un — uncus
unc — uncinate fasciculus
VCl — ventral claustrum

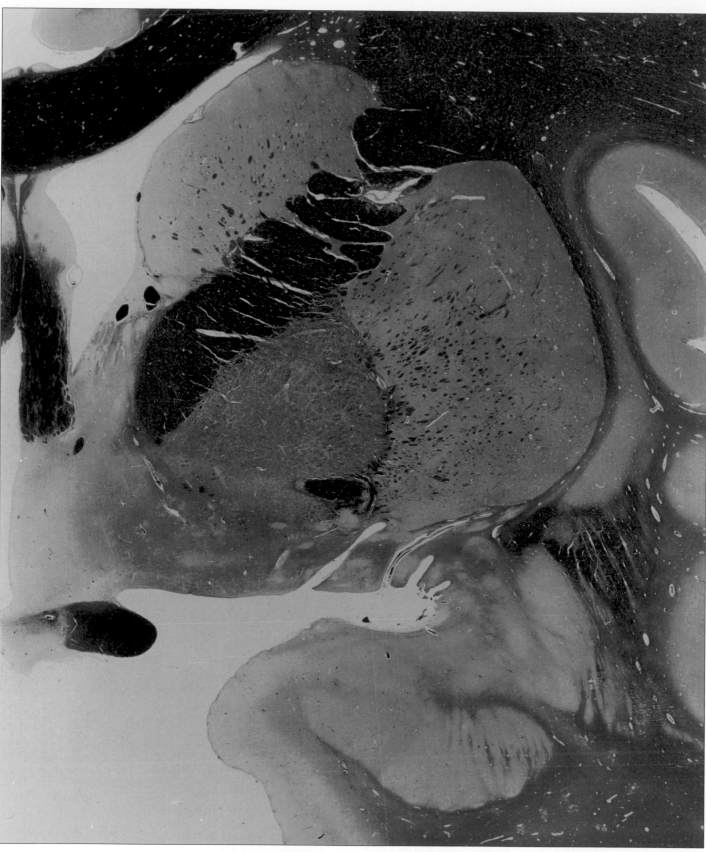

3V	third ventricle		terminalis, central division	CG	cingulate gyrus	fx	fornix
AAA	anterior amygdaloid area	BSTLJ	bed nucleus of the stria	cir	circular insular sulcus	ic	anterior limb of internal capsule
ac	anterior commissure		terminalis ,lateral division,	CoCl	compact insular claustrum	IG	insular gyrus
ACo	anterior cortical amygdaloid nucleus		juxtacapsular part	DiCl	diffuse insular claustrum	IGr	indusium griseum
BC	basal nucleus, compact part	BSTP	bed nucleus of the stria	Do	dorsal hypothalamic nucleus	ilf	inferior longitudinal fasciculus
bcc	body of the corpus callosum		terminalis, posterior part	ec	external capsule	InfS	infundibular stalk
BL	basolateral amygdaloid nucleus	BSTV	bed nucleus of the stria	EGP	external globus pallidus	La	lateral amygdaloid nucleus
BLVM	basolateral amygdaloid nucleus,		terminalis, ventral division	Ent	entorhinal cortex	LHA	lateral hypothalamic area
	ventromedial part	CdL	lateral caudate nucleus	ex	extreme capsule	LiCl	limitans claustrum
BM	basomedial amygdaloid nucleus	CdM	medial caudate nucleus	FOp	frontal operculum	lml	external medullary lamina of the
BSTC	bed nucleus of the stria	CdV	ventral caudate nucleus	FPu	putaminal fundus		globus pallidus

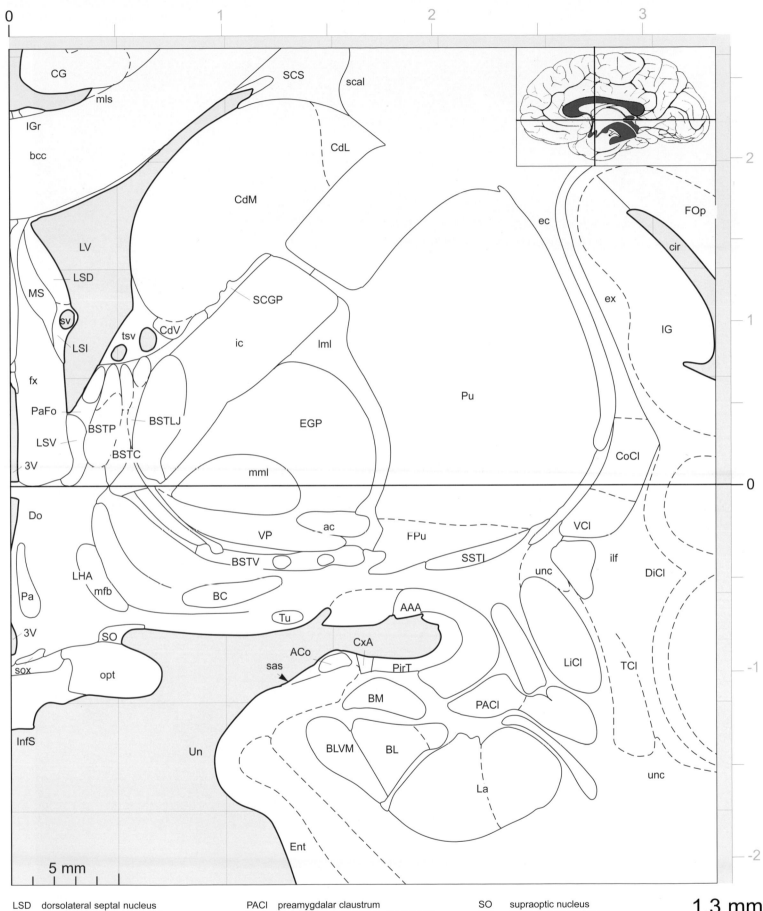

0 1 2 3

CG
mls
IGr
bcc

SCS
scal
CdL
CdM

LV

LSD
MS
sv
LSI
tsv CdV
SCGP
ic
lml
EGP
BSTLJ
BSTP
BSTC
mml

fx
PaFo
LSV
3V

Do

LHA
mfb
Pa
BC
3V
SO
sox
opt
InfS
Un

Tu
AAA
CxA
ACo
sas
PirT
BM
BLVM BL
La
Ent

VP ac
BSTV
Pu

FPu
SSTI
unc
ilf

Un

ec
FOp
cir
ex
IG

CoCl

VCl
DiCl
LiCl TCl
PACl
unc

5 mm

LSD   dorsolateral septal nucleus
LSI   intermediolateral septal nucleus
LSV   ventral septal nucleus
LV   lateral ventricle
mfb   medial forebrain bundle
mls   medial longitudinal stria
mml   medial medullary lamina of the globus pallidus
MS   medial septal nucleus
opt   optic tract
Pa   paraventricular hypothalamic nucleus

PACl preamygdalar claustrum
PaFo paraventricular hypothalamic nucleus,
       fornical part
PirT (pre-)piriform cortex, temporal area
Pu   putamen
PuV   ventral putamen
sas   semiannular sulcus
scal subcallosal bundle
SCGP supracapsular part of the globus pallidus
SCS   subcallosal stratum

SO   supraoptic nucleus
sox   supraoptic commissure
SSTl substriatal terminal island
sv   septal vein
TCl   temporal claustrum
tsv   thalamostriate vein
Tu   olfactory tubercle
Un   uncus
unc   uncinate fasciculus
VCl   ventral claustrum

1,3 mm

23

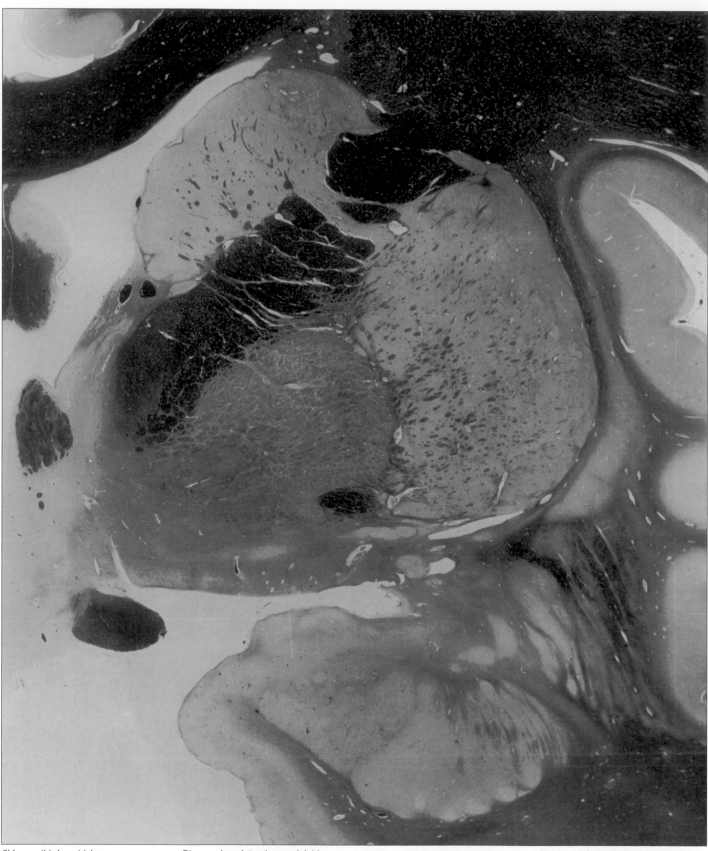

3V	third ventricle	BL	basolateral amygdaloid	DiCl	diffuse insular claustrum	ithp	inferior thalamic peduncle
AAA	anterior amygdaloid area		nucleus	ec	external capsule	IVF	interventricular foramen
ac	anterior commissure	BLVM	basolateral amygdaloid	EGP	external globus pallidus	La	lateral amygdaloid nucleus,
ACoD	anterior cortical amygdaloid		nucleus, ventromedial part	Ent	entorhinal cortex		dorsolateral part
	nucleus, dorsal part	BM	basomedial amygdaloid nucleus	ex	extreme capsule	LaDL	lateral amygdaloid nucleus
ACoV	anterior cortical amygdaloid	CdL	lateral caudate nucleus	FOp	frontal operculum	LHA	lateral hypothalamic area
	nucleus, ventral part	CdM	medial caudate nucleus	fx	fornix	LiCl	limitans claustrum
AI	amygdaloid island	Ce	central amygdaloid nucleus	ic	internal capsule	LSD	dorsolateral septal nucleus
	(extended amygdala)	CG	cingulate gyrus	IG	insular gyrus	LSI	lateral septal nucleus,
AStr	amygdalostriatal transition area	cir	circular insular sulcus	IGP	internal globus pallidus		intermediate part
BC	basal nucleus, compact part	CoCl	compact insular claustrum	IGr	indusium griseum	LV	lateral ventricle
bcc	body of the corpus callosum	DH	dorsal hypothalmic area	ilf	interior longitudinal fasciculus	mfb	medial forebrain bundle

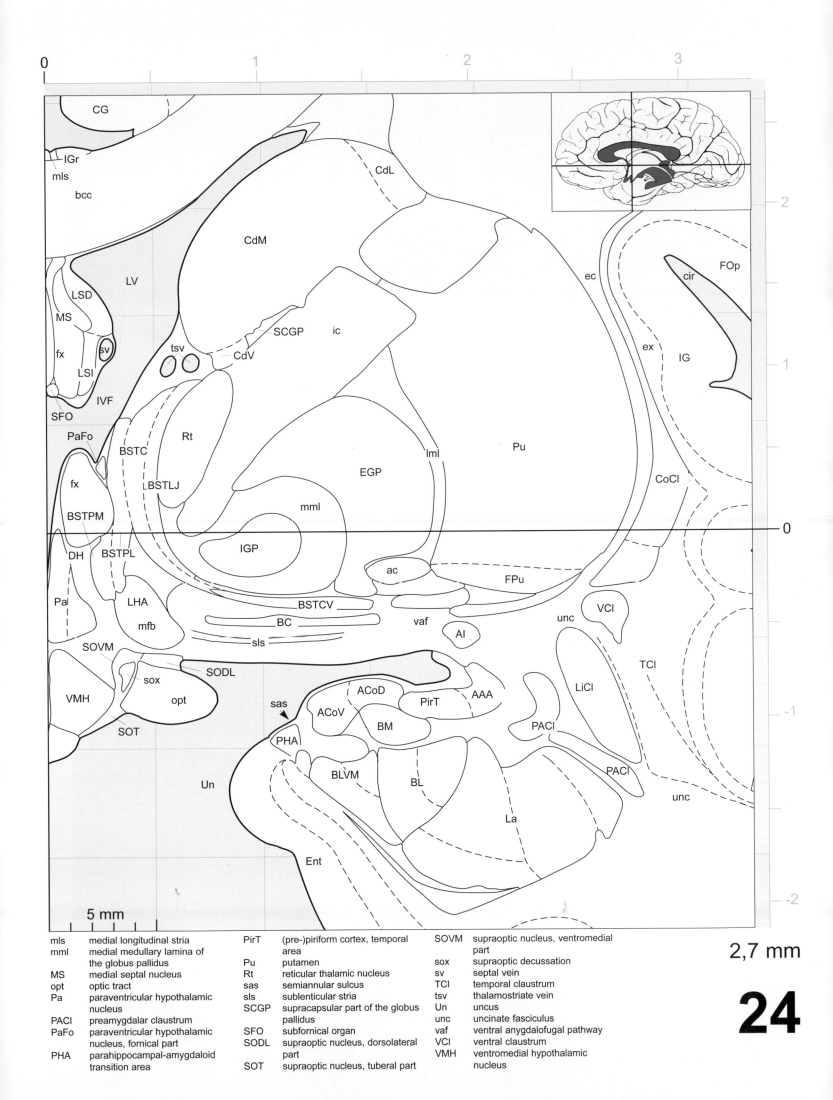

mls	medial longitudinal stria	PirT	(pre-)piriform cortex, temporal area	SOVM	supraoptic nucleus, ventromedial part
mml	medial medullary lamina of the globus pallidus	Pu	putamen	sox	supraoptic decussation
MS	medial septal nucleus	Rt	reticular thalamic nucleus	sv	septal vein
opt	optic tract	sas	semiannular sulcus	TCl	temporal claustrum
Pa	paraventricular hypothalamic nucleus	sls	sublenticular stria	tsv	thalamostriate vein
		SCGP	supracapsular part of the globus pallidus	Un	uncus
PACl	preamygdalar claustrum			unc	uncinate fasciculus
PaFo	paraventricular hypothalamic nucleus, fornical part	SFO	subfornical organ	vaf	ventral anygdalofugal pathway
		SODL	supraoptic nucleus, dorsolateral part	VCl	ventral claustrum
PHA	parahippocampal-amygdaloid transition area	SOT	supraoptic nucleus, tuberal part	VMH	ventromedial hypothalamic nucleus

2,7 mm

24

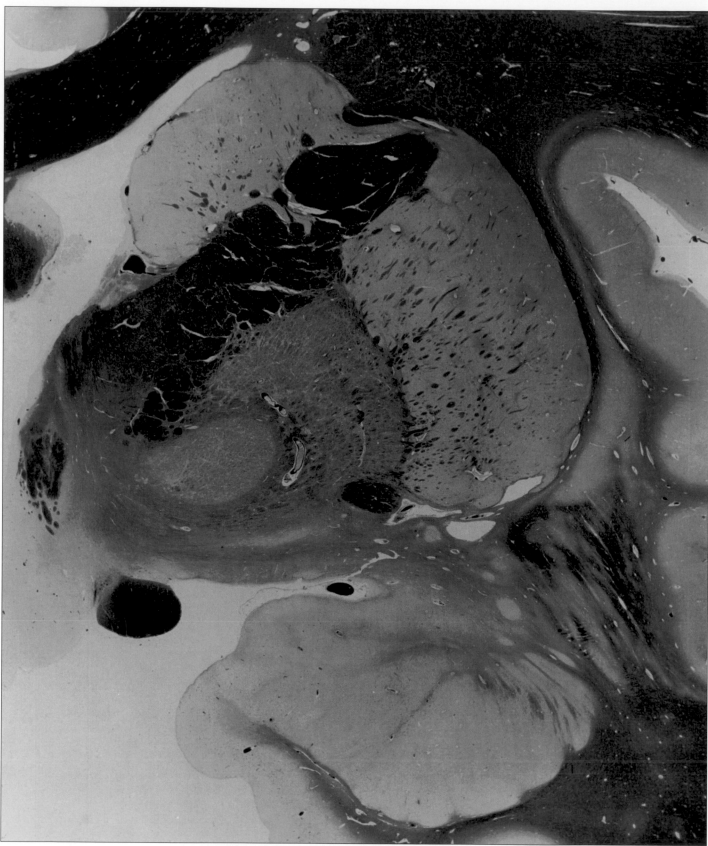

3V	third ventricle	BL	basolateral amygdaloid nucleus	DMC	dorsomedial hypothalamic	ilf	inferior longitudinal fasciculus
AAA	anterior amygdaloid area	BLVM	basolateral amygdaloid nucleus,		nucleus, compact part	ithp	inferior thalamic peduncle
ac	anterior commissure		ventromedial part	ec	external capsule	IVF	interventricular foramen
ACoD	anterior cortical amygdaloid	BM	basomedial amygdaloid nucleus	EGP	external globus pallidus	La	lateral amygdaloid nucleus
	nucleus, dorsal part	CdL	lateral caudate nucleus	Ent	entorhinal cortex	LaDL	lateral amygdaloid nucleus,
ACoV	anterior cortical amygdaloid	CdM	medial caudate nucleus	ex	extreme capsule		dorsolateral part
	nucleus, ventral part	Ce	central amygdaloid nucleus	FOp	frontal operculum	LHA	lateral hypothalamic area
AI	amygdaloid island (extended	CG	cingulate gyrus	fx	fornix	LiCl	limitans claustrum
	amygdala)	cir	circular insular sulcus	ic	internal capsule	lml	external medullary lamina of the
AStr	amygdalostriatal transition area	CoCl	compact insular claustrum	IG	insular gyrus		globus pallidus
BC	basal nucleus, compact part	DH	dorsal hypothalamic area	IGP	internal globus pallidus	LSD	dorsolateral septal nucleus
bcc	body of the corpus callosum	DiCl	diffuse insular claustrum	IGr	indusium griseum	LSI	intermediolateral septal nucleus

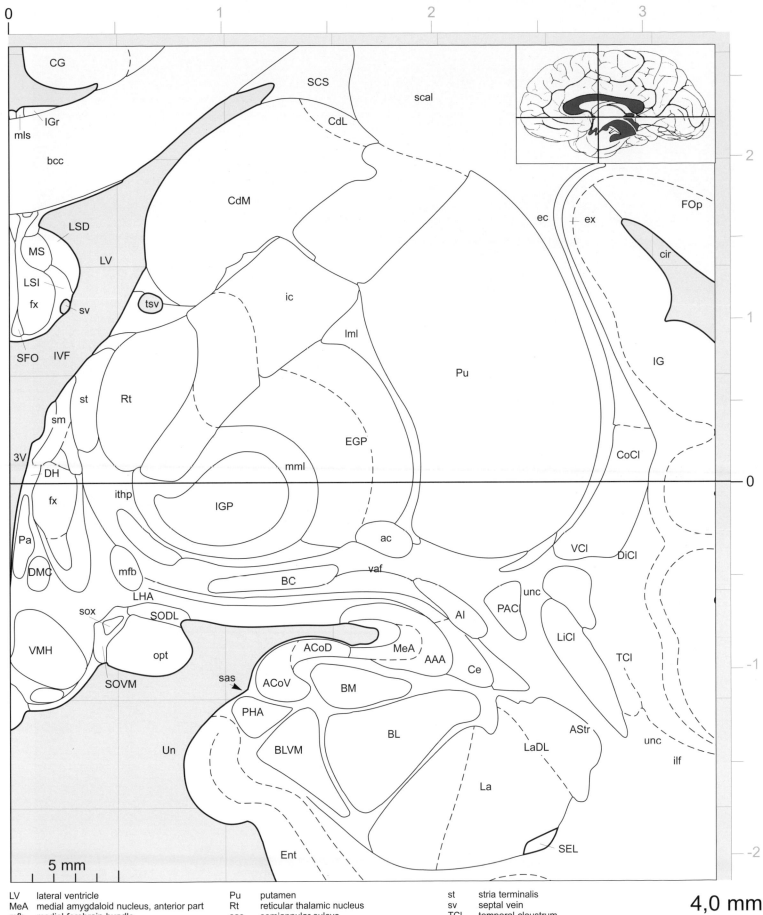

LV	lateral ventricle	Pu	putamen	st	stria terminalis
MeA	medial amygdaloid nucleus, anterior part	Rt	reticular thalamic nucleus	sv	septal vein
mfb	medial forebrain bundle	sas	semiannular sulcus	TCl	temporal claustrum
mls	medial longitudinal stria	scal	subcallosal bundlc	tsv	thalamostriate vein
mml	internal medullary lamina of the globus pallidus	SCS	subcallosal stratum	Un	uncus
		SEL	subependymal layer	unc	uncinate fasciculus
MS	medial septal nucleus	SFO	subfornical organ	vaf	ventral anygdalofugal pathway
opt	optic tract	sm	stria medullaris of the thalamus	VCl	ventral claustrum
Pa	paraventricular hypothalamic nucleus	SODL	supraoptic nucleus, dorsolateral part	VCo	ventral cortical nucleus
PACl	preamygdalar claustrum	SOVM	supraoptic nucleus, ventromedial part	VMH	ventromedial hypothalamic nucleus
PHA	parahippocampal-amygdaloid transition area	sox	supraoptic decussation		

4,0 mm

25

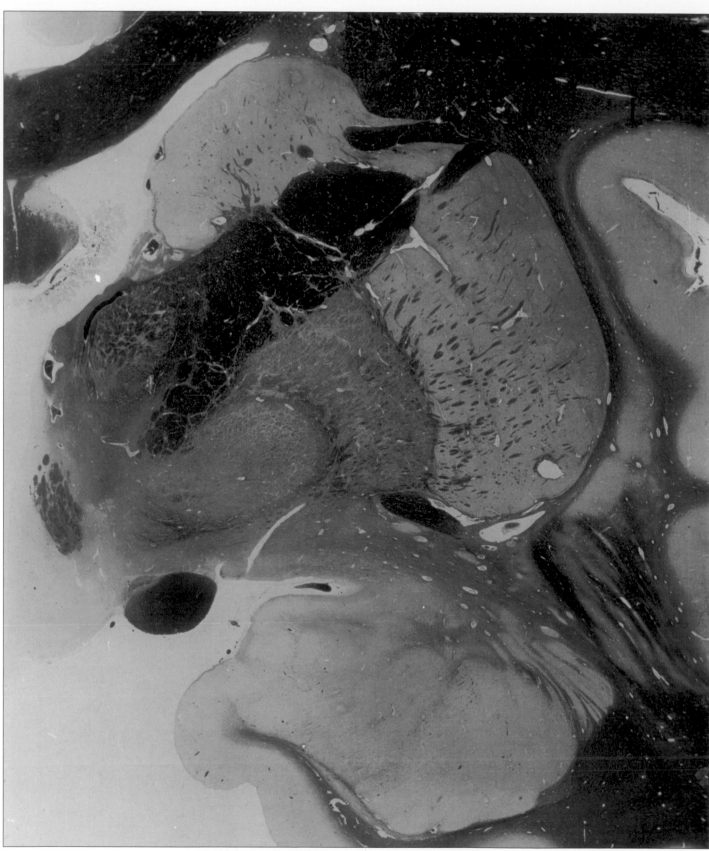

3V	third ventricle	BLVL	basolateral amygdaloid nucleus,	DMH	dorsomedial hypothalamic nucleus	ithp	inferior thalamic peduncle
AAA	anterior amygdaloid area		ventrolateral part	Ent	entorhinal cortex	ithp	inferior thalamic peduncle
ac	anterior commissure	BLVM	basolateral amygdaloid nucleus,	Fa	fasciculosus nucleus	La	lateral amygdaloid nucleus
ACo	anterior cortical amygdaloid nucleus		ventromedial part	FOp	frontal operculum	LaDL	lateral amygdaloid nucl., dorsolat. part
al	ansa lenticularis	BM	basomedial amygdaloid nucleus	fx	fornix	LaDM	lat. amygdaloid nucl., dorsomed. part
BC	basal nucleus, compact part	BSTP	bed nucleus of the stria terminalis,	ic	internal capsule	LaI	lat. amygdaloid nucl., intermed. part
BLD	basolateral amygdaloid nucleus,		posterior division	icml	incomplete medullary lamina of the	LHA	lateral hypothalamic area
	dorsal (magnocellular) part	CdL	lateral caudate nucleus		globus pallidus	LiCl	limitans claustrum
BLI	basolateral amygdaloid nucleus,	CdM	medial caudate nucleus	IGP	internal globus pallidus	lml	external medullary lamina of the
	intermediate part	Ce	central amygdaloid nucleus	IGr	indusium griseum		globus pallidus
BLPL	basolateral amygdaloid nucleus,	CoCl	(compact) insular claustrum	ilf	inferior longitudinal fasciculus	LSD	dorsolateral septal nucleus
	paralaminar part	DiCl	diffuse insular claustrum	Inf	infundibular nucleus	LSI	intermediolateral septal nucleus

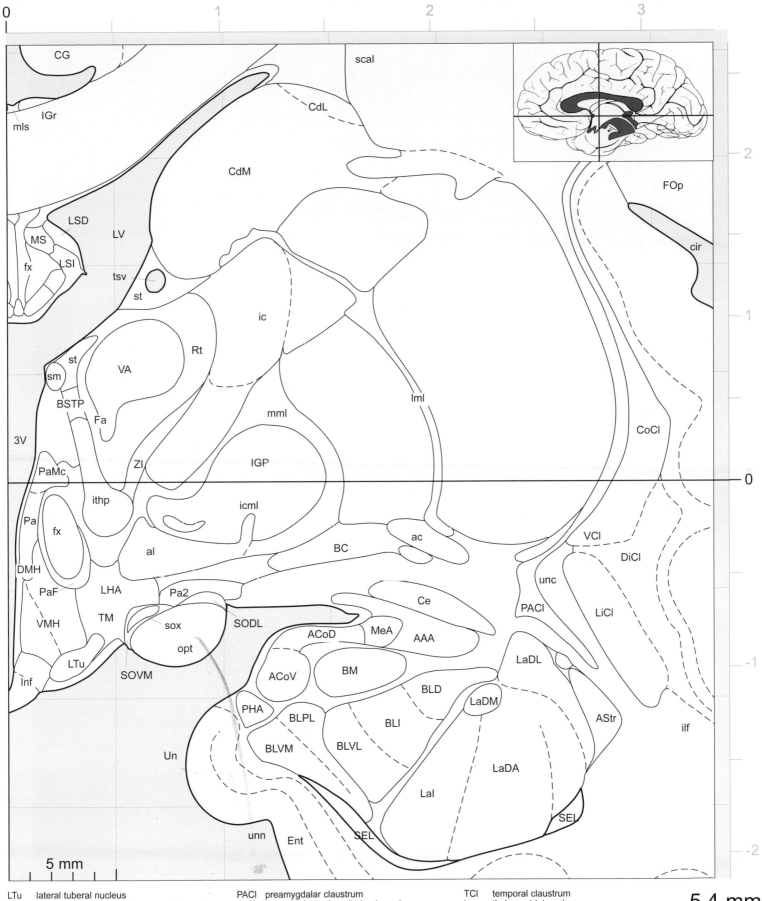

0   1   2   3

CG
scal
IGr
mls
CdL
CdM
FOp
LSD
LV
MS
cir
fx
LSI
tsv
st
ic
st
VA
Rt
sm
lml
BSTP
Fa
mml
CoCl
3V
ZI
IGP
PaMc
ithp
icml
Pa
fx
ac
al
BC
VCl
DMH
unc
DiCl
PaF
LHA
Pa2
Ce
PACl
LiCl
VMH
TM
sox
SODL
ACoD
MeA
AAA
LaDL
LTu
opt
ACoV
BM
BLD
LaDM
Inf
SOVM
PHA
BLPL
BLI
AStr
ilf
Un
BLVM
BLVL
LaDA
LaI
SEL
unn
Ent
SEL

5 mm

5,4 mm

26

LTu	lateral tuberal nucleus	
MeA	medial amygdaloid nucleus, anterior part	
mfb	medial forebrain bundle	
mls	medial longitudinal stria	
mml	internal medullary lamina of the globus pallidus	
MS	medial septal nucleus	
MTu	medial tuberal nucleus	
opt	optic tract	
Pa	paraventricular hypothalamic nucleus	
Pa2	paraoptic nucleus	
PAA	periamygdalar area	
PaAP	paraventricular hypothalamic nucleus, anterior parvocellular part	

PACl	preamygdalar claustrum
PaMc	paraventricular hypothalamic nucleus, magnocellular part
PHA	parahippocampal-amygdaloid transit. area
Rt	reticular thalamic nucleus
scal	subcallosal bundle
SCGP	supracapsular part of the globus pallidus
SEL	subependymal layer
sm	stria medullaris of the thalamus
SO	supraoptic nucleus
sox	supraoptic decussation
SPF	subparafascicular thalamic nucleus
st	stria terminalis

TCl	temporal claustrum
tsv	thalamostriate vein
Un	uncus
unn	uncal notch (intrarhinal sulcus)
unc	uncinate fasciculus
VA	ventral anterior thalamic nucleus
VCl	ventral claustrum
VCo	ventral cortical nucleus
ZI	zona incerta

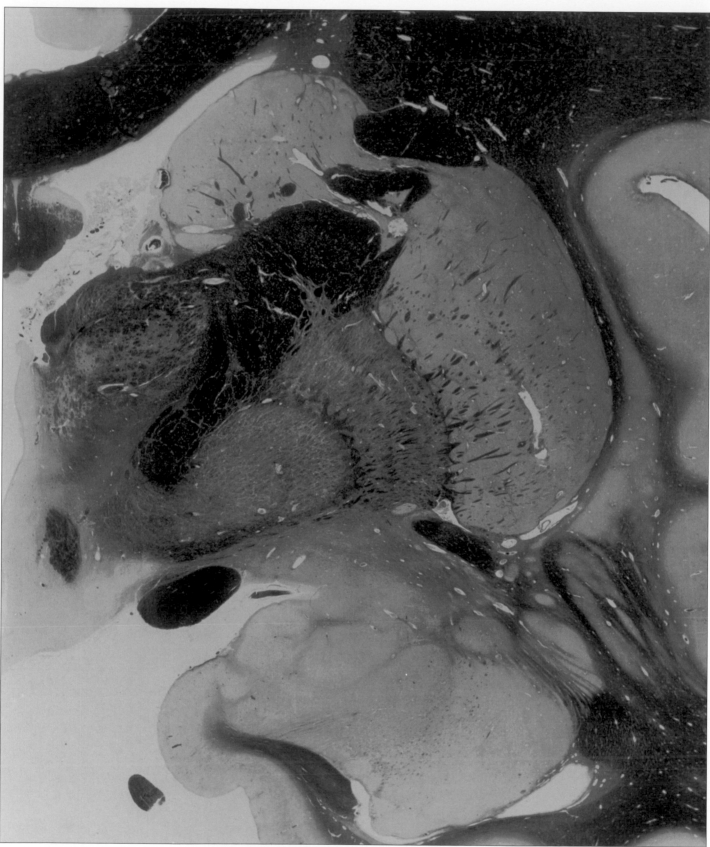

3n	oculomotor nerve	BLVM	basolateral amygdaloid nucleus,	Ent	entorhinal cortex	ithp	inferior thalamic peduncle
3V	third ventricle		ventromedial part	ex	extreme capsule	LaDA	lateral amygdaloid nucleus, dorsal
AAA	anterior amygdaloid area	BM	basomedial amygdaloid nucleus	Fa	fasciculosus nucleus		anterior part
ac	anterior commissure	CdM	medial caudate nucleus	fx	fornix	LADL	lateral amygdaloid nucleus, dorsal
ACo	anterior cortical amygdaloid nucleus	Ce	central amygdaloid nucleus	HiH	hippocampal head		lateral part
al	ansa lenticularis	cir	circular insular sulcus	ic	internal capsule	LHA	lateral hypothalamic area
AM	anteromedial thalamic nucleus	CoCl	(compact) insular claustrum	icml	incomplete medullary lamina of	LiCl	limitans claustrum
ap	ansa peduncularis	DHA	dorsal hypothalamic area		the globus pallidus	liml	limiting medullary lamina of the globus
APr	anteroprincipal thalamic nucleus	DiCl	diffuse insular claustrum	IG	insular gyrus		pallidus
AStr	amygdalo-striatal transition area	DMH	dorsomedial hypothalamic nucleus	IGP	internal globus pallidus	LSD	dorsolateral septal nucleus
bcc	body of the corpus callosum	ec	external capsule	IGr	indusium griseum	LSI	intermediolateral septal nucleus
BL	basolateral amygdaloid nucleus	EGP	external globus pallidus	ilf	inferior longitudinal fasciculus	LTu	lateral tuberal nucleus
		eml	external medullary lamina	Inf	infundibular nucleus	LV	lateral ventricle

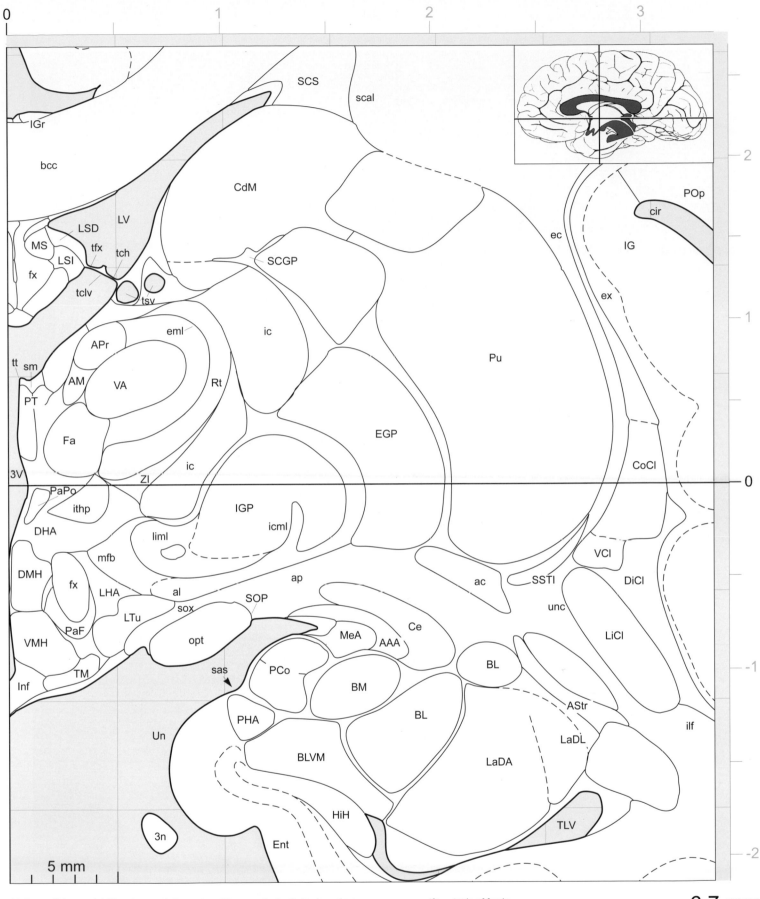

0 1 2 3

SCS
scal

IGr

bcc

CdM

LSD
LV
MS
tfx tch
LSI
fx
tclv
tsv

POp
cir
ec
IG

ex

tt sm
APr eml ic
AM VA Rt
PT
Fa
Pu

EGP

CoCl

3V
ZI ic
PaPo
ithp
IGP icml
DHA liml
VCl
mfb
DMH fx ac SSTI DiCl
LHA al unc
LTu sox SOP LiCl
VMH PaF opt MeA Ce
TM AAA
Inf sas PCo BL
BM AStr
Un PHA BL LaDL
BLVM LaDA
3n HiH TLV
Ent

5 mm

6,7 mm

27

MeA medial amygdaloid nucleus, anterior part
mfb medial forebrain bundle
MS medial septal nucleus
opt optic tract
PaF parafornical nucleus
PaPo paraventricular hypothalamic nucleus, posterior part
PCo posterior cortical amygdaloid nucleus
PHA parahippocampo-amygdaloid transit. area
POp parietal operculum
PT paratenial thalamic nucleus
Pu putamen

Rt reticular thalamic nucleus
sas semiannular sulcus
scal subcallosal bundle
SCGP supracapsular part of the globus pallidus
sm stria medullaris of the thalamus
SOP supraoptic nucleus, posterior part
sox supraoptic decussation
SSTI substriatal terminal island
tch tenia of choroid plexus
tclv tela choroides of lateral ventricle
TLV temporal horn of lateral ventricle

tfx tenia of fornix
TM tuberomammillary nucleus
tsv thalamostriate vein
tt tenia thalamus
Un uncus
unc uncinate fasciculus
VA ventroanterior thalamic nucleus
VCl ventral claustrum
VMH ventromedial hypothalamic nucleus
ZI zona incerta

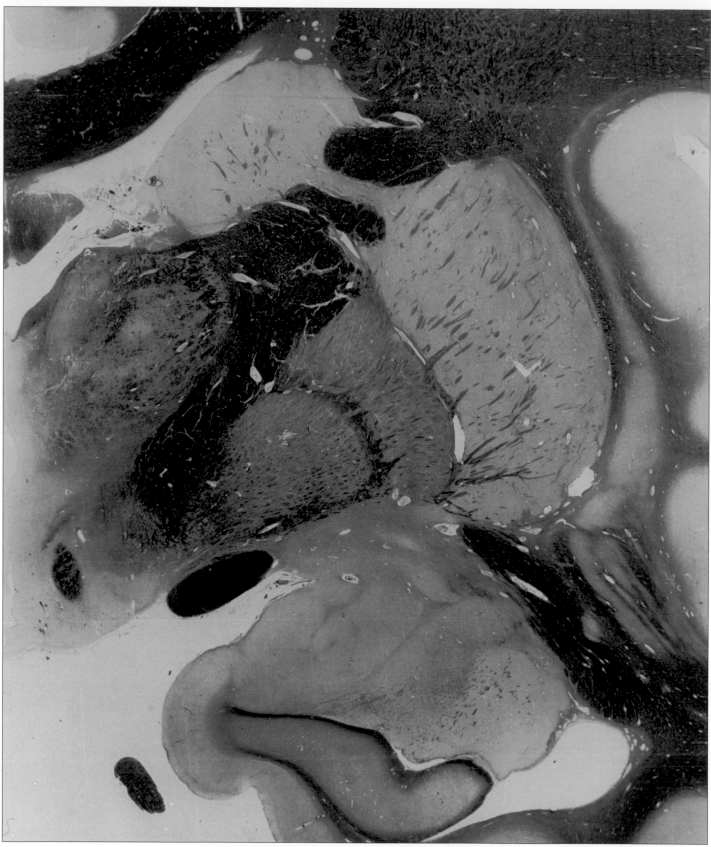

3n	oculomotor nerve	BC	basal nucleus, compact part	CeL	central amygdaloid nucl., lateral part	HiH	hippocampal head
3V	third ventricle	BLD	basolateral amygd. nucl., dorsal part	CeM	central amygdaloid nucl., medial part	ic	internal capsule
AAA	anterior amygdaloid area	BLI	basolateral amygdaloid nucleus,	cir	circular insular sulcus	icml	incomplete medullary lamina of the
ac	anterior commissure		intermediate part	CoCl	(compact) insular claustrum		globus pallidus
AD	anterodorsal thalamic nucleus	BLPL	basolateral amygdaloid nucleus,	DHA	dorsal hypothalamic area	IGP	internal globus pallidus
AI	amygdaloid island (extended		paralaminar part	DiCl	diffuse insular claustrum	inf	infundibular nucleus
	amygdala)	BLVM	basolateral amygdaloid nucleus,	DMH	dorsomedial hypothalamic nucleus	ithp	inferior thalamic peduncle
al	ansa lenticularis		ventromedial part	eml	external medullary lamina	LaDA	lateral amygd. nucl., dorsal anterior
AM	anteromedial thalamic nucleus	BMDM	basomedial amygdaloid nucleus,	Ent	entorhinal cortex		part
ap	ansa peduncularis		dorsomedial part	Fa	fasciculosus nucleus	LaI	lateral amygdaloid nucl., intermediate
APr	anteroprincipal thalamic nucleus	BMVM	basomedial amygdaloid nucleus,	fx	fornix		part
AStr	amygdalo-striatal transition area		ventromedial part	H2	lenticular fasciculus (field H2)	LaV	lateral amygdaloid nucl., ventral part

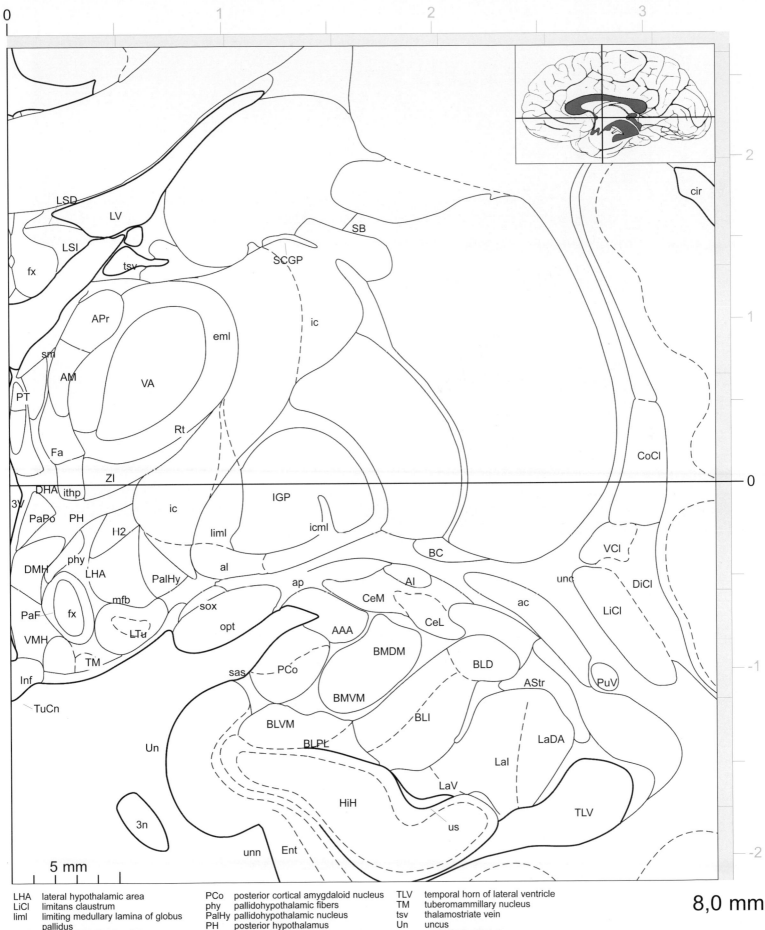

5 mm

8,0 mm

28

LHA	lateral hypothalamic area	PCo	posterior cortical amygdaloid nucleus	TLV	temporal horn of lateral ventricle
LiCl	limitans claustrum	phy	pallidohypothalamic fibers	TM	tuberomammillary nucleus
liml	limiting medullary lamina of globus pallidus	PalHy	pallidohypothalamic nucleus	tsv	thalamostriate vein
		PH	posterior hypothalamus	Un	uncus
LSD	dorsolateral septal nucleus	PuV	ventral putamen	unc	uncinate fasciculus
LSI	intermediolateral septal nucleus	PT	paratenial thalamic nucleus	unn	uncal notch
LTu	lateral tuberal nucleus	Rt	reticular thalamic nucleus	us	uncal sulcus (diverticulum unci)
LV	lateral ventricle	sas	semiannular sulcus	VA	ventral anterior thalamic nucleus
mfb	medial forebrain bundle	SB	striatal cell bridges	VCl	ventral claustrum
opt	optic tract	TuCn	tuber cinereum	VMH	ventromedial hypothalamic nucleus
PaF	parafornical nucleus	SCGP	supracapsular part of globus pallidus	ZI	zona incerta
PaPo	paraventricular hypothalamic nucleus, posterior part	sm	stria medullaris of the thalamus		
		sox	supraoptic decussation		

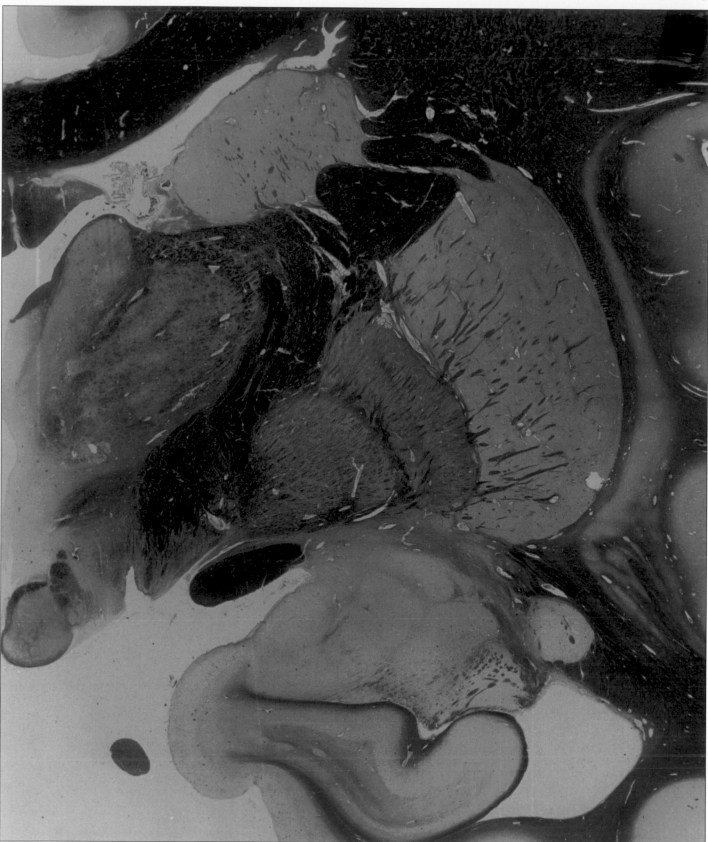

3n	oculomotor nerve	BLD	basolateral amygdaloid nucleus,	Cd	caudate nucleus	Fa	fasciculosus nucleus
3V	third ventricle		dorsal part	CeL	central amygdaloid nucleus, lat. part	H2	lenticular fasciculus (field H2)
AAA	anterior amygdaloid area	BLI	basolateral amygdaloid nucleus,	CeM	central amygdaloid nucl., medial part	HiH	hippocampal head
ac	anterior commissure		intermediate part	CG	cingulate gyrus	ic	internal capsule
afx	anterior column of fornix	BLPL	basolateral amygdaloid nucleus,	CoCl	(compact) insular claustrum	icml	incomplete medullary lamina of the
al	ansa lenticularis		paralaminar part	DHA	dorsal hypothalamic area		globus pallidus
AM	anteromedial thalamic nucleus	BLVL	basolateral amygdaloid nucleus,	DiCl	diffuse insular claustrum	IG	insular gyrus
ap	ansa peduncularis		ventrolateral part	DMH	dorsomedial hypothalamic nucleus	IGP	internal globus pallidus
APr	anteroprincipal thalamic nucleus	BLVM	basolateral amygdaloid nucleus,	EGP	external globus pallidus	iml	internal medullary lamina of thalamus
BC	basal nucleus, compact part		ventromedial part	eml	external medullary lamina	IthA	interthalamic adhesion
bcc	body of the corpus callosum	BM	basomedial amygdaloid nucleus	Ent	entorhinal cortex	ithp	inferior thalamic peduncle
bfx	body of fornix	CA1	CA1 field of the hippocampus	EP	entopeduncular nucleus	LHA	lateral hypothalamic area

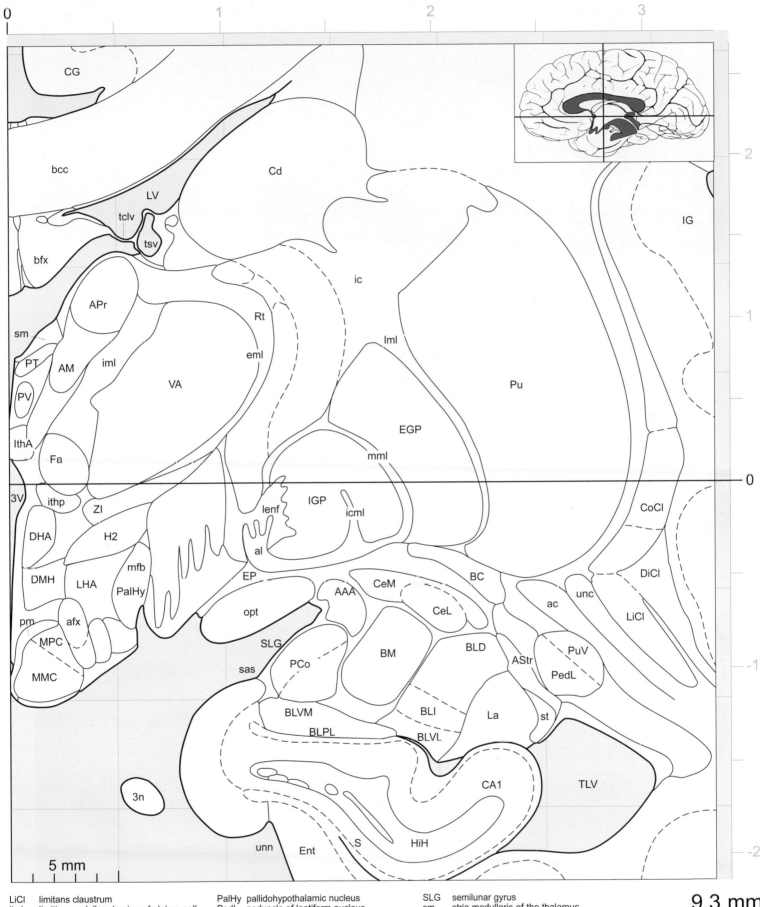

LiCl	limitans claustrum	PalHy	pallidohypothalamic nucleus
liml	limiting medullary lamina of globus pall.	PedL	peduncle of lentiform nucleus
lml	lateral medullary lamina of globus pall.	PCo	posterior cortical amygdaloid nucleus
La	lateral amygdaloid nucleus	pm	principal mammillary fasciculus
lenf	lenticular fasciculus	PuLi	limitans putamen
LV	lateral ventricle	PT	paratenial thalamic nucleus
MMC	mammillary nucleus, magnocellular part	Pu	putamen
MPC	mammillary nucleus, parvocellular part	PuV	ventral putamen
mfb	medial forebrain bundle	PV	paraventricular thalamic nucleus
mml	medial medullary lamina of globus pall.	Rt	reticular thalamic nucleus
opt	optic tract	S	subiculum
PaF	parafornical nucleus	sas	semianular sulcus

SLG	semilunar gyrus
sm	stria medullaris of the thalamus
st	stria terminalis
sth	subthalamic fascicle
TCd	tail of caiudate nucleus
tclv	tela choroides of lateral ventricle
TLV	temporal horn of lateral ventricle
tsv	thalamostriate vein
unc	uncinate fasciculus
unn	uncal notch (Duvernoy)
VA	ventroanterior thalamic nucleus
ZI	zona incerta

29

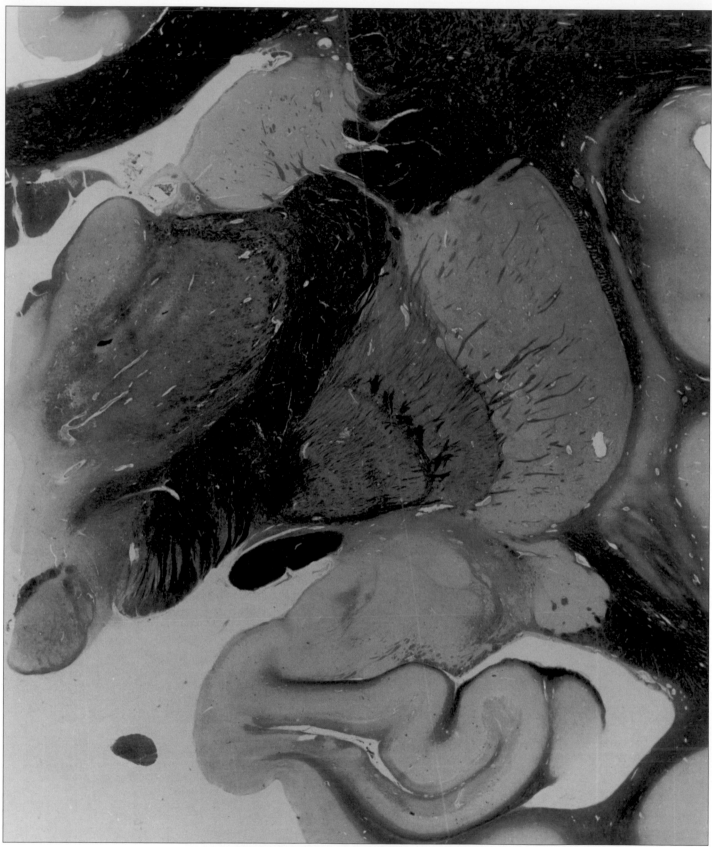

3n	oculomotor nerve	BLPL	basolat. amygdaloid n.,	CA1	CA1 field of the hippocampus	Ent	entorhinal cortex
3V	third ventricle		paralam. part	Cd	caudate nucleus	EP	entopeduncular nucleus
ac	anterior commissure	BLVL	basolat. amygdaloid n.,	CeL	central amygdaloid nucleus, lateral p.	ers	endorhinal sulcus
AG	ambiens gyrus		ventrolat. part	CeM	central amygdaloid nucleus, medial p.	Fa	fasciculosus nucleus
AHi	amygdalohippocampal area	BMCM	basomedial amygdaloid	CoCl	(compact) insular claustrum	gic	genu of the internal capsule
al	ansa lenticularis		nucleus,centromedial part	comb	comb system	H2	lenticular fasciculus (field H2)
AM	anteromedial thalamic nucleus	BMDL	basomed. amygdaloid n.,	cp	cerebral peduncle	IGP	internal globus pallidus
APr	anteroprincipal thalamic nucleus		dorsolat. part	DiCl	diffuse insular claustrum	iml	internal medullary lamina of thalamus
AStr	amygdalostriatal transition area	BMDM	basomedial amygdaloid	DHA	dorsal hypothalamic area	IthA	interthalamic adhesion
bfx	body of fornix		nucleus,dorsomedial part	DMH	dorsomedial hypothalamic nucleus	ithp	inferior thalamic peduncle
BLD	basolateral amygdaloid n., dorsal part	BMVM	basomedial amygdaloid n.,	EGP	external globus pallidus	La	lateral amygdaloid nucleus
BLI	basolat. amygdaloid n., intermed. part		ventromedial part	eml	external medullary lamina (thalamus)	lenf	lenticular fascicle

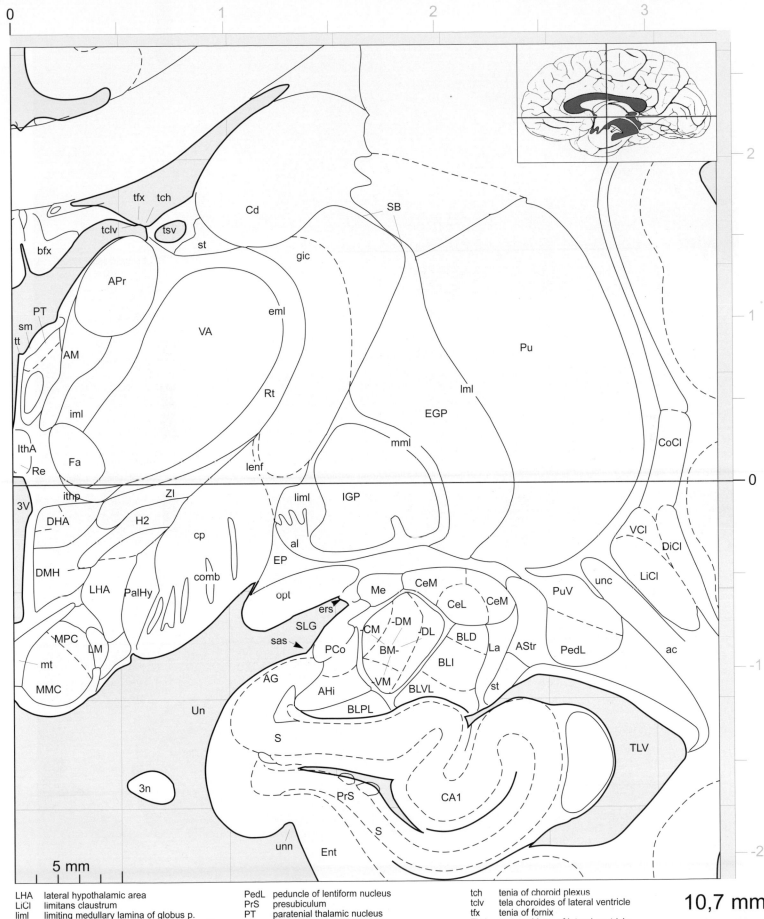

0   1   2   3

5 mm

LHA	lateral hypothalamic area	PedL	peduncle of lentiform nucleus	tch	tenia of choroid plexus
LiCl	limitans claustrum	PrS	presubiculum	tclv	tela choroides of lateral ventricle
liml	limiting medullary lamina of globus p.	PT	paratenial thalamic nucleus	tfx	tenia of fornix
LM	lateral mammillary n. (and intercalatus n.)	Pu	putamen	TLV	temporal horn of lateral ventricle
lml	lateral medullary lamina of the globus pall.	PuV	ventral putamen	tsv	thalamostriate vein
Me	medial amygdaloid nucleus	Re	reuniens thalamic nucleus	tt	tenia thalamus
MPC	medial mammillary n., parvocellular part	Rt	reticular thalamic nucleus	Un	uncus
MMC	medial mammillary n., magnocellular part	S	subiculum	unc	uncinate fasciculus
mml	medial medullary lamina of the globuspallidus	sas	semiannular sulcus	unn	uncal notch (Duvernoy)
mt	mammillo-thalamic tract	SB	striatal cell bridges	VA	ventroanterior thalamic nucleus
opt	optic tract	SLG	semilunar gyrus	VCl	ventral claustrum
PalHy	pallidohypothalamic nucleus	sm	stria medullaris of the thalamus	ZI	zona incerta
PCo	posterior cortical amygdaloid nucleus	st	stria terminalis		

10,7 mm

30

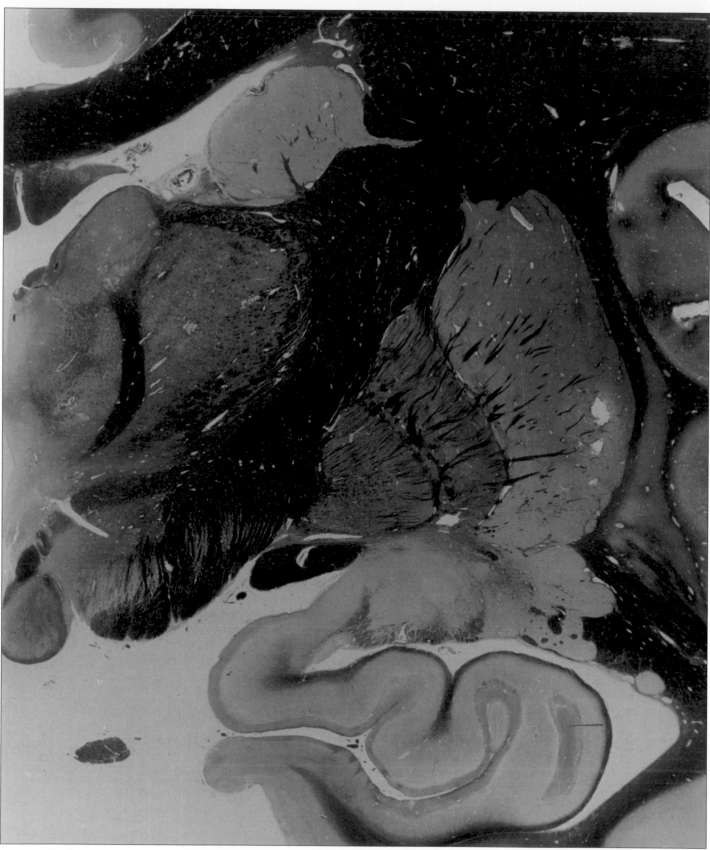

3n	oculomotor nerve	BM	basomedial amygdaloid nucleus	DiCl	diffuse insular claustrum	iml	internal medullary lamina (thalamus)
3V	third ventricle	CA1	CA1 field of the hippocampus	EGP	external globus pallidus	LHA	lateral hypothalamic area
AG	ambiens gyrus	Cd	caudate nucleus	eml	external medullary lamina	LiCl	limitans claustrum
AHi	amygdalohippocampal area	CeL	central amygdaloid nucleus,		(thalamus)	LM	lateral mamillary nucleus
al	ansa lenticularis		lateral part	Ent	entorhinal cortex	lml	lateral medullary lamina of the globus
APr	anteroprincipal thalamic nucleus	CeM	central amygdaloid nucleus,	EP	entopeduncular nucleus		pallidus
AStr	amygdalostriate transition area		medial part	Fa	fasciculosus nucleus	LV	lateral ventricle
BC	basal nucleus, compact part	comb	comb system	gic	genu of the internal capsule	MD	medial dorsal thalamic nucleus
bcc	body of the corpus callosum	cp	cerebral peduncle	H2	lenticular fasciculus (field H2)	Me	medial amygdaloid nucleus
bfx	body of fornix	Cuc	cucullaris nucleus	HiH	hippocampal head	mfb	medial forebrain bundle
BL	basolateral amygdaloid nucleus	DG	dentate gyrus	IGP	internal globus pallidus	MMC	medial mammillary n., magnocellular p.

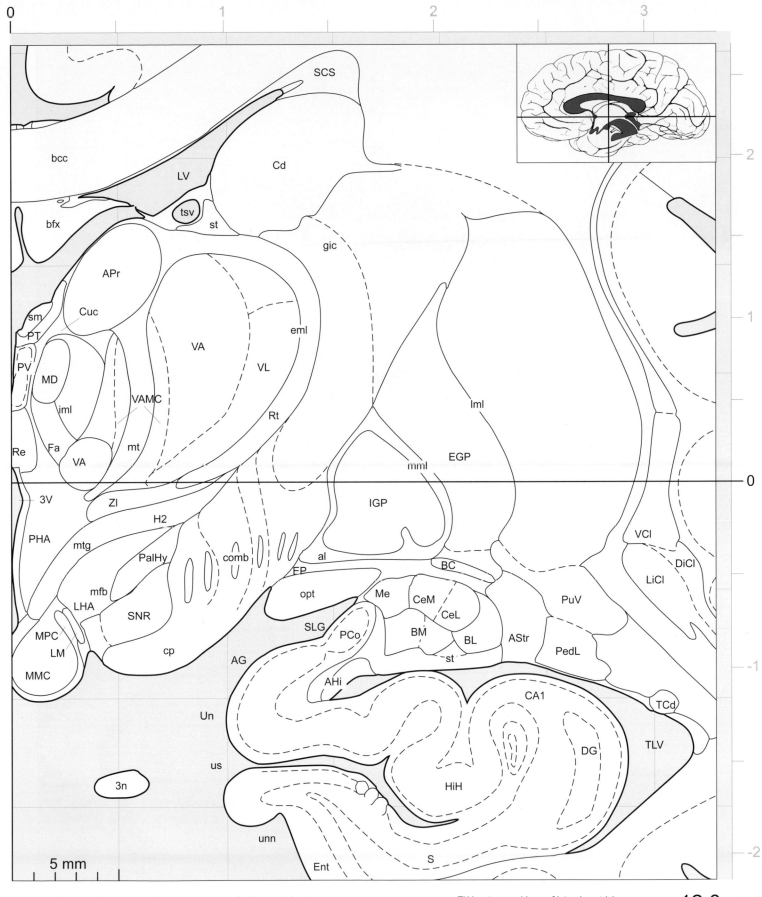

0   1   2   3

5 mm

mml	medial medullary lamina of the globus pallidus	PuV	ventral putamen	TLV	temporal horn of lateral ventricle
MPC	medial mammillary n., parvocellular part	PV	paraventricular thalamic nucleus	tsv	thalamostriate vein
mt	mammillo-thalamic tract	Re	reuniens thalamic nucleus	Un	uncus
mtg	mammillo-tegmental tract	Rt	reticular thalamic nucleus	unn	uncal notch (Duvernoy)
opt	optic tract	S	subiculum	us	uncal sulcus
PalHy	pallidohypothalamic nucleus	SCS	subcallosal stratum	VA	ventroanterior thalamic nucleus
PCo	posterior cortical amygdaloid nucleus	SLG	semilunar gyrus	VAMC	ventroanterior thalamic nucleus, magnocellular part
PedL	peduncle of lentiform nucleus	sm	stria medullaris of the thalamus		
PHA	posterior hypothalamic area	SNR	substantia nigra, reticular part	VCl	ventral claustrum
PT	paratenial thalamic nucleus	st	stria terminalis	VL	ventral lateral thalamic nucleus
		TCd	tail of caudate nucleus	ZI	zona incerta

12,0 mm

31

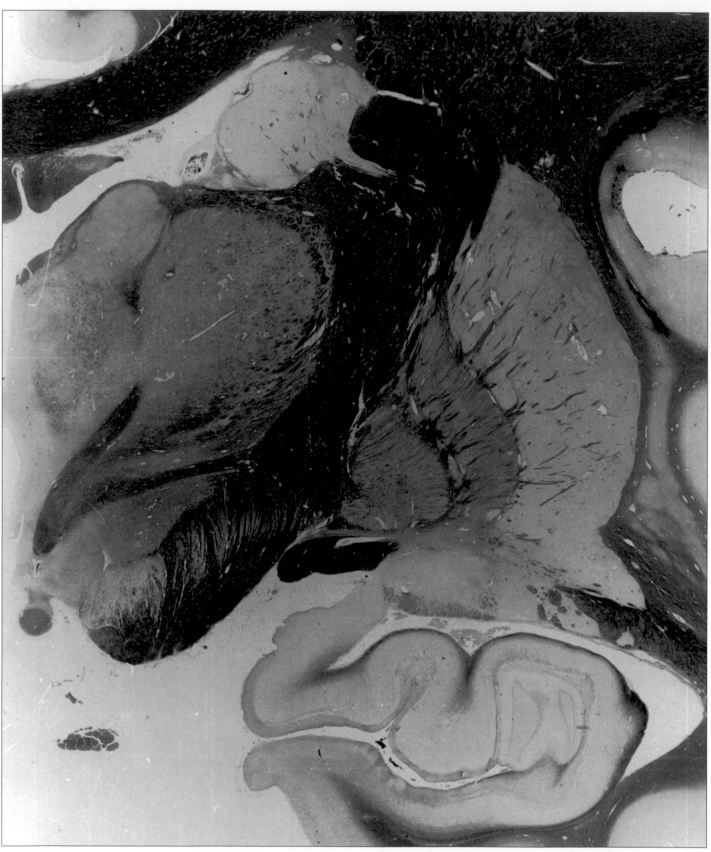

3n	oculomotor nerve	Cd	caudate nucleus	Ent	entorhinal cortex	lenf	lentiform fibers
3V	third ventricle	CeL	central amygdaloid nucl., lateral part	ex	extreme capsule	LHA	lateral hypothalamic area
AD	anterodorsal thalamic nucleus	CeM	central amygdaloid nucl., medial part	Fas	fasciculosus nucleus	LiCl	limitans claustrum
al	ansa lenticularis	comb	comb system	H1	thalamic fasciculus (field H1)	lml	lateral medullary lamina of the
APr	anteroprincipal thalamic nucleus	cp	cerebral peduncle	H2	lenticular fasciculus (field H2)		globus pallidus
AStr	amygdalostriate transition area	Cuc	cucullaris nucleus	HiH	hippocampal head	LV	lateral ventricle
bcc	body of corpus callosum	DCl	dorsal claustrum	IG	insular gyrus	MD	medial dorsal thalamic nucleus
bfx	body of fornix	DG	dentate gyrus	IGP	internal globus pallidus	Me	medial amygdaloid nucleus
bG	band of Giacomini (Duv. 85)	DiCl	diffuse insular claustrum	iml	internal medullary lamina with cell	MM	medial mamillary nucleus
BL	basolateral amygdaloid nucleus	ec	external capsule		clusters (thalamus)	mml	medial medullary lamina of the globus
BM	basomedial amygdaloid nucleus	EGP	external globus pallidus	IthA	interthalamic adhesion		pallidus
CA1	CA1 field of the hippocampus	eml	external medullary lamina (thalamus)	LDO	laterodorsal nucleus, oral part	mt	mammillo-thalamic tract

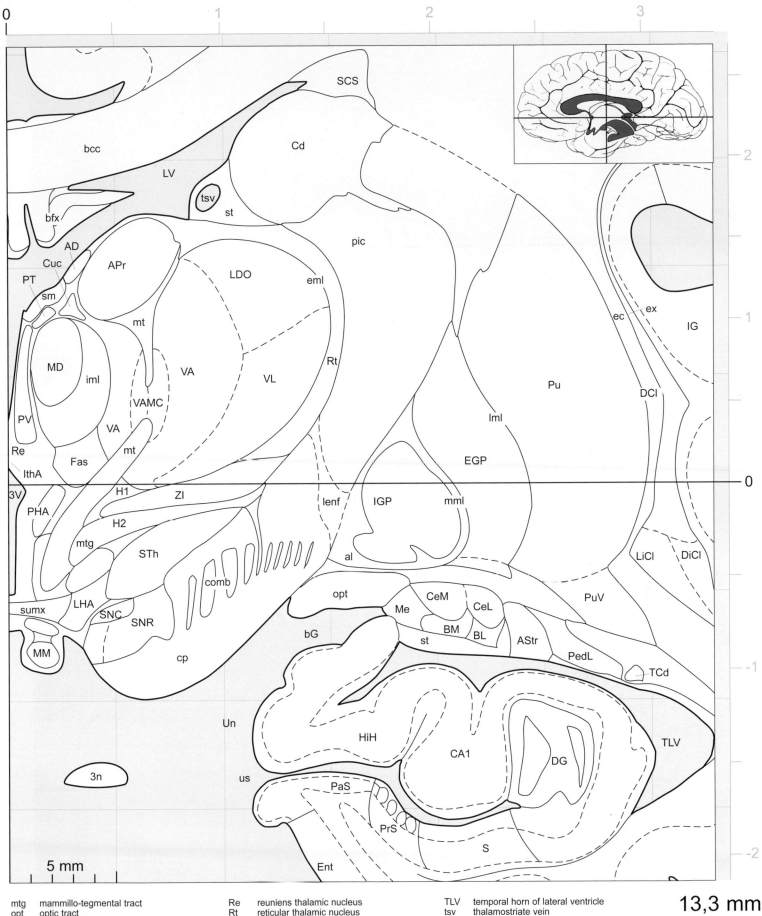

0 1 2 3

SCS

bcc

Cd

LV

tsv

st

bfx

pic

AD

Cuc

APr

LDO

eml

PT

sm

mt

ec

ex

IG

MD

iml

VA

VL

Rt

Pu

DCl

PV

VAMC

VA

lml

Re

mt

Fas

EGP

IthA

3V

H1

ZI

lenf

IGP

mml

PHA

H2

LiCl

DiCl

mtg

STh

al

PuV

comb

opt

CeM

CeL

sumx

LHA

SNC

SNR

Me

BM

CeL

BL

AStr

MM

cp

bG

st

PedL

TCd

Un

HiH

CA1

DG

TLV

3n

us

PaS

PrS

S

Ent

5 mm

13,3 mm

mtg	mammillo-tegmental tract	Re	reuniens thalamic nucleus	TLV	temporal horn of lateral ventricle
opt	optic tract	Rt	reticular thalamic nucleus	tsv	thalamostriate vein
PaS	parasubiculum	S	subiculum	Un	uncus
PedL	peduncle of lentiform nucleus	SCS	subcallosal stratum	us	uncal sulcus
PHA	posterior hypothalamic area	sm	stria medullaris of the thalamus	VA	ventroanterior thalamic nucleus
pic	posterior part of the internal capsule	SNC	substantia nigra, pars compacta	VAMC	ventroanterior thalamic nucleus,
PrS	presubiculum	SNR	substantia nigra, pars reticulata		magnocellular part
PT	paratenial thalamic nucleus	st	stria terminalis	VL	ventrolateral thalamic nucleus
Pu	putamen	STh	subthalamic nucleus	VCl	ventral claustrum
PuV	ventral putamen	sumx	supramammillary commissure	ZI	zona incerta
PV	paraventricular thalamic nucleus	TCd	tail of caudate nucleus		

32

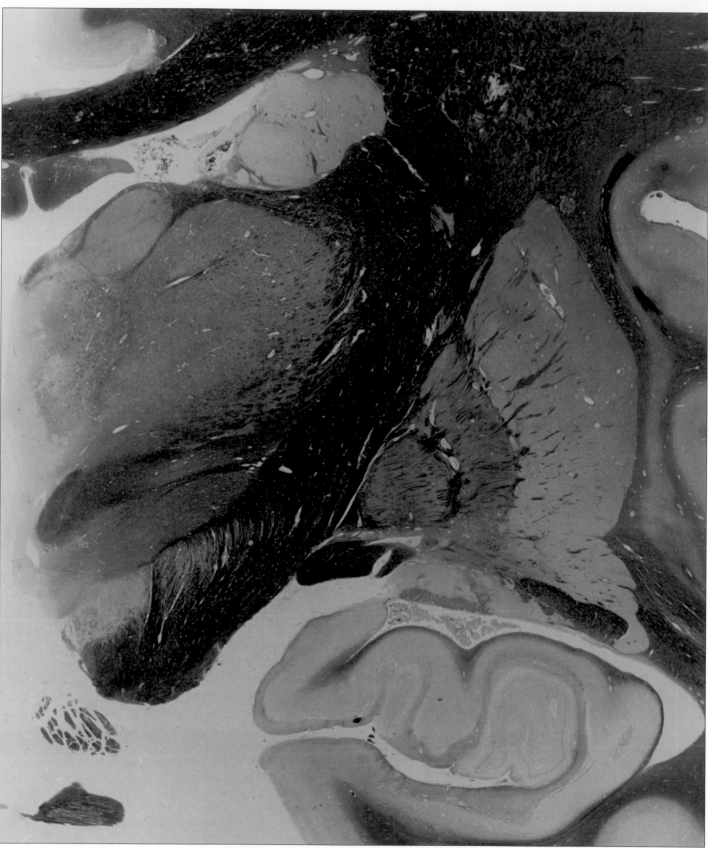

3n	oculomotor nerve	CG	cingulate gyrus	IGP	internal globus pallidus	MDV	medial dorsal thalamic nucl., ventral part
3V	third ventricle	comb	comb system	iml	internal medullary lamina with intra-laminar cell clusters (thalamus)		
AD	anterodorsal thalamic nucleus	cp	cerebral peduncle			Me	medial amygdaloid nucleus
al	ansa lenticularis	Cuc	cucullaris nucleus	IthA	interthalamic adhesion	mls	medial longitudinal stria
APr	anteroprincipal thalamic nucleus	DG	dentate gyrus	LD	lateral dorsal thalamic nucleus	mml	med. medull. lamina of globus pallidus
AStr	amygdalostriate transition area	ec	external capsule	lls	lateral longitudinal stria		
bcc	body of the corpus callosum	EGP	external globus pallidus	lml	lat. medull. lamina of globus pallidus	mt	mammillo-thalamic tract
bfx	body of fornix	eml	external medullary lamina of thalamus	LV	lateral ventricle	opt	optic tract
bG	band of Giacomini	Ent	entorhinal cortex	MD	medial dorsal thalamic nucleus	PaS	parasubiculum
CA1	CA1 field of the hippocampus	ex	extreme capsule	MDFa	medial dorsal thalamic nucl., fasciculosus part	pic	posterior part of the internal capsule
CA2	CA2 field of the hippocampus	H1	thalamic fasciculus (field H1)				
Cd	caudate nucleus	H2	lenticular fasciculus (field H2)	MDFi	medial dorsal thalamic nucl., fibrosus part	Pons	pons
Ce	central amygdaloid nucleus	IG	insular gyrus			PrS	presubiculum

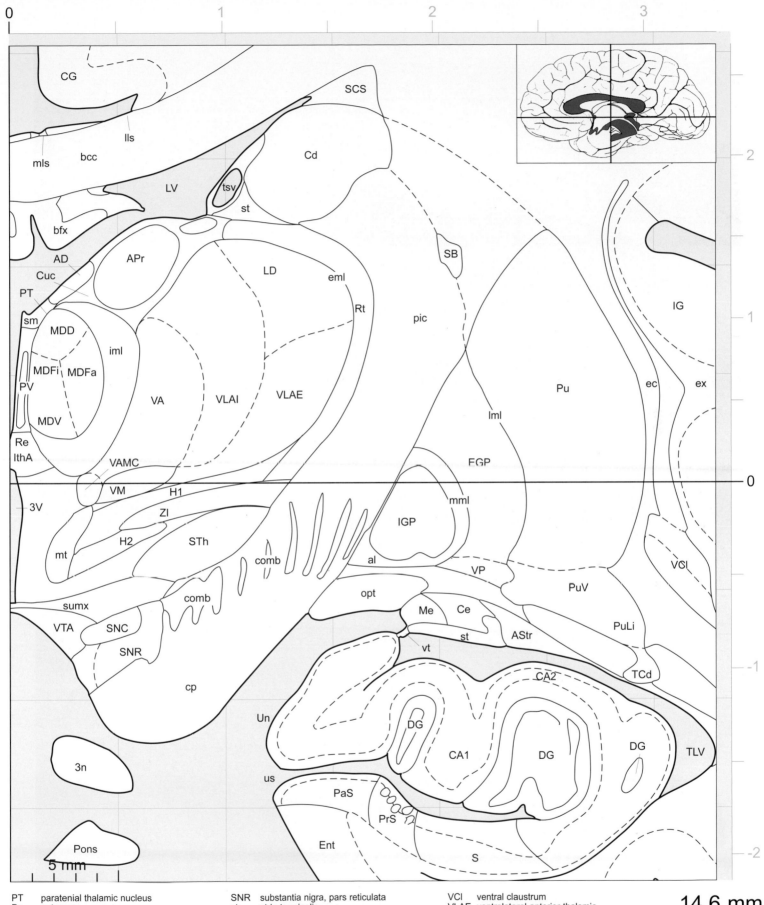

PT	paratenial thalamic nucleus	SNR	substantia nigra, pars reticulata	VCl	ventral claustrum
Pu	putamen	st	stria terminalis	VLAE	ventrolateral anterior thalamic
PuLi	limitans putamen	STh	subthalamic nucleus		nucleus, external part
PuV	ventral putamen	sumx	supramammillary commissure	VLAI	ventrolateral anterior thalamic
PV	paraventricular thalamic nucleus	TCd	tail of caudate nucleus		nucleus, internal part
Re	reuniens thalamic nucleus	TLV	temporal horn of lateral ventricle	VM	ventromedial thalamic nucleus
Rt	reticular thalamic nucleus	tsv	thalamostriate vein	VP	ventral pallidum
S	subiculum	Un	uncus	vt	velum terminale
SB	striatal cell bridge	us	uncal sulcus	VTA	ventral tegmental area
SCS	subcallosal stratum	VA	ventroanterior thalamic nucleus	ZI	zona incerta
sm	stria medullaris of the thalamus	VAMC	ventroanterior thalamic nucleus,		
SNC	substantia nigra, pars compacta		magnocellular part		

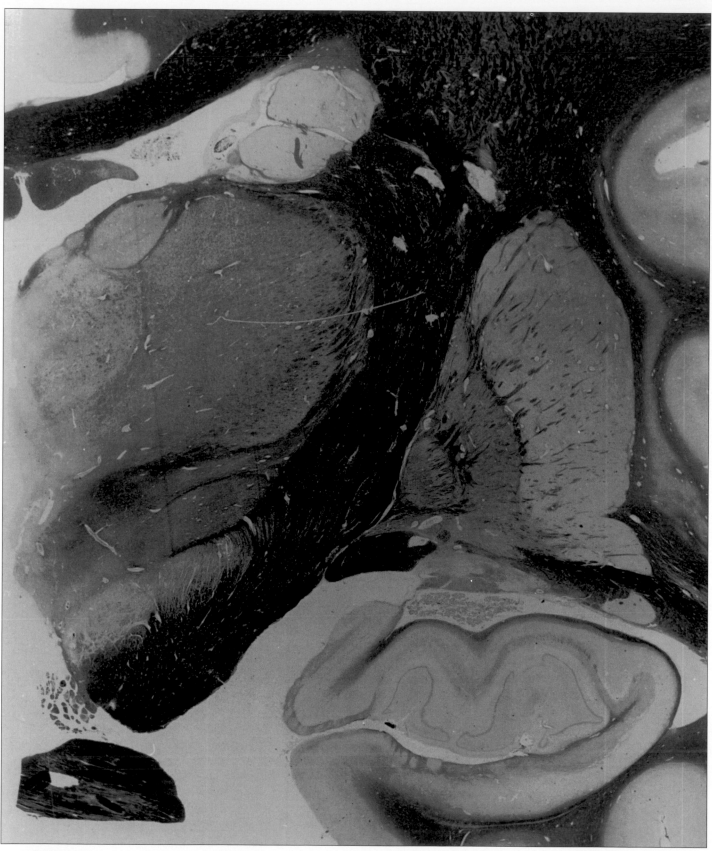

3n	oculomotor nerve			ex	extreme capsule	MDFa	medial dorsal thalamic n.,
3V	third ventricle	CA3	CA3 field of the hippocampus	H1	thalamic fasciculus (field H1)		fasciculosus part
AD	anterodorsal thalamic nucleus	Cd	caudate nucleus	H2	lenticular fasciculus (field H2)	MDFi	medial dorsal thalamic n., fibrosus part
al	ansa lenticularis	comb	comb system	IG	insular gyrus	MDV	medial dorsal thalamic n., ventral part
Amg	amygdala	cp	cerebral peduncle	IGP	internal globus pallidus	mml	medial medullary lamina of the globus
APr	anteroprincipal thalamic nucleus	Cuc	cucullaris nucleus	iml	internal medullary lamina of thalamus		pallidus
AStr	amygdalostriate transition area	DG	dentate gyrus	LD	lateral dorsal thalamic nucleus	opt	optic tract
bcc	body of the corpus callosum	ec	external capsule	lml	lateral medullary lamina of the globus	PF	parafascicular thalamic nucleus
bfx	body of fornix	EGP	external globus pallidus		pallidus	pic	posterior part of the internal capsule
bG	band of Giacomini	eml	external medullary lamina of	LV	lateral ventricle	Pons	pons
CA1	CA1 field of the hippocampus		thalamus	MDD	medial dorsal thalamic n., dorsal part	PT	paratenial thalamic nucleus
CA2	CA2 field of the hippocampus	Ent	entorhinal cortex				

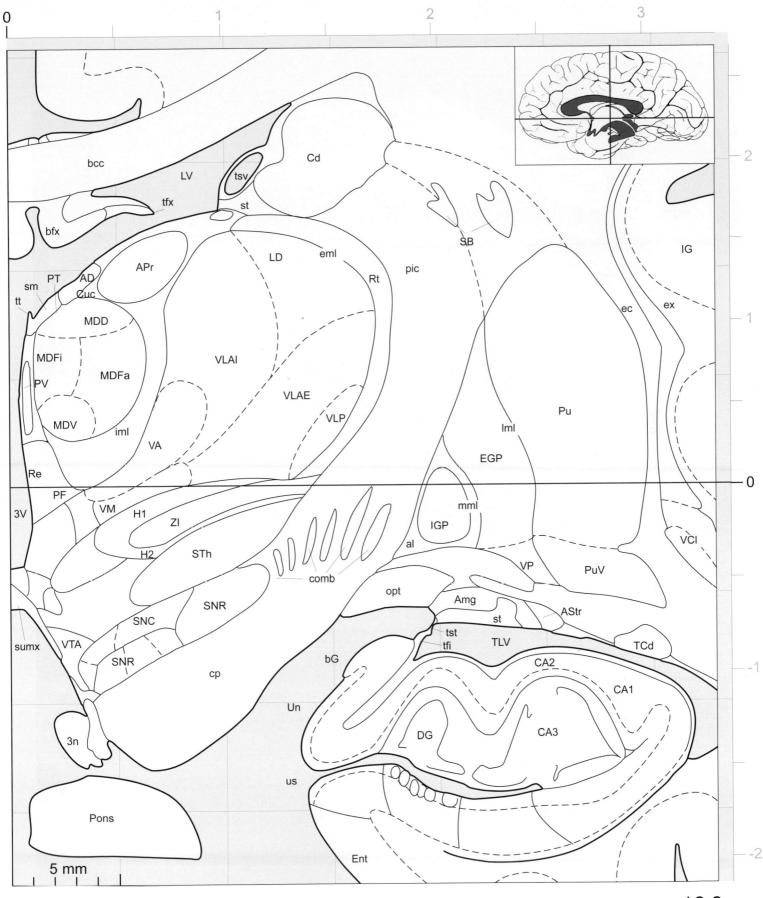

0　　　　　1　　　　　2　　　　　3

bcc
LV
tsv
Cd
tfx
st
SB
IG
bfx
LD
eml
Rt
pic
ec
ex
APr
sm　PT　AD
tt　Cuc
MDD
MDFi
VLAI
PV
MDFa
VLAE
Pu
MDV
VLP
lml
iml
VA
EGP
Re
mml
PF
3V
VM
IGP
VCI
H1
ZI
H2
STh
al
VP
PuV
comb
opt
Amg
AStr
SNR
tst
st
SNC
tfi
TLV
TCd
sumx
VTA
SNR
bG
CA2
cp
CA1
Un
DG
CA3
3n
us
Pons
Ent

5 mm

16,0 mm

34

Pu　putamen
PuV　ventral putamen
PV　paraventricular thalamic nucleus
Re　reuniens thalamic nucleus
Rt　reticular thalamic nucleus
SB　striatal cell bridge
sm　stria medullaris of the thalamus
SNC　substantia nigra, pars compacta
SNR　substantia nigra, pars reticulata
st　stria terminalis
STh　subthalamic nucleus

sumx　supramammillary commissure
TCd　tail of caudate nucleus
tfi　tenia of fimbria
tfx　tenia of fornix
TLV　temporal horn of lateral ventricle
tst　tenia of stria terminalis
tsv　thalamostriate vein
tt　tenia of thalamus
Un　uncus
us　uncal sulcus
VA　ventroanterior thalamic nucleus

VCI　ventral claustrum
VM　ventromedial thalamic nucleus
VLAE　ventrolateral anterior thalamic
　　　nucleus, external part
VLAI　ventrolateral anterior thalamic
　　　nucleus, internal part
VLP　ventrolateral posterior thalamic
　　　nucleus
VP　ventral pallidum
VTA　ventral tegmental area
ZI　zona incerta

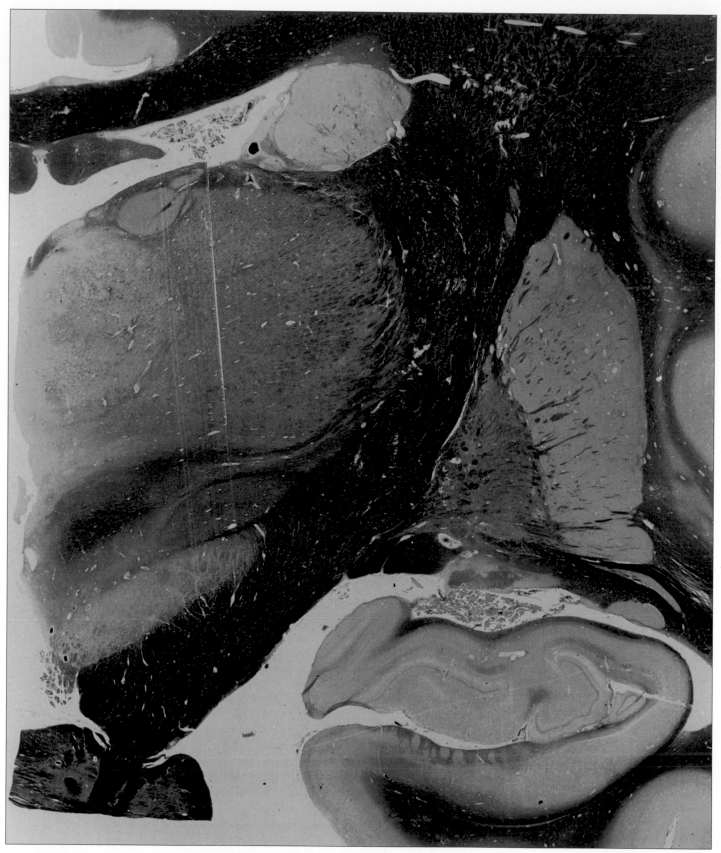

3n	oculomotor root	CA3	CA3 field of the hippocampus	EGP	external globus pallidus	LD	lateral dorsal thalamic nucleus
3V	third ventricle	Cd	caudate nucleus	eml	external medullary lamina of thalamus	LDSF	laterodorsal nucleus, superficial part
AD	anterodorsal thalamic nucleus	CG	cingulate gyrus	Ent	entorhinal cortex	lml	lateral medullary lamina
al	ansa lenticularis	CM	centromedian thalamic nucleus	ex	extreme capsule	LV	lateral ventricle
Amg	amygdala	CoCl	(compact) insular claustrum	FD	fascia dentata	MDD	medial dorsal thalamic n., dorsal part
APr	anteroprincipal thalamic nucleus	comb	comb system	H1	thalamic fasciculus (field H1)	MDFa	medial dorsal thalamic n., fasciculosus part
AStr	amygdalostriate transition area	cos	collateral sulcus	H2	lenticular fasciculus (field H2)		
bcc	body of the corpus callosum	cp	cerebral peduncle	IG	insular gyrus	MDFi	medial dorsal thalamic n., fibrosus p.
bfx	body of fornix	cr	capsule of red nucleus	IGP	internal globus pallidus	MDV	medial dorsal thalamic n., ventral part
bG	band of Giacomini	crt	cerebello-rubro-thalamic fibers	IGr	indusium griseum	mls	medial longitudinal stria
CA1	CA1 field of the hippocampus	DG	dentate gyrus	lml	internal medullary lamina of thalamus	mml	medial medullary lamina
CA2	CA2 field of the hippocampus	ec	external capsule	IPCi	interpeduncular cistern	opt	optic tract

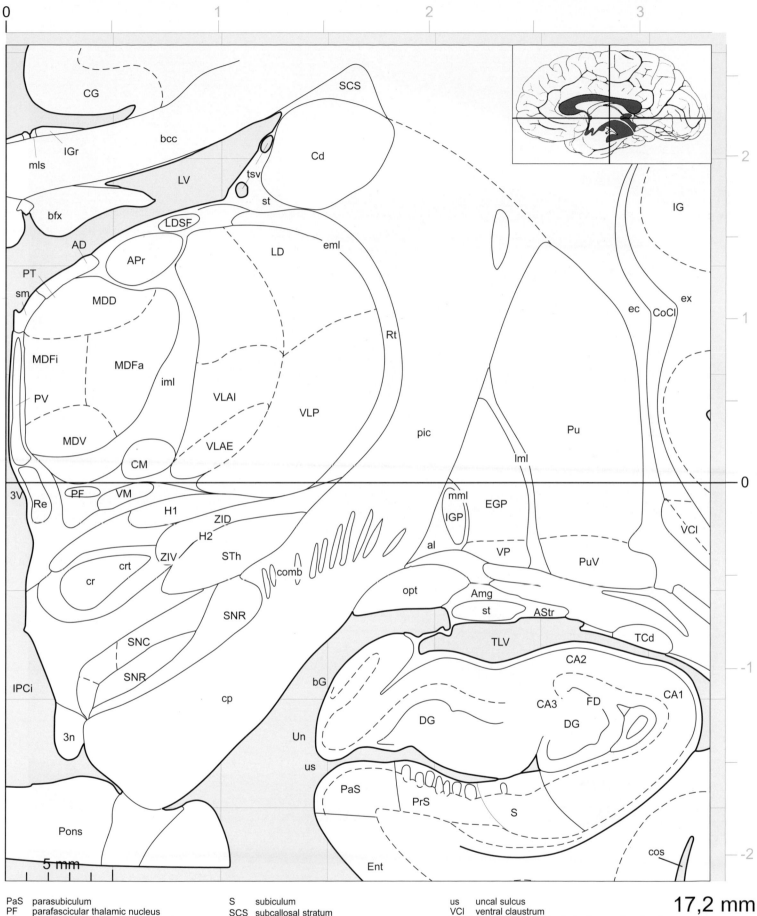

17,2 mm

35

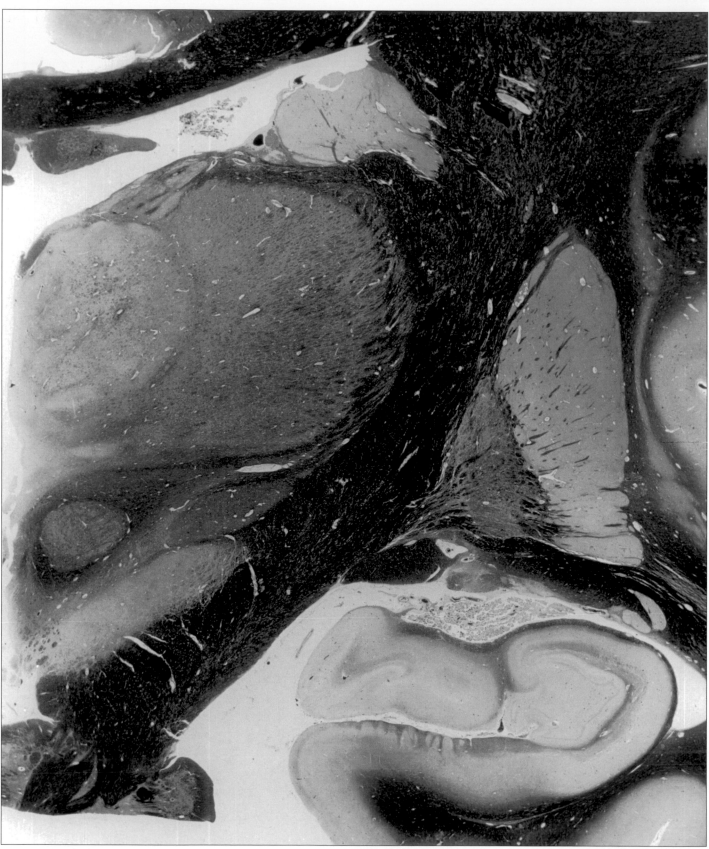

3n	oculomotor fibers	Cd	caudate nucleus	eml	external medullary lamina of		part
al	ansa lenticularis	chf	choroidal fissure		thalamus	lml	lateral medullary lamina of the globus
Amg	amygdala	CM	centromedian thalamic nucleus	Ent	entorhinal cortex		pallidus
APr	anteroprincipal thalamic nucleus	comb	comb system	ex	extreme capsule	LV	lateral ventricle
AStr	amygdalostriate transition area	cos	collateral sulcus	FD	fascia dentata	MDCe	medial dorsal thalamic n., central part
bcc	body of the corpus callosum	cp	cerebral peduncle	fi	fimbria of the hippocampus	MDD	medial dorsal thalamic n., dorsal part
bfx	body of fornix	cr	capsule of red nucleus	H1	thalamic fasciculus (field H1)	MDFa	medial dorsal thalamic n.,
CA1	CA1 field of the hippocampus	crt	cerebello-rubro-thalamic fibers	iml	internal medullary lamina of		fasciculosus part
CA2	CA2 field of the hippocampus	DCl	dorsal claustrum		thalamus	MDFi	medial dorsal thalamic n., fibrosus part
CA3	CA3 field of the hippocampus	DG	dentate gyrus	LD	lateral dorsal thalamic nucleus	MDV	medial dorsal thalamic n., ventral part
		EGP	external globus pallidus	LDSF	laterodorsal nucleus, superficial	opt	optic tract

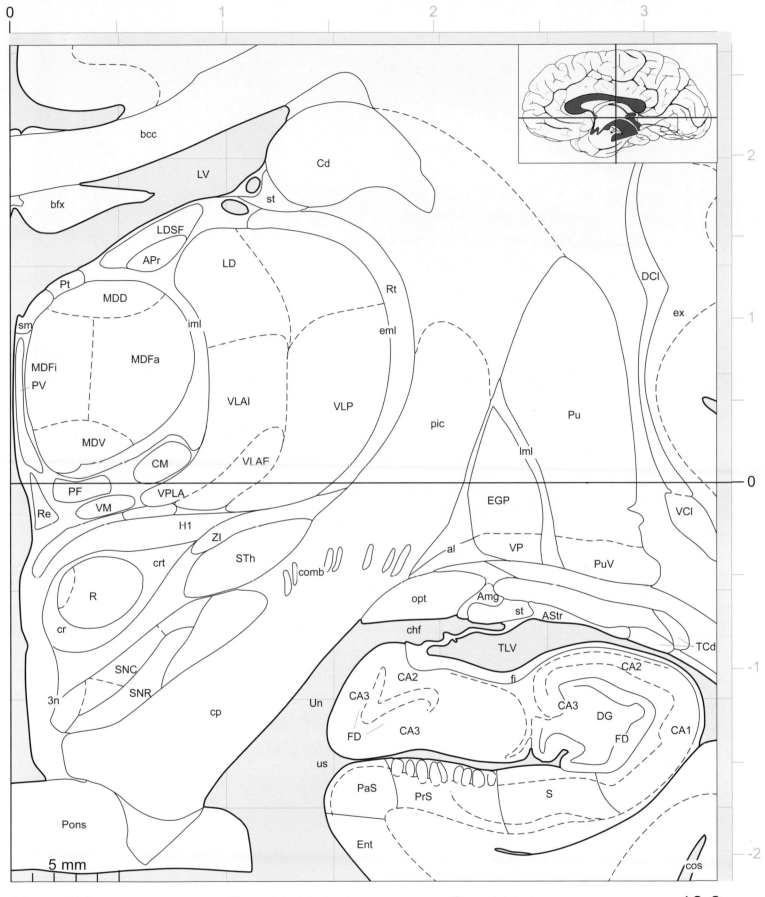

0   1   2   3

5 mm

18,6 mm

36

PaS	parasubiculum
PF	parafascicular thalamic nucleus
pic	posterior part of the internal capsule
Pons	pons
PrS	presubiculum
Pt	paratenial thalamic nucleus
Pu	putamen
PuV	ventral putamen
PV	paraventricular thalamic nucleus
R	red nucleus
Re	reuniens thalamic nucleus

Rt	reticular thalamic nucleus
S	subiculum
sm	stria medullaris of the thalamus
SNC	substantia nigra, pars compacta
SNR	substantia nigra, reticular part
st	stria terminalis
STh	subthalamic nucleus
TCd	tail of caudate nucleus
TLV	temporal horn of lateral ventricle
Un	uncus
us	uncal sulcus

VCl	ventral claustrum
VLAE	ventrolateral anterior thalamic nucleus, external part
VLAI	ventrolateral anterior thalamic nucleus, internal part
VLP	ventrolateral posterior thalamic nucleus
VM	ventromedial thalamic nucleus
VP	ventral pallidum
VPLA	ventral posterolateral thalamic nucleus, anterior part
ZI	zona incerta

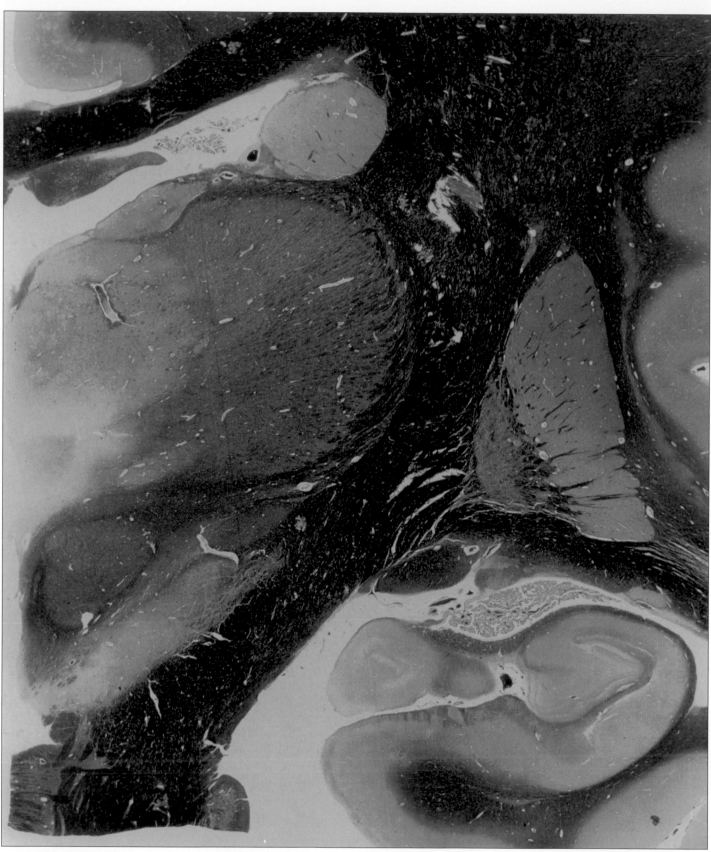

3n	oculomotor fibers	CI	claustrum	Ent	entorhinal cortex	LDSF	laterodorsal nucleus, superficial part
al	ansa lenticularis	CM	centromedian thalamic	ex	extreme capsule	lml	lateral medullary lamina of the
alv	alveus of the hippocampus		nucleus	FD	fascia dentata		globus pallidus
AStr	amygdalostriate transition area	cp	cerebral peduncle	fi	fimbria of the hippocampus	LV	lateral ventricle
bcc	body of the corpus callosum	cr	capsule of red nucleus	fr	fasciculus retroflexus	MD	mediodorsal thalamic nucleus
bfx	body of fornix	crt	cerebello-rubro-thalamic fibers	H1	thalamic fasciculus (field H1)	opt	optic tract
CA1	CA1 field of the hippocampus	DG	dentate gyrus	IG	insular gyrus	PaS	parasubiculum
CA2	CA2 field of the hippocampus	ec	external capsule	IGr	indusium griseum	PF	parafascicular thalamic nucleus
CA3	CA3 field of the hippocampus	EGP	external globus pallidus	iml	internal medullary lamina of	pic	posterior part of the internal capsule
Cd	caudate nucleus	eml	external medullary lamina of		thalamus		
CG	cingulate gyrus		thalamus	LD	lateral dorsal thalamic nucleus		

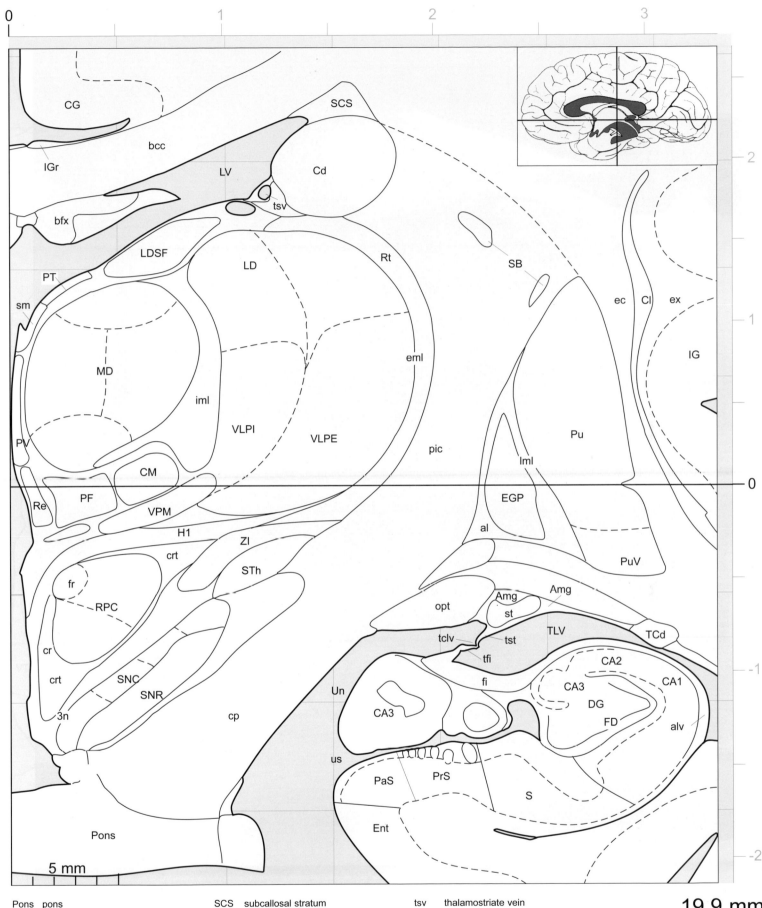

5 mm

19,9 mm

37

Pons	pons		SCS	subcallosal stratum		tsv	thalamostriate vein
PrS	presubiculum		sm	stria medullaris of the thalamus		Un	uncus
PT	paratenial thalamic nucleus		SNC	substantia nigra, pars compacta		us	uncal sulcus
Pu	putamen		SNR	substantia nigra, pars reticulata		VLPE	ventrolateral posterior thalamic nucleus, external part
PuV	ventral putamen		st	stria terminalis			
PV	paraventricular thalamic nucleus		STh	subthalamic nucleus		VLPI	ventrolateral posterior thalamic nucleus, internal part
Re	reuniens thalamic nucleus		TCd	tail of caudate nucleus			
RPC	red nucleus, parvocellular part		tclv	tela choroides of lateral ventricle		VPM	ventroposterior medial thalamic nucleus
Rt	reticular thalamic nucleus		tfi	tenia of fimbria			
S	subiculum		TLV	temporal horn of lateral ventricle		ZI	zona incerta
SB	striatal cell bridges		tst	tenia of stria terminalis			

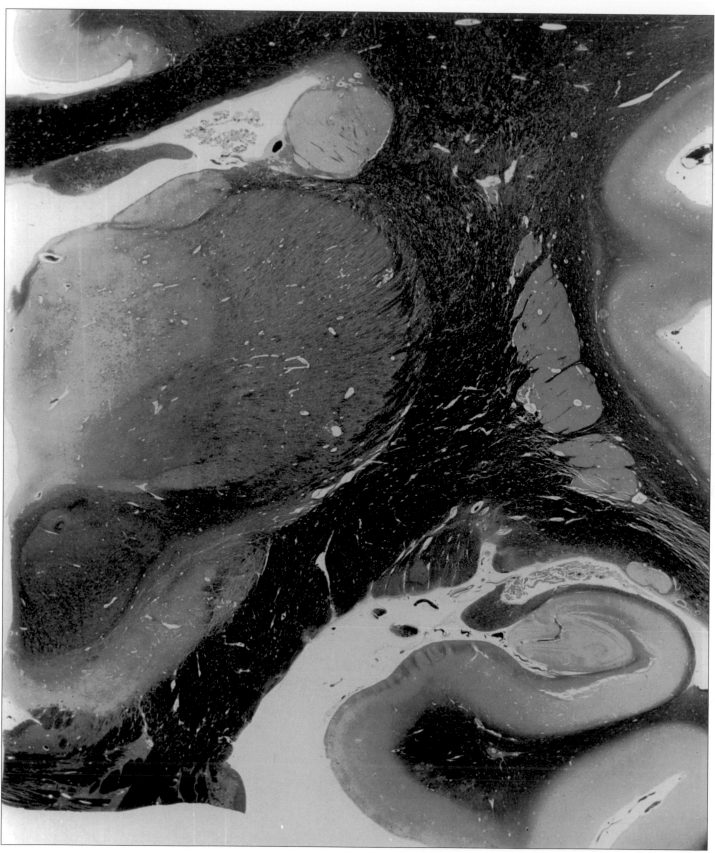

AD	anterodorsal thalamic nucleus	CM	centromedian thalamic nucleus	Ent	entorhinal cortex	IP	interpeduncular nucleus
al	ansa lenticularis	CMMC	centromedian thalamic nucleus,	ex	extreme capsule	LD	laterodorsal thalamic nucleus
alv	alveus of the hippocampus		magnocellular part	FD	fascia dentata	LDSF	laterodorsal nucleus, superficial
bcc	body of the corpus callosum	cos	collateral sulcus	fi	fimbria of the hippocampus		part
bfx	body of fornix	cp	cerebral peduncle	fr	fasciculus retroflexus	LG	lateral geniculate nucleus
CA1	CA1 field of the hippocampus	crt	cerebello-rubro-thalamic fibers	FuG	fusiform gyrus	lml	lateral medullary lamina (globus
CA2	CA2 field of the hippocampus		(superior cerebellar peduncle)	H1	thalamic fasciculus (field H1)		pall.)
CA3	CA3 field of the hippocampus	Cuc	cucullaris nucleus	his	hippocampal sulcus	LV	lateral ventricle
Cd	caudate nucleus	ec	external capsule	IG	insular gyrus	MD	medial dorsal thalamic nucleus
CG	cingulate gyrus	eml	external medullary lamina of	iml	internal medullary lamina of	PaS	parasubiculum
Cl	claustrum		thalamus		thalamus	PBP	parabrachial pigmented nucleus

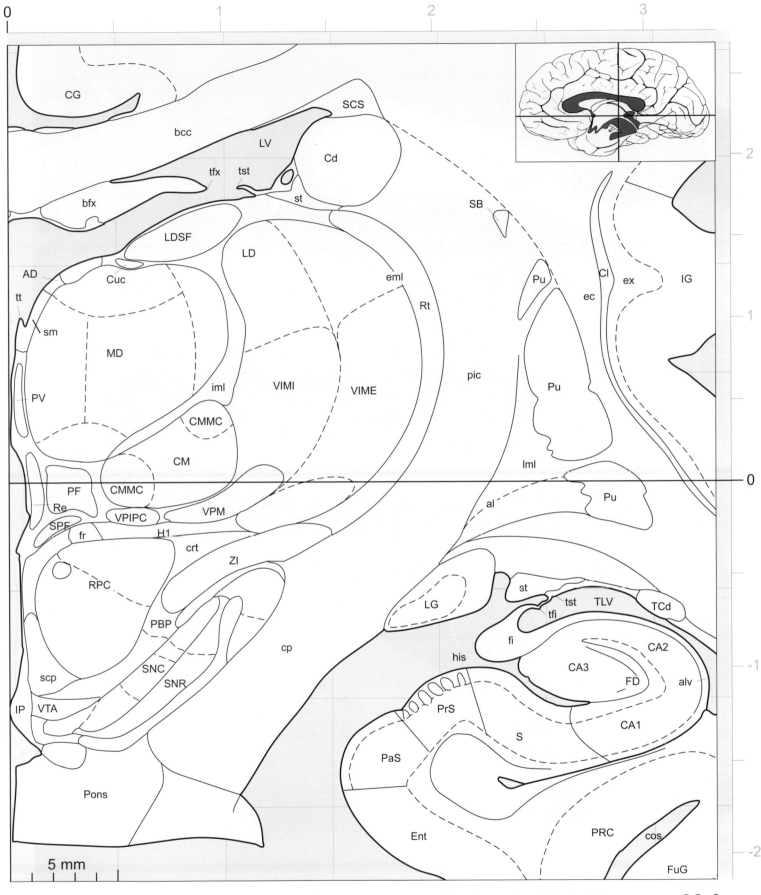

PF	parafascicular thalamic nucleus	SB	striatal cell bridge	TLV	temporal horn of lateral ventricle
pic	posterior part of the internal capsule	scp	superior cerebellar peduncle	tst	tenia of stria terminalis
Pons	pons	SCS	subcallosal stratum	tt	tenia of thalamus
PRC	perirhinal cortex	sm	stria medullaris of the thalamus	VIME	ventrointermedius nucl., external part
PrS	presubiculum	SNC	substantia nigra, pars compacta	VIMI	ventrointermedius nucl., internal part
Pu	putamen	SNR	substantia nigra, pars reticulata	VPIPC	ventroposterior internus nucleus,
PV	paraventricular thalamic nucleus	SPF	subparafascicular thalamic nucleus		parvocellular part
Re	reuniens thalamic nucleus	st	stria terminalis	VPM	ventroposterior medial thalamic nucleus
RPC	red nucleus, parvocellular part	TCd	tail of caudate nucleus	VTA	ventral tegmental area
Rt	reticular thalamic nucleus	tfi	tenia of fimbria	ZI	zona incerta
S	subiculum	tfx	tenia of fornix		

22,6 mm

39

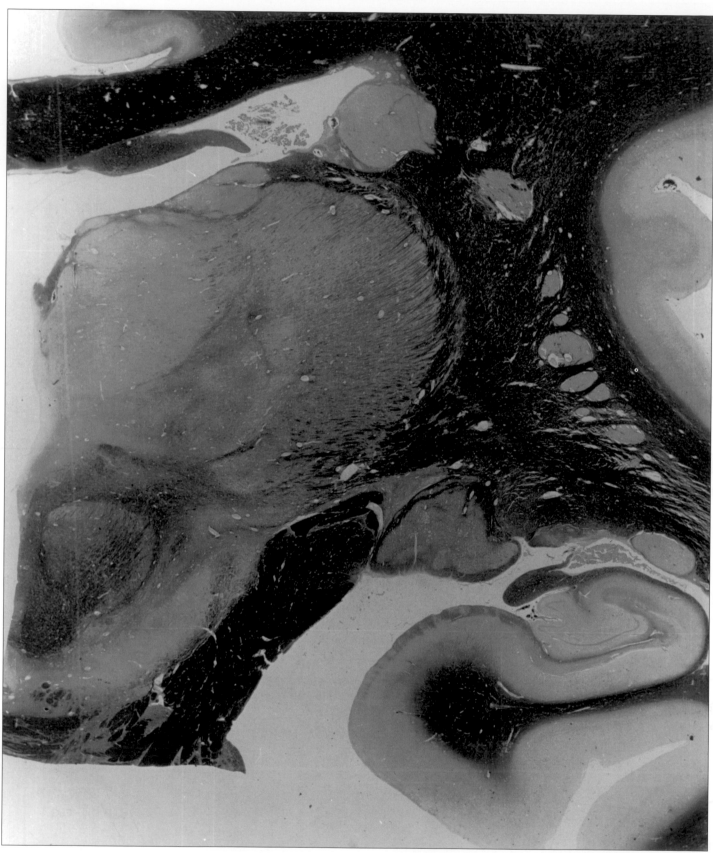

AD	anterodorsal thalamic nucleus	CA1	CA1 field of the hippocampus	FuG	fusiform gyrus	LV	lateral ventricle
alv	alveus of the hippocampus	CA2	CA2 field of the hippocampus	H1	thalamic fasciculus (field H1)	MDD	medial dorsal thalamic n., dorsal part
bcc	body of the corpus callosum	CA3	CA3 field of the hippocampus	his	hippocampal sulcus		
bfx	body of fornix	Cd	caudate nucleus	IG	insular gyrus	MDFa	medial dorsal thalamic n., fasciculosus part
		CG	cingulate gyrus	iml	internal medullary lamina of thalamus		
		CM	centromedian thalamic nucleus			MDFi	medial dorsal thalamic n., fibrosusp.
		cp	cerebral peduncle	IP	interpeduncular nucleus		
		eml	external medullary lamina of thalamus	LD	laterodorsal thalamic nucleus	MDMC	medial dorsal thalamic n., magnocellular part
				LDSF	laterodorsal nucleus, superficial part		
208		fi	fimbria of the hippocampus			MDV	medial dorsal thalamic n., ventral part
		fr	fasciculus retroflexus	LG	lateral geniculate nucleus		

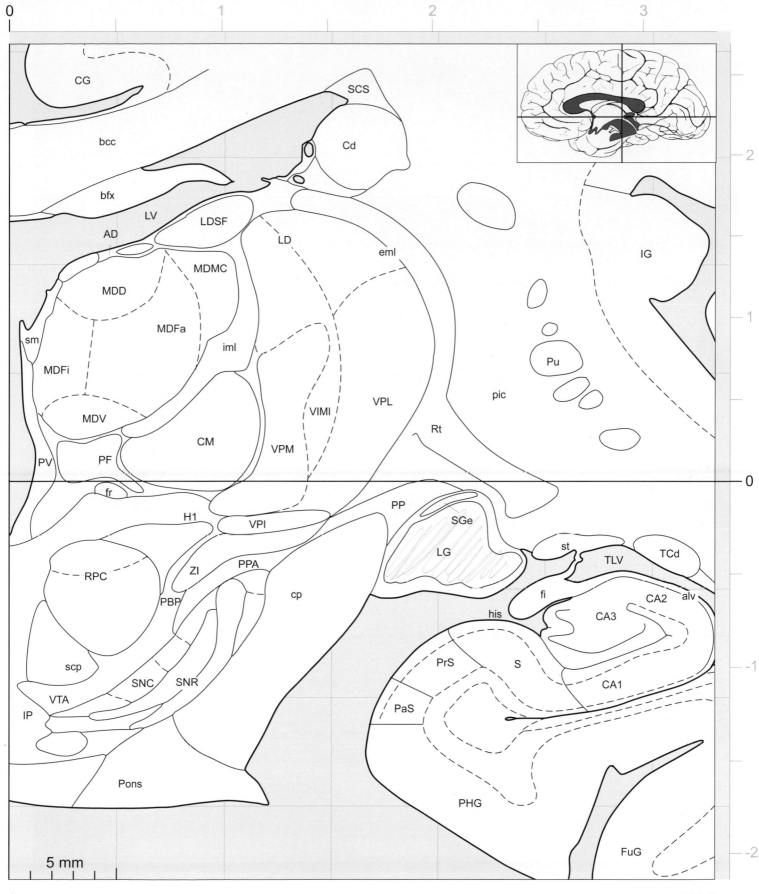

0   1   2   3

CG

bcc

SCS

bfx

Cd

LV

LDSF

AD

LD

eml

IG

MDMC

MDD

MDFa

iml

sm

Pu

MDFi

pic

VPL

VIMI

MDV

Rt

CM

VPM

PV   PF

fr

PP

H1

VPI

SGe

RPC

ZI   PPA

LG

st

TLV   TCd

PBP

cp

fi

CA2   alv

his

CA3

scp

PrS   S   CA1

SNC   SNR

VTA

PaS

IP

Pons

PHG

FuG

5 mm

25,2 mm

PaS	parasubiculum	RPC	red nucleus, parvocellular part
PBP	parabrachial pigmented nucleus	Rt	reticular thalamic nucleus
PF	parafascicular thalamic nucleus	S	subiculum
PHG	parahippocampal gyrus	scp	superior cerebellar peduncle
pic	posterior part of the internal capsule	SCS	subcallosal stratum
Pons	pons	SGe	suprageniculate nucleus
PP	peripeduncular nucleus	sm	stria medullaris of the thalamus
PPA	peripeduncular area	SNC	substantia nigra, pars compacta
PrS	presubiculum	SNR	substantia nigra, pars reticulata
Pu	putamen	st	stria terminalis
PV	paraventricular thalamic nucleus	TCd	tail of caudate nucleus

TLV   temporal horn of lateral ventricle
VIMI ventrointermedius nucleus,
      internal part
VPI   ventroposterolateral thalamic
      nucleus, inferior part
VPL   ventroposterolateral thalamic
      nucleus
VPM   ventroposterior medial thalamic
      nucleus
VTA   ventral tegmental area
ZI   zona incerta

41

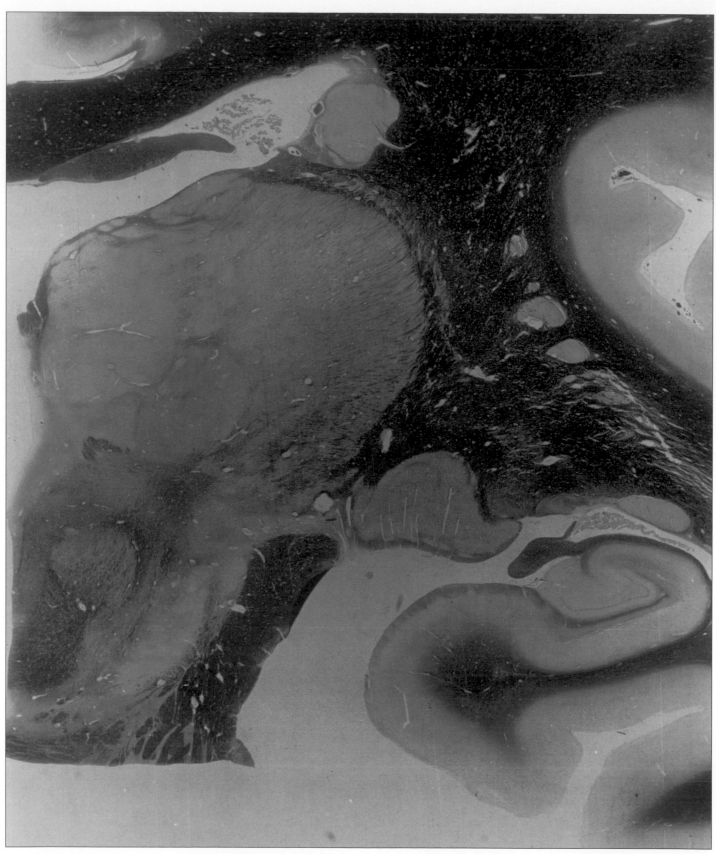

AD	anterodorsal thalamic nucleus	CA2	CA2 field of the hippocampus	fi	fimbria of the hippocampus	LV	lateral ventricle
alv	alveus of the hippocampus	CA3	CA3 field of the hippocampus	fr	fasciculus retroflexus	MDD	medial dorsal thalamic n., dorsal part
bcc	body of the corpus callosum	Cd	caudate nucleus	FuG	fusiform gyrus		
bfx	body of fornix	CG	cingulate gyrus	his	hippocampal sulcus	MDFa	medial dorsal thalamic n., fasciculosus part
CA1	CA1 field of the hippocampus	CM	centromedian thalamic nucleus	IG	insular gyrus		
		CMMC	centromedian thalamic n., magnocelular part	iml	internal medullary lamina of thalamus	MDFi	medial dorsal thalamic n., fibrosus part
		cos	collateral sulcus	LD	lateral dorsal thalamic nucleus		
		cp	cerebral peduncle	LDSF	laterodorsal nucleus, superficial part	MDMC	medial dorsal thalamic n., magnocellular part
		eml	external medullary lamina of thalamus	LG	lateral geniculate nucleus		

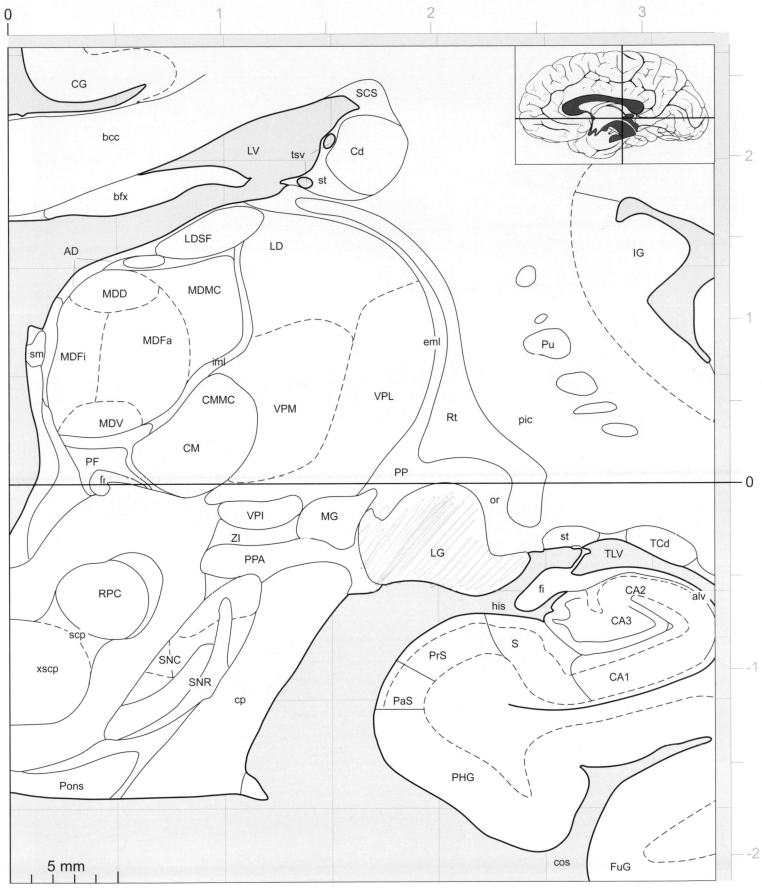

MDV	medial dorsal thalamic n., ventral part	RPC	red nucleus, parvocellular part	tsv	thalamostriate vein
MG	medial geniculate nucleus	Rt	reticular thalamic nucleus	VPI	ventroposterior thalamic
or	optic radiation	S	subiculum		nucleus, inferior part
PaS	parasubiculum	scp	superior cerebellar peduncle	VPL	ventroposterolateral thalamic
PF	parafascicular thalamic nucleus	SCS	subcallosal stratum		nucleus
PHG	parahippocampal gyrus	sm	stria medullaris of the thalamus	VPM	ventroposterior medial thalamic
pic	posterior part of the internal capsule	SNC	substantia nigra, pars compacta		nucleus
Pons	pons	SNR	substantia nigra, reticular part	xscp	decussation of the superior
PPA	peripeduncular area	st	stria terminalis		cerebellar peduncle
PrS	presubiculum	TCd	tail of caudate nucleus	ZI	zona incerta
Pu	putamen	TLV	temporal horn of lateral ventricle		

26,5 mm

42

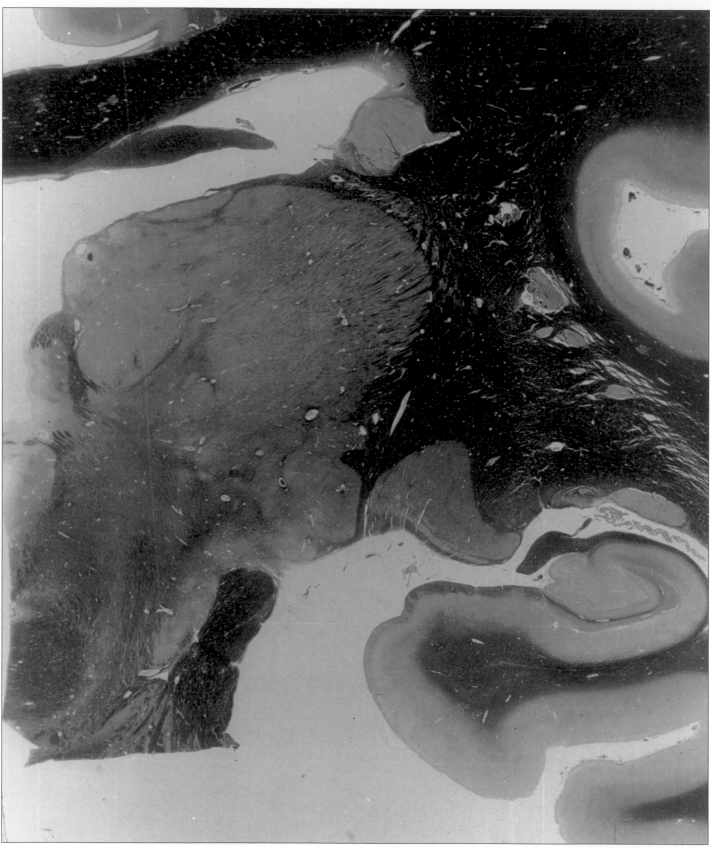

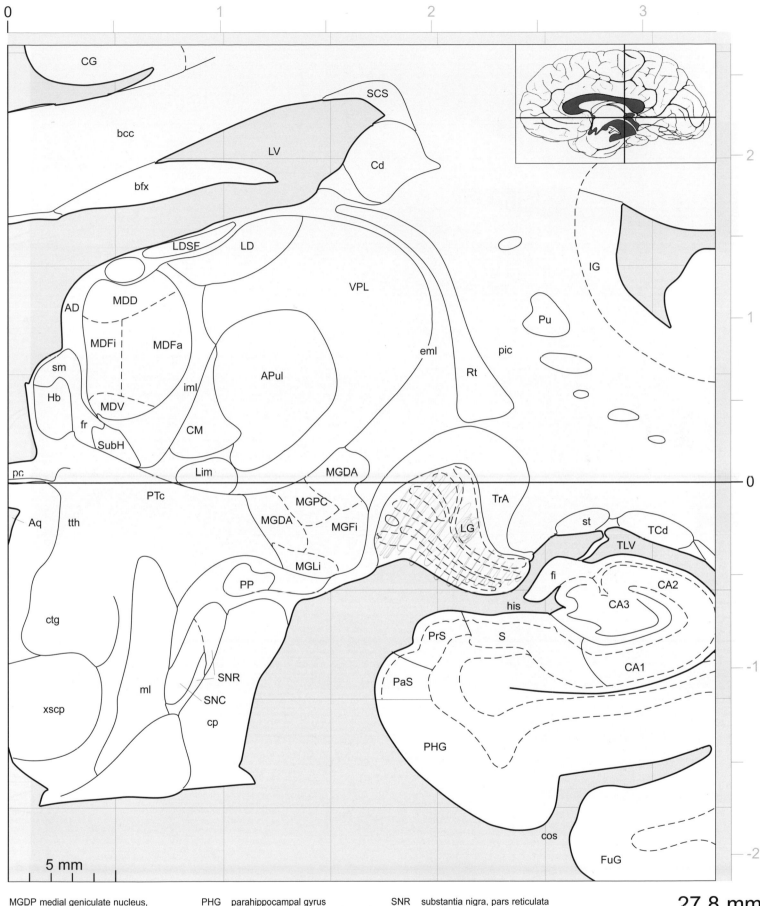

0   1   2   3

CG

SCS

bcc

LV

bfx   Cd

LDSF   LD

VPL

MDD   IG

AD

MDFi   MDFa   Pu

sm   eml   pic

Hb   APul   Rt

MDV   iml

fr   CM

SubH

Lim   MGDA

pc   TrA   st   TCd

PTc   MGPC   LG   TLV

Aq   tth   MGDA   MGFi   fi   CA2

his   CA3

MGLi

PP   PrS   S   CA1

ctg   PaS

SNR

ml   CA1

SNC

xscp   cp   PHG

cos

FuG

5 mm

MGDP	medial geniculate nucleus, dorsoposterior part	PHG	parahippocampal gyrus
MGFi	medial geniculate nucleus, fibrosus part	pic	posterior part of the internal capsule
		PP	peripeduncular nucleus
MGLi	medial geniculate nucleus, limitans part	PrS	presubiculum
		PTc	pretectal area
MGPC	medial geniculate nucleus, parvocellular part	Pu	putamen
		Rt	reticular thalamic nucleus
ml	medial lemniscus	S	subiculum
PaS	parasubiculum	SCS	subcallosal stratum
pc	posterior commissure	sm	stria medullaris of the thalamus
		SNC	substantia nigra, pars compacta

SNR substantia nigra, pars reticulata
st   stria terminalis
SubH subhabenular nucleus
TCd tail of caudate nucleus
TLV temporal horn of lateral ventricle
TrA triangular area (Wernicke)
tth dorsal trigemino-thalamic tract
VPL ventroposterolateral thalamic nucleus
xscp decussation of the superior cerebellar peduncle

27,8 mm

43

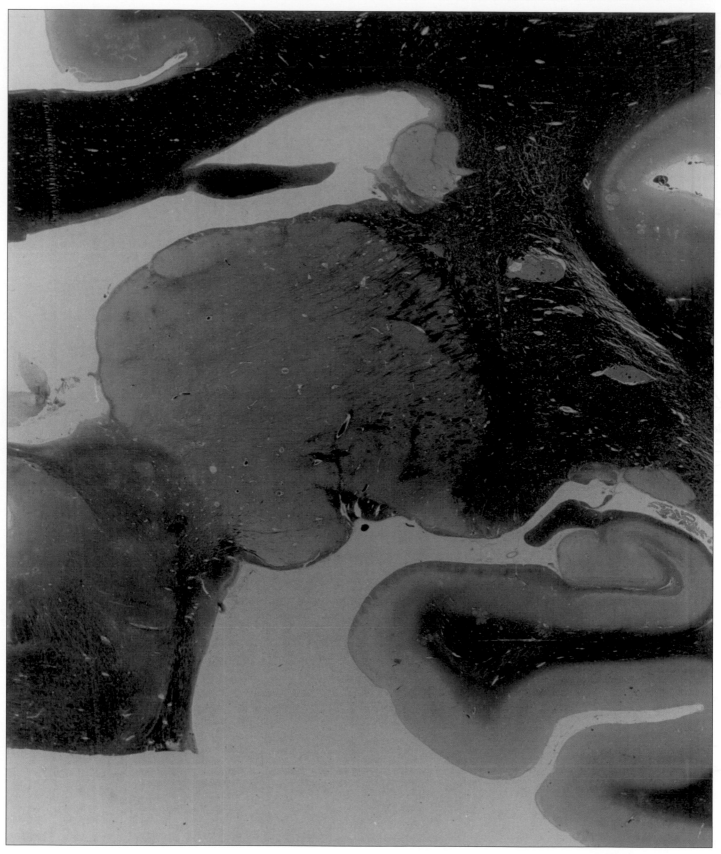

AD	anterodorsal thalamic nucleus	CG	cingulate gyrus	fi	fimbria of the hippocampus	Lim	limitans nucleus
Aq	cerebral aqueduct (Sylvius)	cos	collateral sulcus	FuG	fusiform gyrus	ILPul	inferior pulvinar nucleus
bcc	body of the corpus callosum	csc	commissure of the superior	ILPul	inferior pulvinar nucleus	LV	lateral ventricle
bic	brachium of the inferior colliculus		colliculi	IG	insular gyrus	MD	mediodorsal thalamic nucleus
CA1	CA1 field of the hippocampus	ctg	central tegmental tract	IGPul	intergeniculate pulvinar	MDe	margo denticulatus
CA2	CA2 field of the hippocampus	DG	dentate gyrus	ILPul	inferior pulvinar nucleus	MGDP	medial geniculate nucleus,
CA3	CA3 field of the hippocampus	dhc	dorsal hippocampal commissure	liml	internal medullary lamina of		dorsoposterior part
Cd	caudate nucleus	eml	external medullary lamina of		thalamus	MGFi	medial geniculate nucleus,
			thalamus	LG	lateral geniculate nucleus		fibrosus part
						MGLi	medial geniculate nucleus,

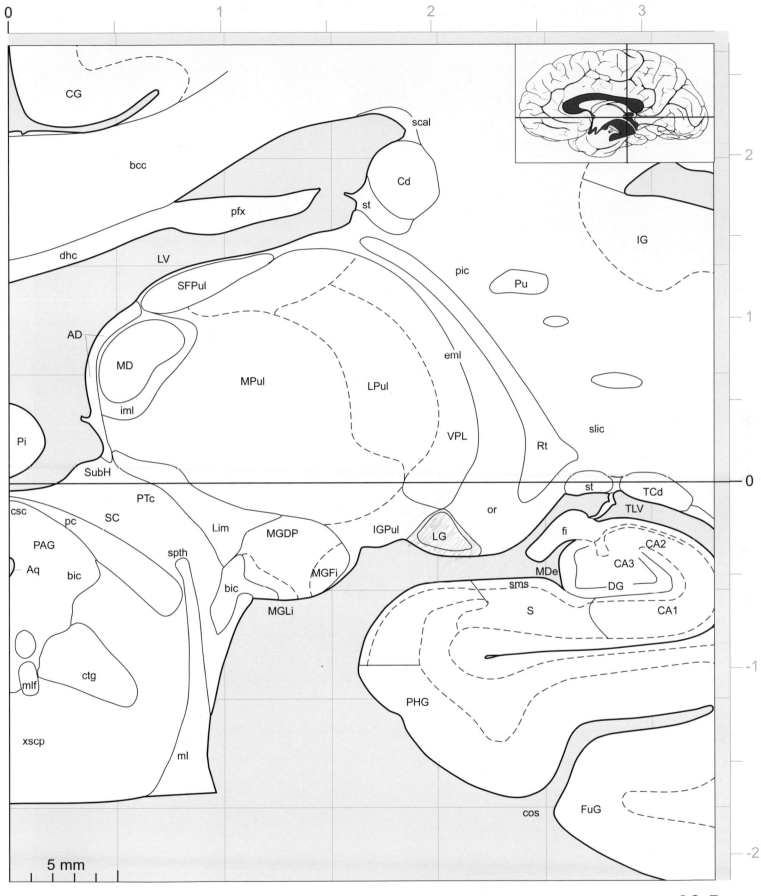

	limitans part	pic	posterior part of internal capsule	spth	spino-thalamic tract
ml	medial lemniscus	PTc	pretectal area	st	stria terminalis
mlf	medial longitudinal fasciculus	Pu	putamen	SubH	subhabenular nucleus
MPul	medial pulvinar nucleus	Rt	reticular thalamic nucleus	TCd	tail of caudate nucleus
or	optic radiation	S	subiculum	TLV	temporal horn of lateral ventricle
PAG	periaqueductal gray	SC	superior colliculus	VPL	ventroposterolateral thalamic nucleus
pc	posterior commissure	scal	subcallosal bundle	xscp	decussation of the superior cerebellar
pfx	posterior column (crus) of fornix	SFPul	superficial pulvinar nucleus		peduncle
PHG	parahippocampal gyrus	slic	sublenticular part of internal capsule		
Pi	pineal gland	sms	superficial medullary stratum		

45

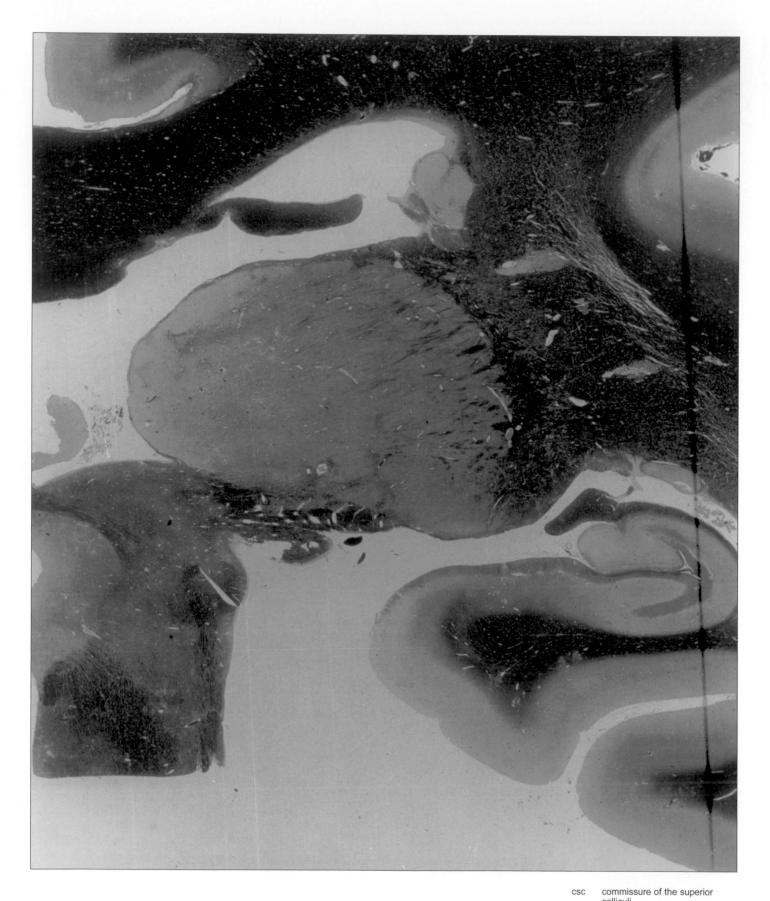

		csc	commissure of the superior colliculi
		CuA	cuneiform area
Aq	cerebral aqueduct (Sylvius)	DG	dentate gyrus
CA1	CA1 field of the hippocampus	dhc	dorsal hippocampal commissure
CA2	CA2 field of the hippocampus	eml	external medullary lamina of thalamus
CA3	CA3 field of the hippocampus		
Cd	caudate nucleus	fi	fimbria of the hippocampus
CG	cingulate gyrus	FuG	fusiform gyrus
cmg	capsule of medial geniculate n.	his	hippocampal sulcus
cos	collateral sulcus	IC	inferior colliculus

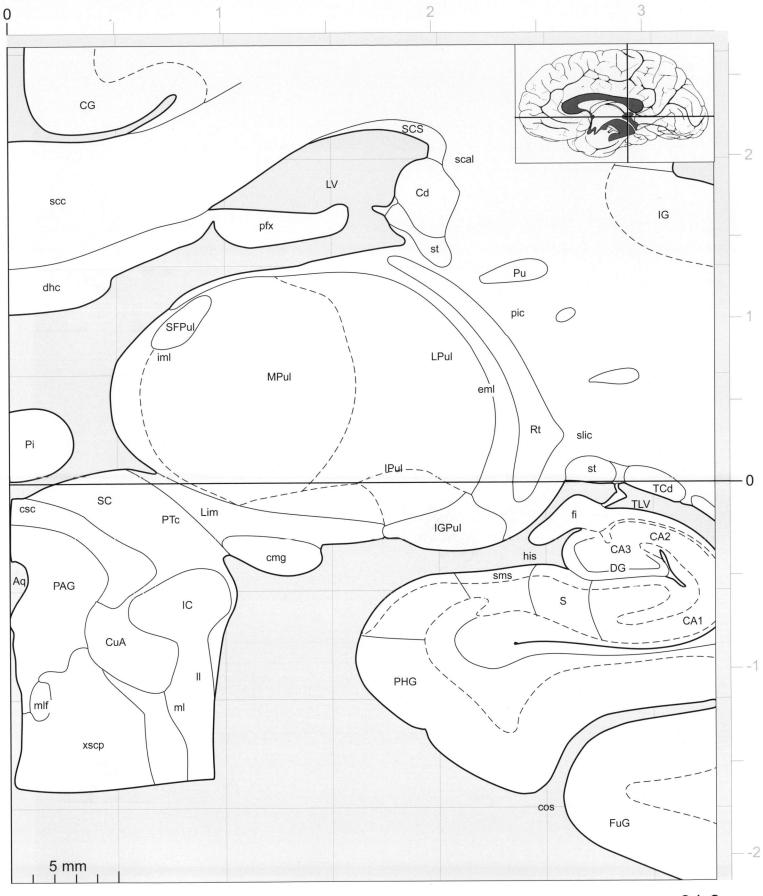

IG	insular gyrus	MPul	medial pulvinar nucleus	scal	subcallosal bundle
IGPul	intergeniculate pulvinar	PAG	periaqueductal gray	scc	splenium of the corpus callosum
iml	internal medullary lamina of thalamus	pfx	posterior column (crus) of fornix	SCS	subcallosal stratum
		PHG	parahippocampal gyrus	SFPul	superficial pulvinar nucleus
IPul	inferior pulvinar nucleus	Pi	pineal gland	slic	sublenticular part of internal capsule
Lim	limitans nucleus	pic	posterior part of internal capsule	sms	superficial medullary stratum
ll	lateral lemniscus	PTc	pretectal area	st	stria terminalis
LPul	lateral pulvinar nucleus	Pu	putamen	TCd	tail of caudate nucleus
LV	lateral ventricle	Rt	reticular thalamic nucleus	TLV	temporal horn of lateral ventricle
ml	medial lemniscus	S	subiculum	xscp	decussation of the superior cerebellar peduncle
mlf	medial longitudinal fasciculus	SC	superior colliculus		

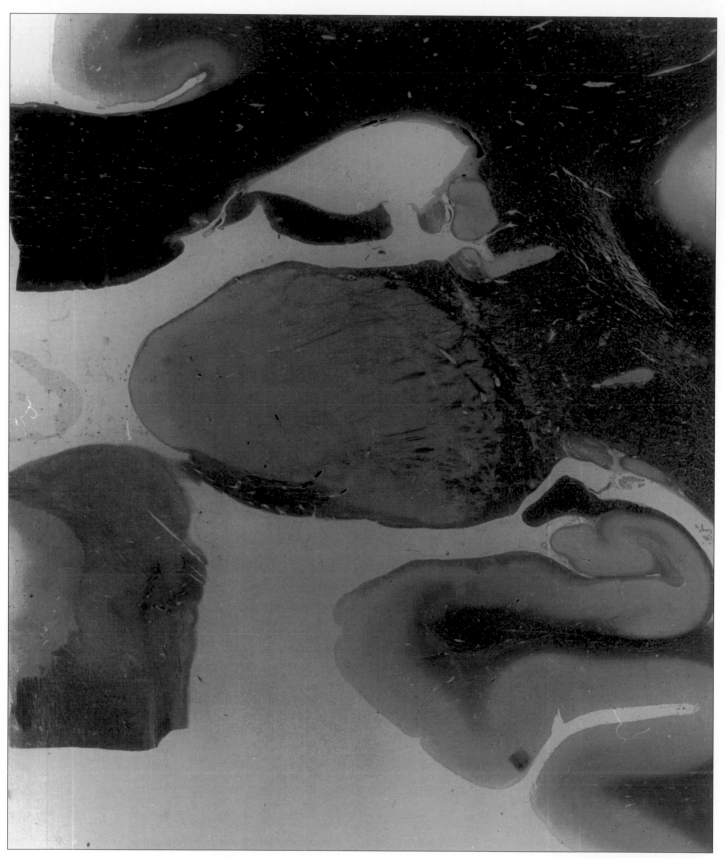

Aq   cerebral aqueduct (Sylvius)
bic   brachium of the inferior colliculus
bsc   brachium of the superior
       colliculus
CA1   CA1 field of the hippocampus
CA2   CA2 field of the hippocampus
CA3   CA3 field of the hippocampus
Cd   caudate nucleus
CG   cingulate gyrus
cg   cingulum
cos   collateral sulcus

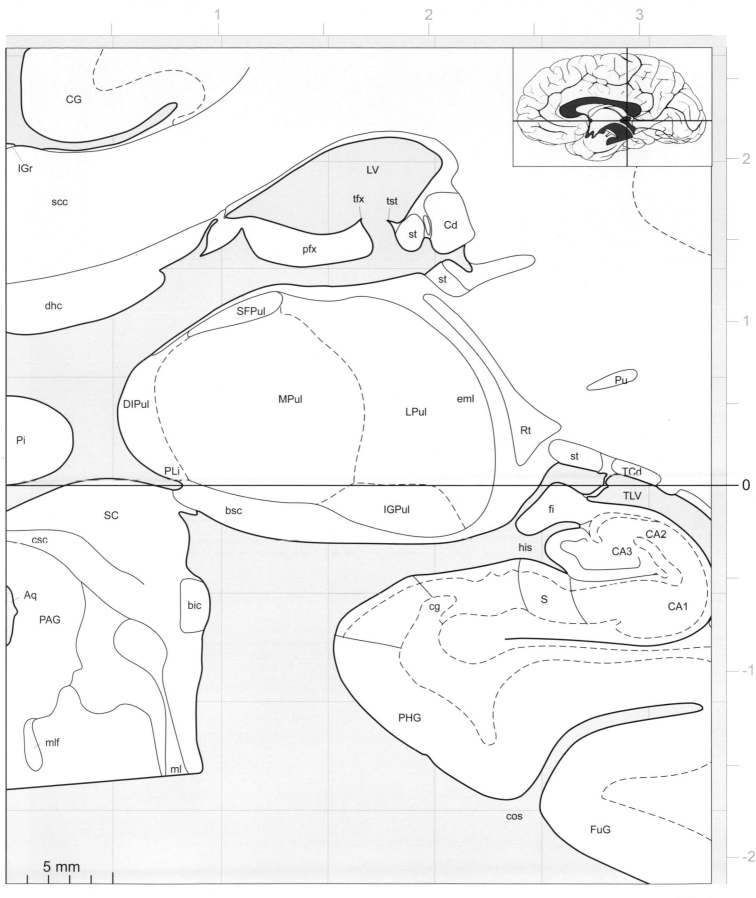

csc	commissure of the superior colliculi	LV	lateral ventricle	S	subiculum	
dhc	dorsal hippocampal commissure	ml	medial lemniscus	SC	superior colliculus	
DiPul	diffuse pulvinar nucleus	mlf	medial longitudinal fasciculus	scc	splenium of the corpus callosum	
eml	external medullary lamina of thalamus	MPul	medial pulvinar nucleus	SFPul	superficial pulvinar nucleus	
fi	fimbria of the hippocampus	PAG	periaqueductal gray	st	stria terminalis	
FuG	fusiform gyrus	pfx	posterior column (crus) of fornix	TCd	tail of caudate nucleus	
his	hippocampal sulcus	PHG	parahippocampal gyrus	tfx	tenia of fornix	
IGPul	intergeniculate pulvinar	Pi	pineal gland	TLV	temporal horn of lateral ventricle	
IGr	indusium griseum	PLi	posterior limitans thalamic nucleus	tst	tenia of stria terminalis (of choroid plexus)	
LPul	lateral pulvinar nucleus	Pu	putamen	Rt	reticular thalamic nucleus	

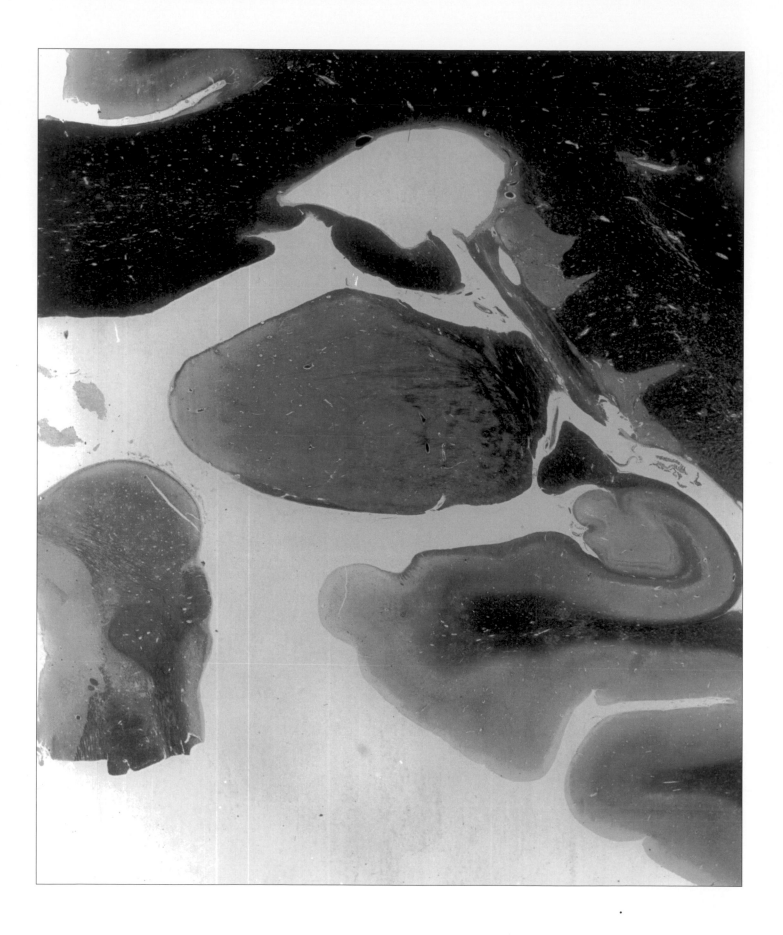

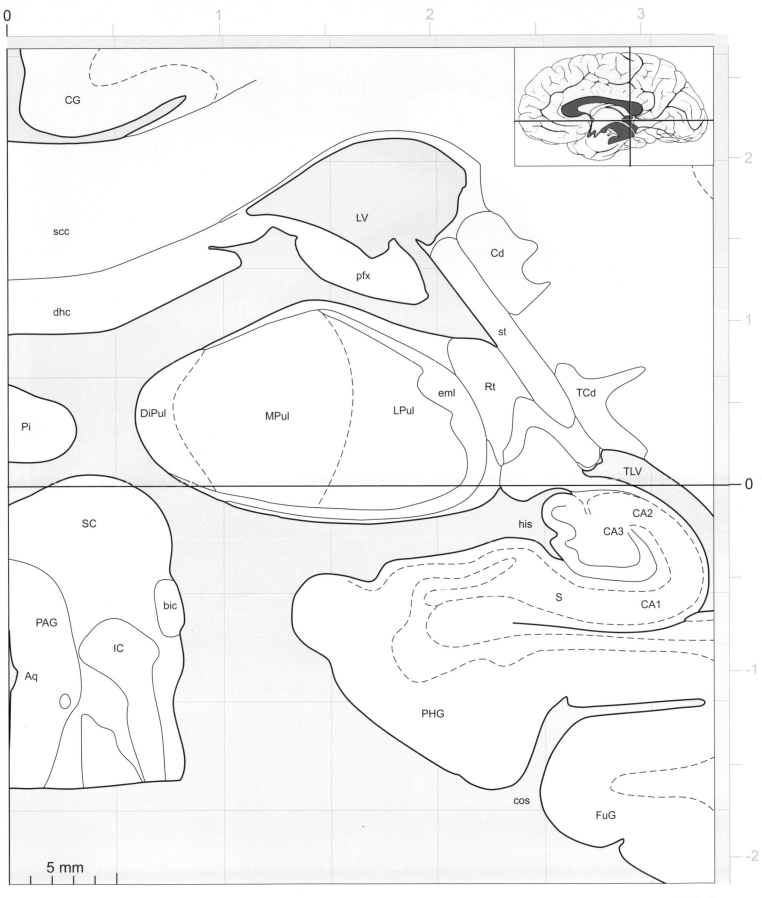

0   1   2   3

CG

scc

dhc

LV

pfx

Cd

st

Pi

DiPul

MPul

LPul

eml

Rt

TCd

TLV

SC

bic

PAG

IC

Aq

his

CA2

CA3

S

CA1

PHG

cos

FuG

5 mm

34,6 mm

cos	collateral sulcus		PAG	perlaqueductal gray
dhc	dorsal hippocampal commissure		pfx	posterior column (crus) of fornix
DiPul	diffuse pulvinar nucleus		PHG	parahippocampal gyrus
eml	external medullary lamina of thalamus		Pi	pineal gland
Aq	cerebral aqueduct (Sylvius)	FuG	fusiform gyrus	Rt	reticular thalamic nucleus
bic	brachium of the inferior colliculus	his	hippocampal sulcus	S	subiculum
CA1	CA1 field of the hippocampus	IC	nucleus of inferior colliculus	SC	superior colliculus
CA2	CA2 field of the hippocampus	LPul	lateral pulvinar nucleus	scc	splenium of the corpus callosum
CA3	CA3 field of the hippocampus	LV	lateral ventricle	st	stria terminalis
Cd	caudate nucleus	MPul	medial pulvinar nucleus	TCd	tail of caudate nucleus
CG	cingulate gyrus			TLV	temporal horn of lateral ventricle

48

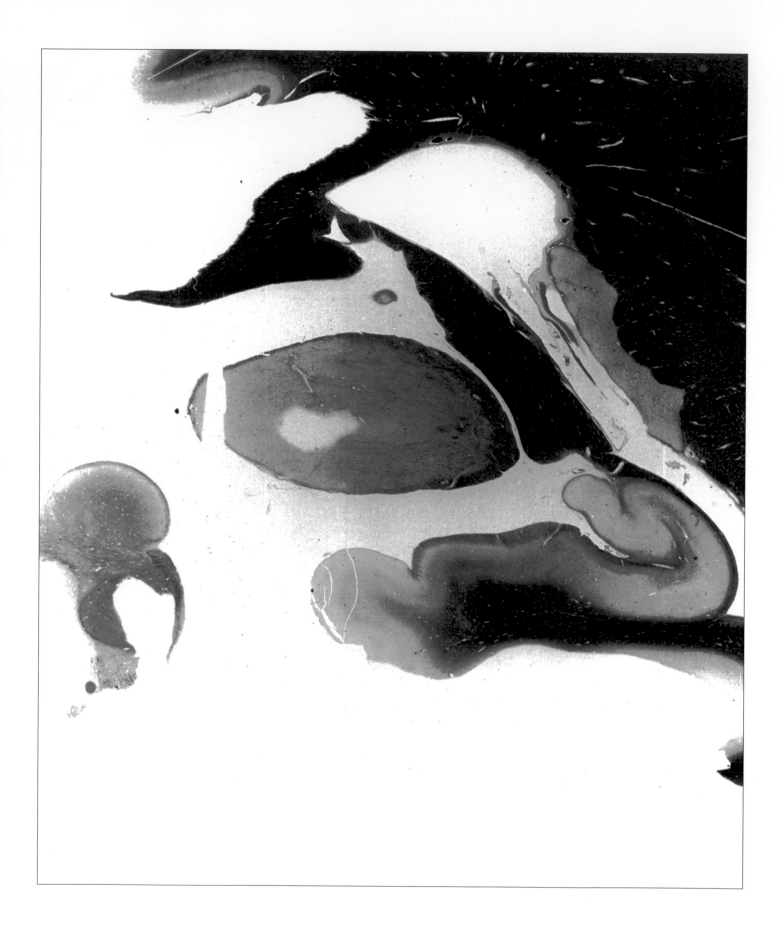

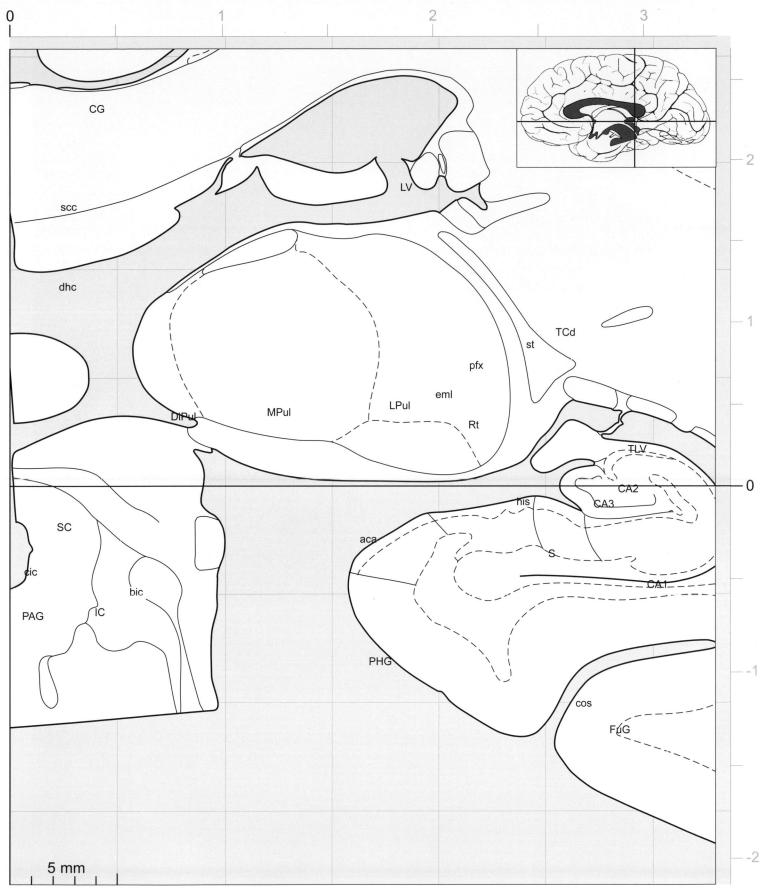

5 mm

36,0 mm

aca	anterior calcarine sulcus
bic	brachium of the inferior colliculus
CA1	CA1 field of the hippocampus
CA2	CA2 field of the hippocampus
CA3	CA3 field of the hippocampus
CG	cingulate gyrus
cic	commissure of the inferior colliculi
cos	collateral sulcus
dhc	dorsal hippocampal commissure
DiPul	diffuse pulvinar nucleus
eml	external medullary lamina of thalamus
FuG	fusiform gyrus
his	hippocampal sulcus
IC	inferior colliculus
LPul	lateral pulvinar nucleus
LV	lateral ventricle
MPul	medial pulvinar nucleus
PAG	periaqueductal gray
pfx	posterior column (crus) of fornix
PHG	parahippocampal gyrus
Rt	reticular thalamic nucleus
S	subiculum
SC	superior colliculus
scc	splenium of the corpus callosum
st	stria terminalis
TCd	tail of caudate nucleus
TLV	temporal horn of lateral ventricle

49

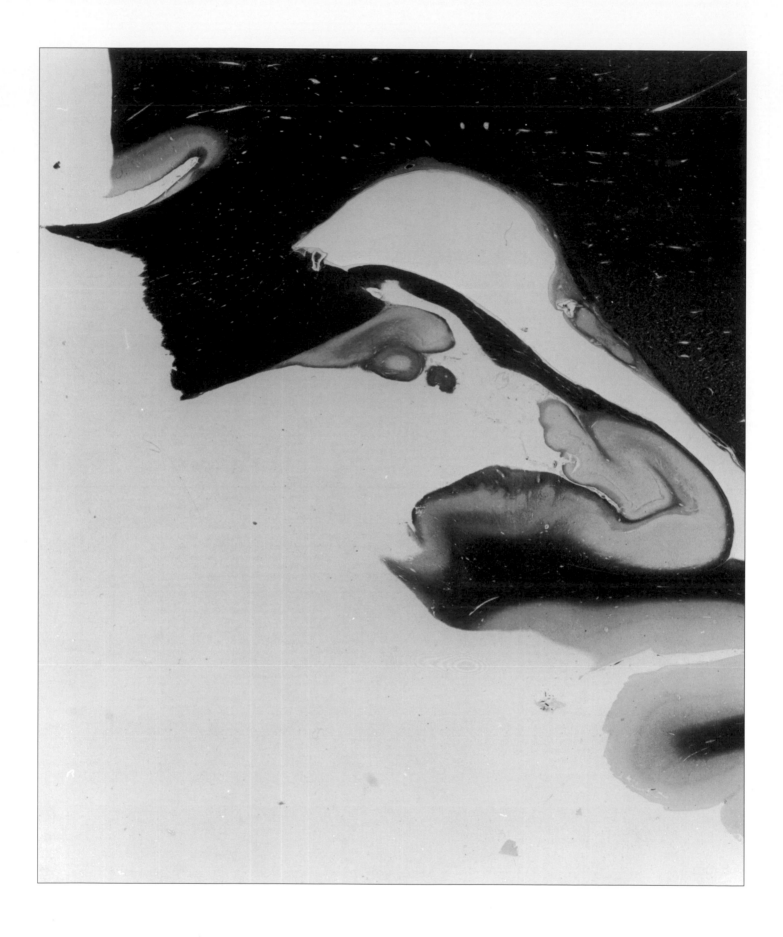

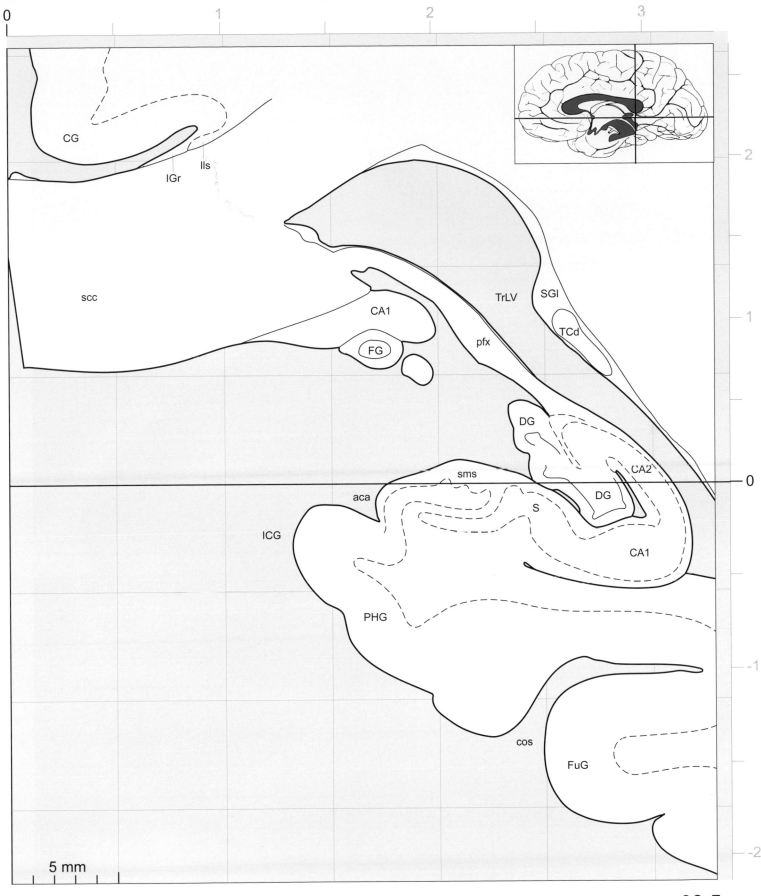

0	... 1 ... 2 ... 3

CG

IGr   Ils

scc

CA1

FG

TrLV   SGl

pfx   TCd

DG

sms   CA2

aca   S   DG

ICG   CA1

PHG

cos

FuG

5 mm

39,5 mm

aca	anterior calcarine sulcus		FuG	fusiform gyrus
CA1	CA1 field of the hippocampus		ICG	isthmus of cingulate gyrus
CA2	CA2 field of the hippocampus		IGr	indusium griseum
CG	cingulate gyrus		pfx	posterior column (crus) of fornix
cos	collateral sulcus		PHG	parahippocampal gyrus
FG	fasciolar gyrus		S	subiculum
			scc	splenium of the corpus callosum
			SGl	substantia gliosa
			sms	superficial medullary stratum
			TCd	tail of caudate nucleus
			TrLV	trigone of lateral ventricle

50

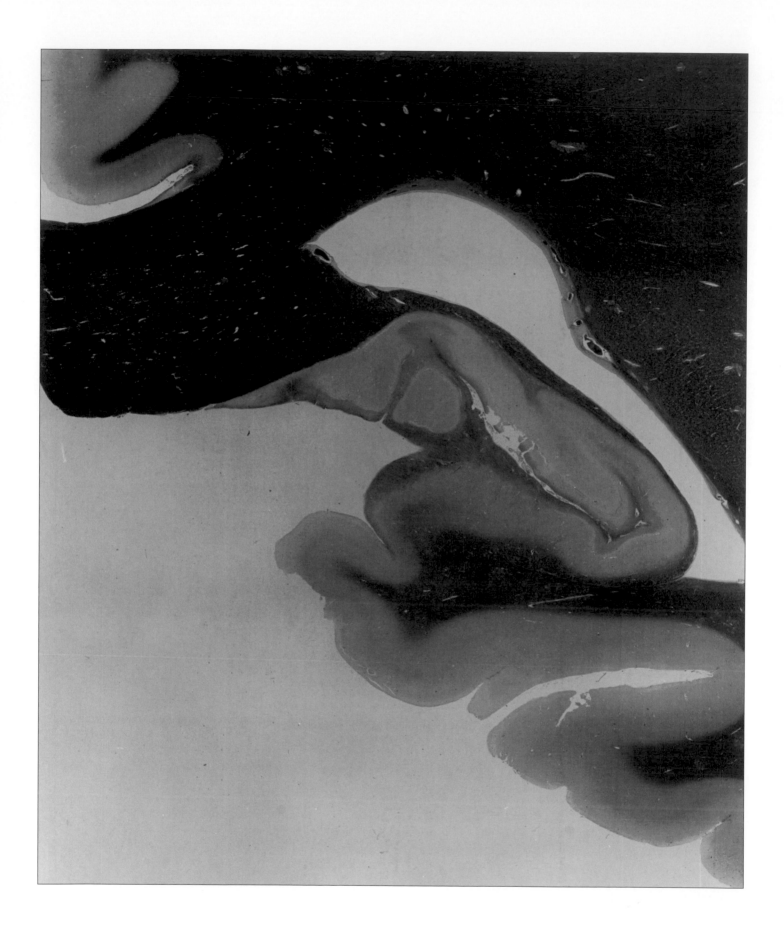

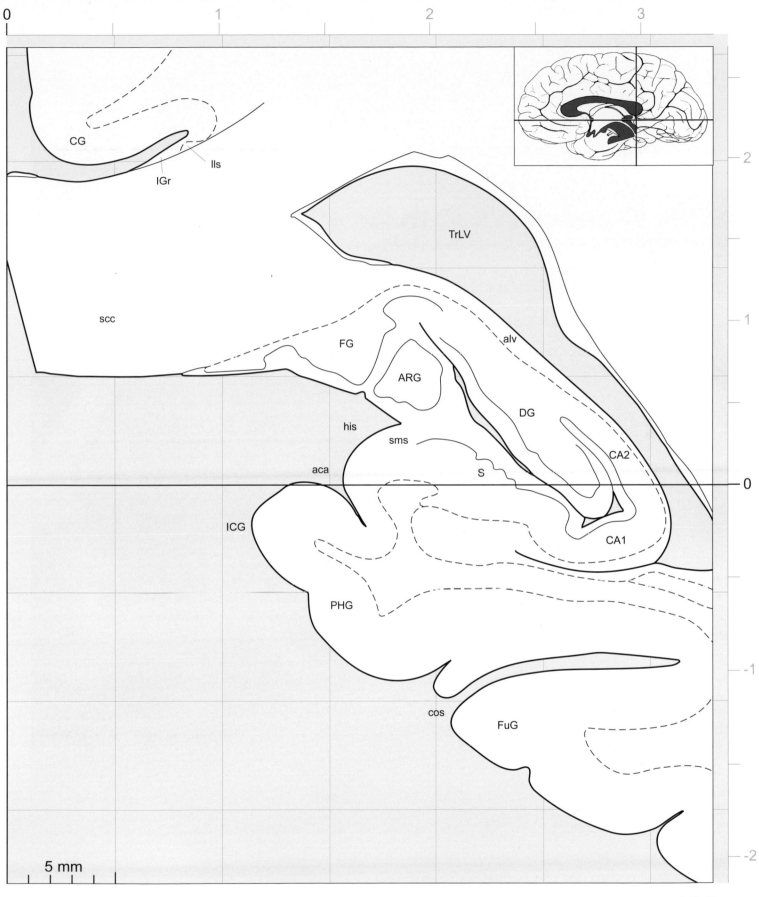

aca	anterior calcarine sulcus	ICG	isthmus of cingulate gyrus
alv	alveus of the hippocampus	IGr	indusium griseum
ARG	Andreas Retzius gyrus	lls	lateral longitudinal stria
CA1	CA1 field of the hippocampus	PHG	parahippocampal gyrus
CA2	CA2 field of the hippocampus	S	subiculum
cfx	crus of the fornix	scc	splenium of the corpus callosum
CG	cingulate gyrus	sms	superficial medullary stratum
cos	collateral sulcus	TrLV	trigone of lateral ventricle
FG	fasciolar gyrus		
FuG	fusiform gyrus		
his	hippocampal sulcus		

40,8 mm

51

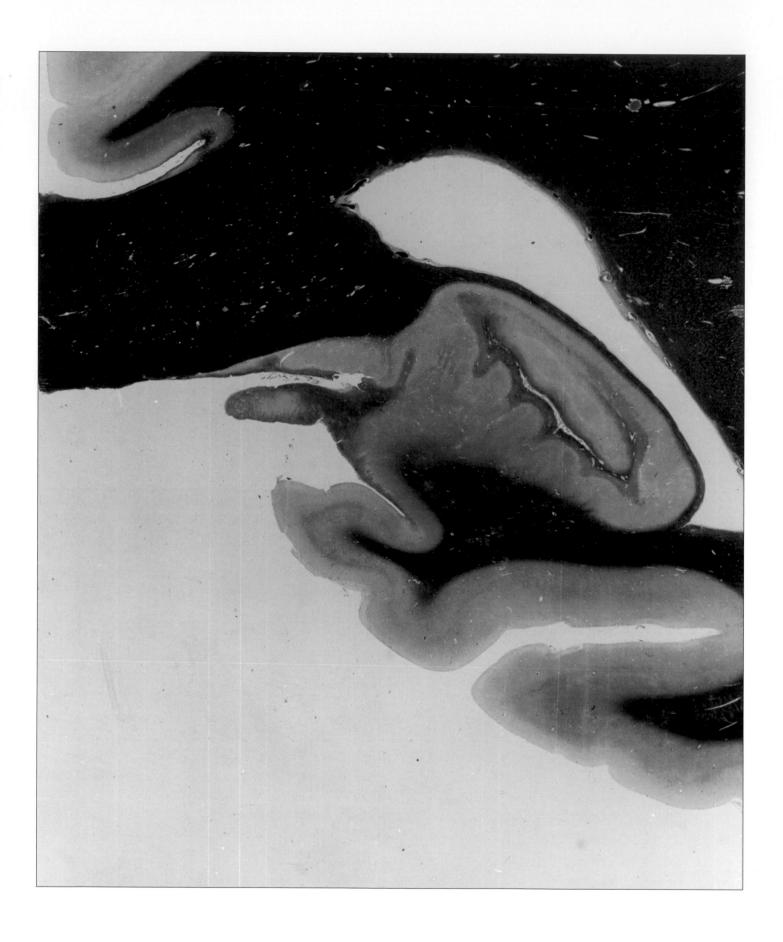

230

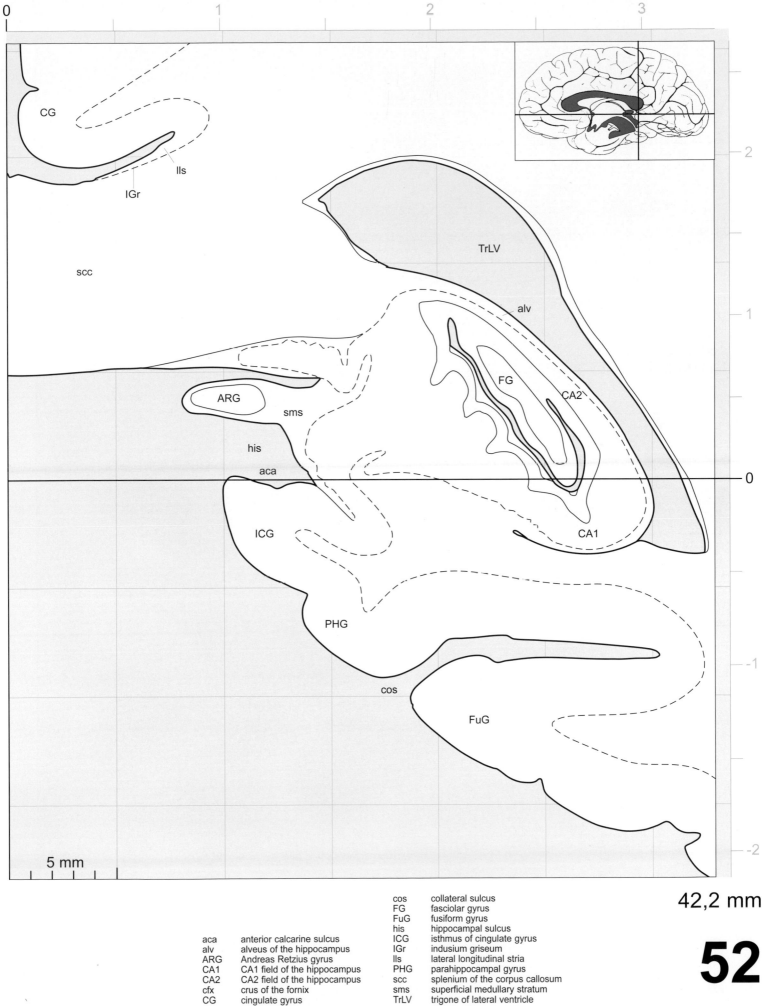

0   1   2   3

CG

lls

IGr

scc

TrLV

alv

FG

CA2

ARG

sms

his

aca

ICG

CA1

PHG

cos

FuG

5 mm

42,2 mm

52

aca	anterior calcarine sulcus
alv	alveus of the hippocampus
ARG	Andreas Retzius gyrus
CA1	CA1 field of the hippocampus
CA2	CA2 field of the hippocampus
cfx	crus of the fornix
CG	cingulate gyrus

cos	collateral sulcus
FG	fasciolar gyrus
FuG	fusiform gyrus
his	hippocampal sulcus
ICG	isthmus of cingulate gyrus
IGr	indusium griseum
lls	lateral longitudinal stria
PHG	parahippocampal gyrus
scc	splenium of the corpus callosum
sms	superficial medullary stratum
TrLV	trigone of lateral ventricle

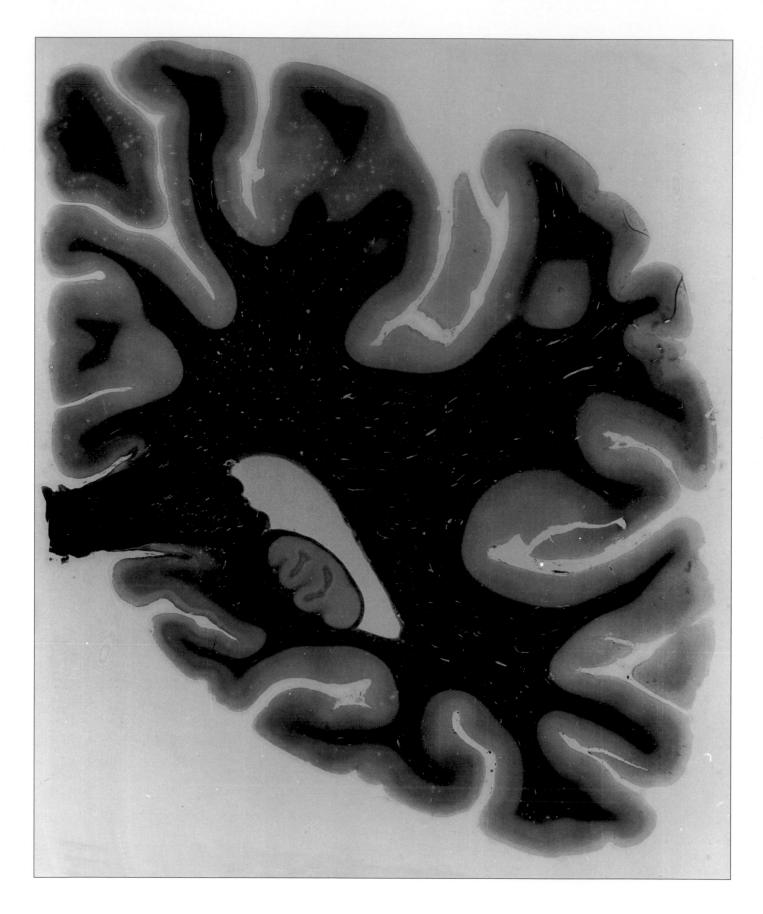

acs   anterior calcarine sulcus
AnG   angular gyrus
cas   callosal sulcus
ccs   calcarine sulcus
CG   cingulate gyrus
FuG   fusiform gyrus
Hi   hippocampus

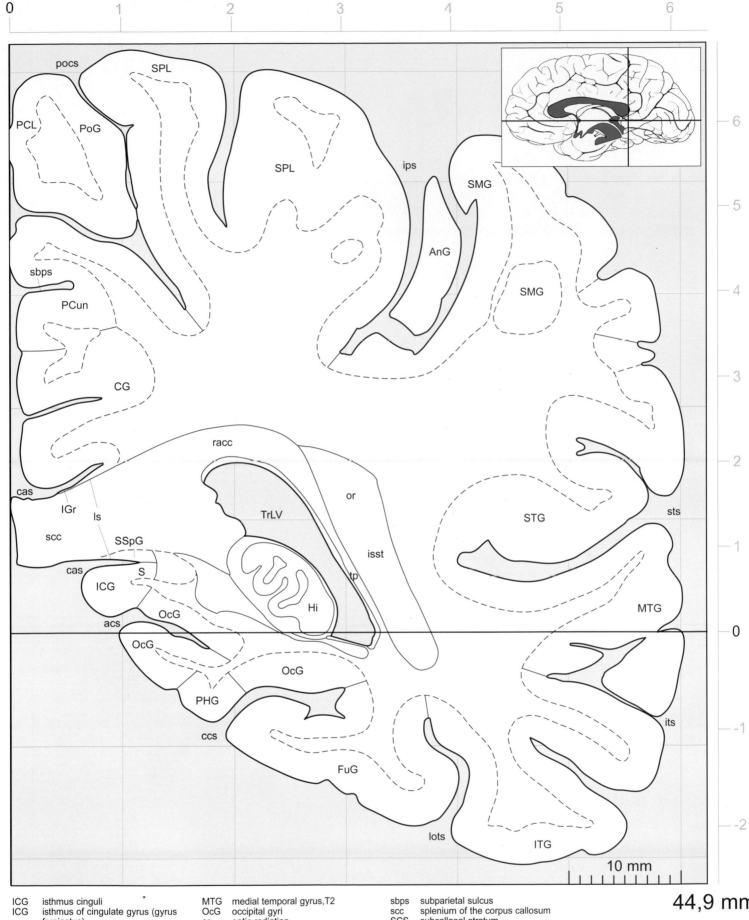

0 1 2 3 4 5 6

SPL
pocs
PCL
PoG
SPL
ips
SMG
sbps
AnG
SMG
PCun
CG
racc
or
cas
sts
IGr
ls
TrLV
STG
scc
SSpG
isst
cas
S
tp
ICG
Hi
acs
OcG
MTG
OcG
OcG
PHG
its
ccs
FuG
lots
ITG

10 mm

44,9 mm

53

ICG	isthmus cinguli	MTG	medial temporal gyrus, T2	sbps	subparietal sulcus
ICG	isthmus of cingulate gyrus (gyrus fornicatus)	OcG	occipital gyri	scc	splenium of the corpus callosum
		or	optic radiation	SCS	subcallosal stratum
IGr	indusium griseum	PCL	paracentral lobule	SMG	supramarginal gyrus
ips	intraparietal sulcus	PCun	precuneus	SPL	superior parietal lobule
isst	internal sagittal stratum	PHG	parahippocampal gyrus	SSpG	subsplenial gyrus
ITG	inferior temporal gyrus, T3	pocs	postcentral sulcus	STG	superior temporal gyrus, T1
its	inferior temporal sulcus	PoG	postcentral gyrus	sts	superior temporal sulcus
lots	lateral occipitotemporal sulcus	racc	radiation of the corpus callosum	tp	tapetum
ls	longitudinal stria	S	subiculum	TrLV	trigone of lateral ventricle

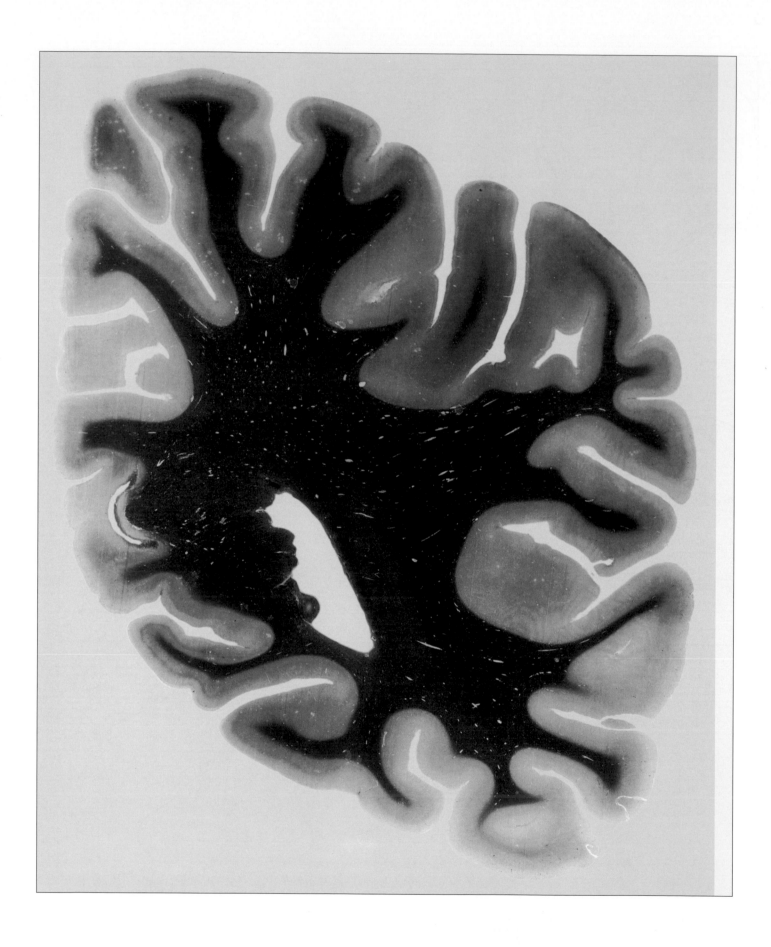

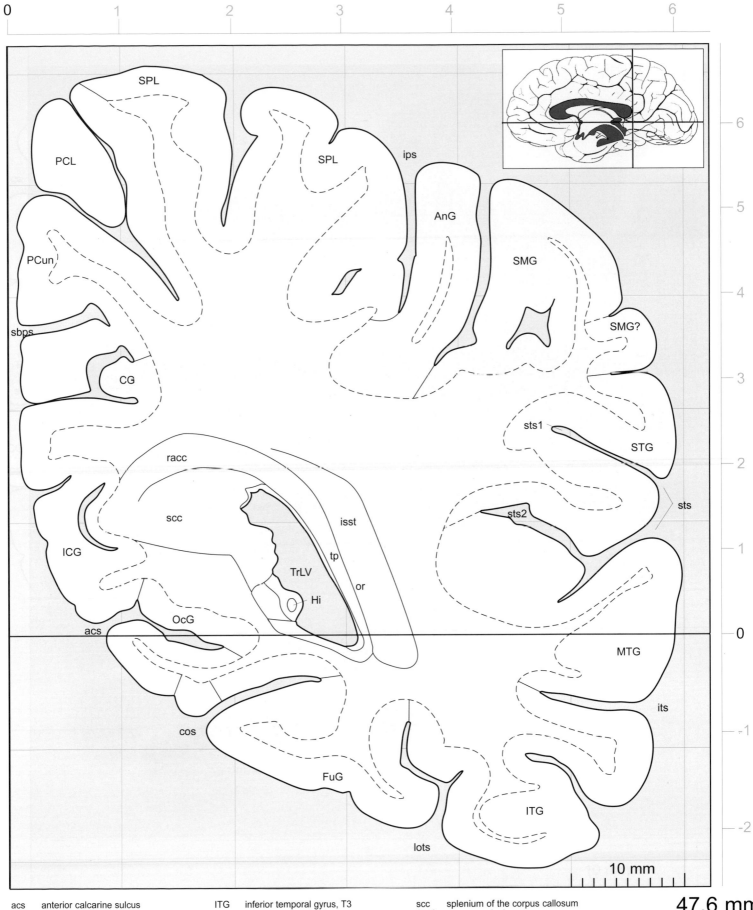

0   1   2   3   4   5   6

10 mm

47,6 mm

54

acs	anterior calcarine sulcus	ITG	inferior temporal gyrus, T3	scc	splenium of the corpus callosum
AnG	angular gyrus	its	inferior temporal sulcus	SMG	supramarginal gyrus
CG	cingulate gyrus	lots	lateral occipitotemporal sulcus	SMG?	part of STG according to Busch, 1960
cos	collateral sulcus	MTG	medial temporal gyrus, T2	SPL	superior parietal lobule
FuG	fusiform gyrus	OcG	occipital gyri	STG	superior temporal gyrus, T1
Hi	hippocampus	or	optic radiation	sts	superior temporal sulcus
ICG	isthmus of cingulate gyrus (gyrus fornicatus)	PCL	paracentral lobule	tp	tapetum
		PCun	precuneus	TrLV	trigone of lateral ventricle
ips	intraparietal sulcus	racc	radiation of the corpus callosum		
isst	internal sagittal stratum	sbps	subparietal sulcus		

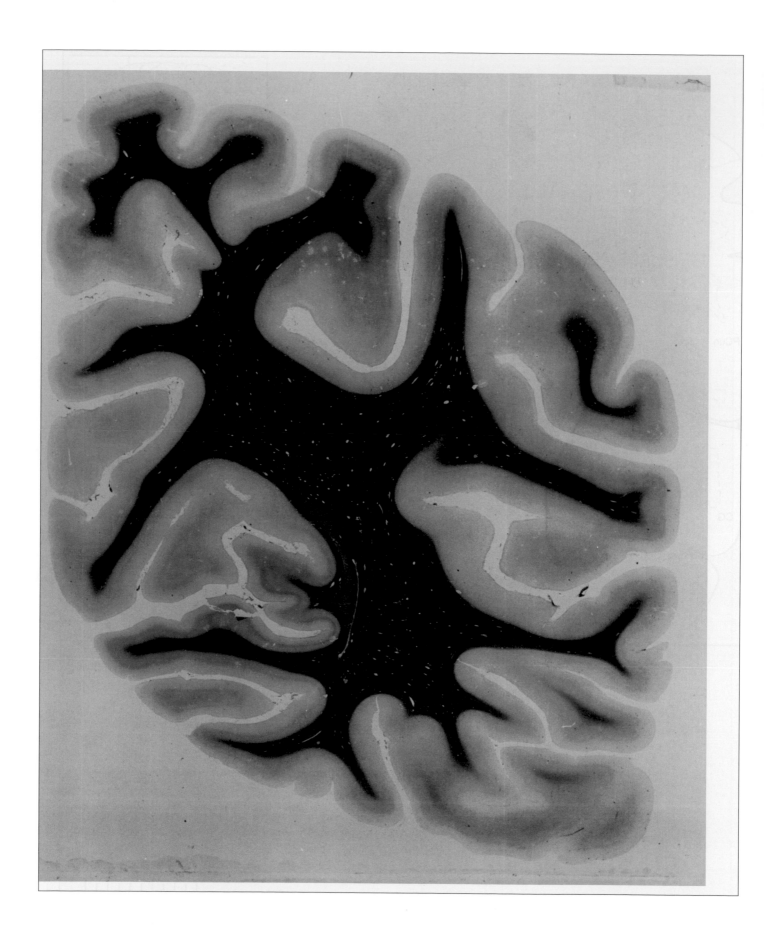

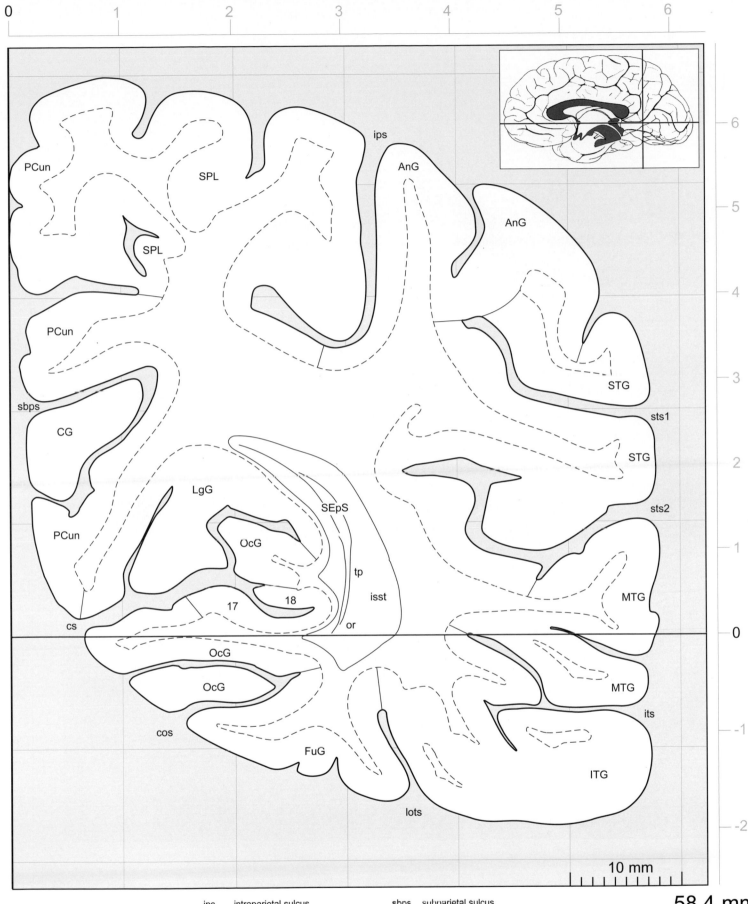

58,4 mm

58

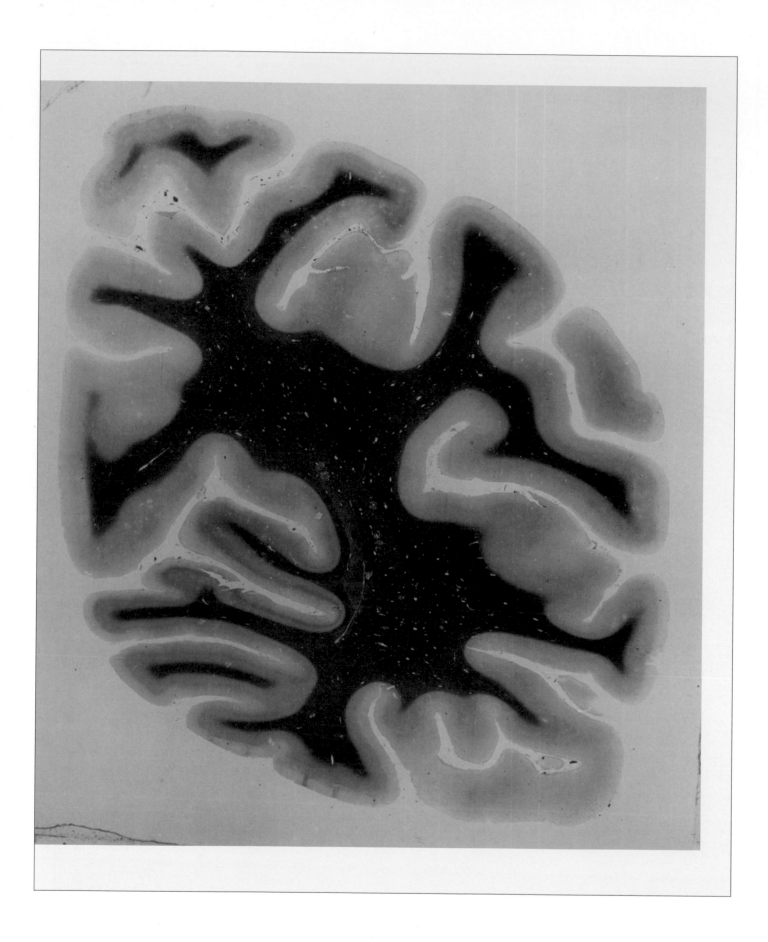

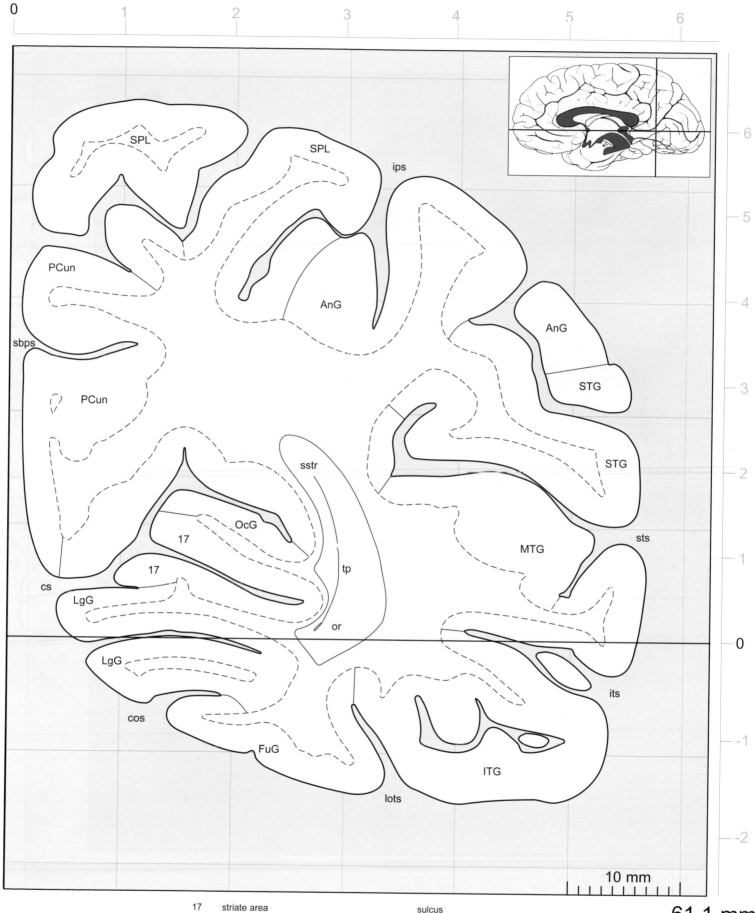

0   1   2   3   4   5   6

10 mm

61,1 mm

17	striate area		sulcus
AnG	angular gyrus	MTG	medial temporal gyrus, T2
cos	collateral sulcus	OcG	occipital gyri
cs	calcarine sulcus	or	optic radiation
FuG	fusiform gyrus	PCun	precuneus
ips	intraparietal sulcus	sbps	subparietal sulcus
ITG	inferior temporal gyrus, T3	sstr	sagittal stratum
its	inferior temporal sulcus	STG	superior temporal gyrus,T1
LgG	lingual gyrus (O5)	sts	superior temporal sulcus
lots	lateral occipitotemporal	tp	tapetum

59

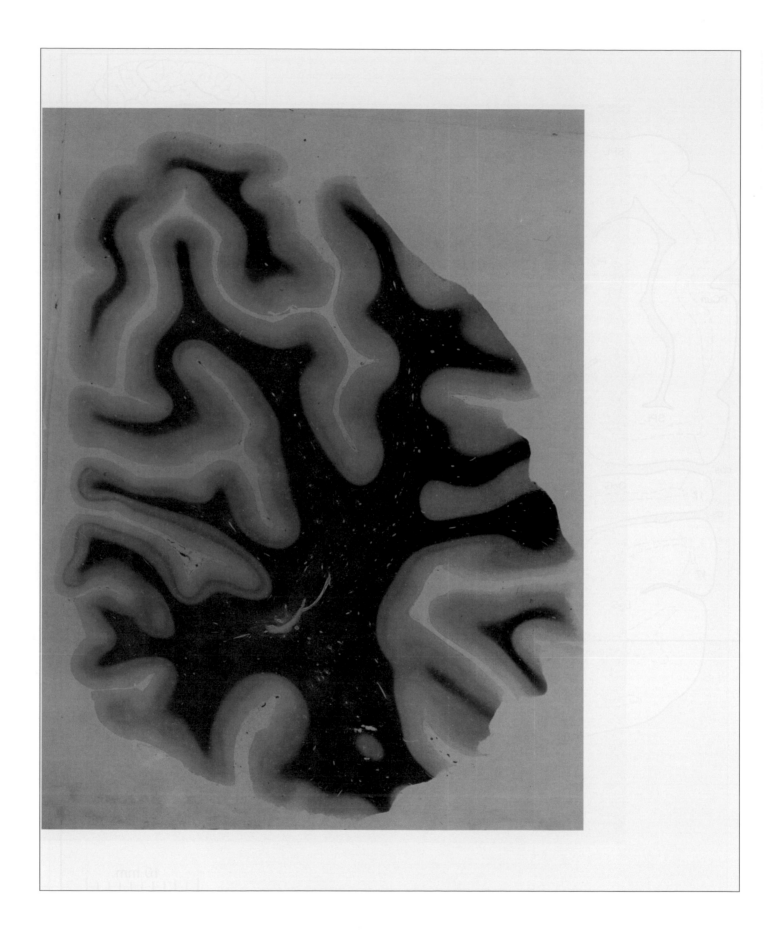

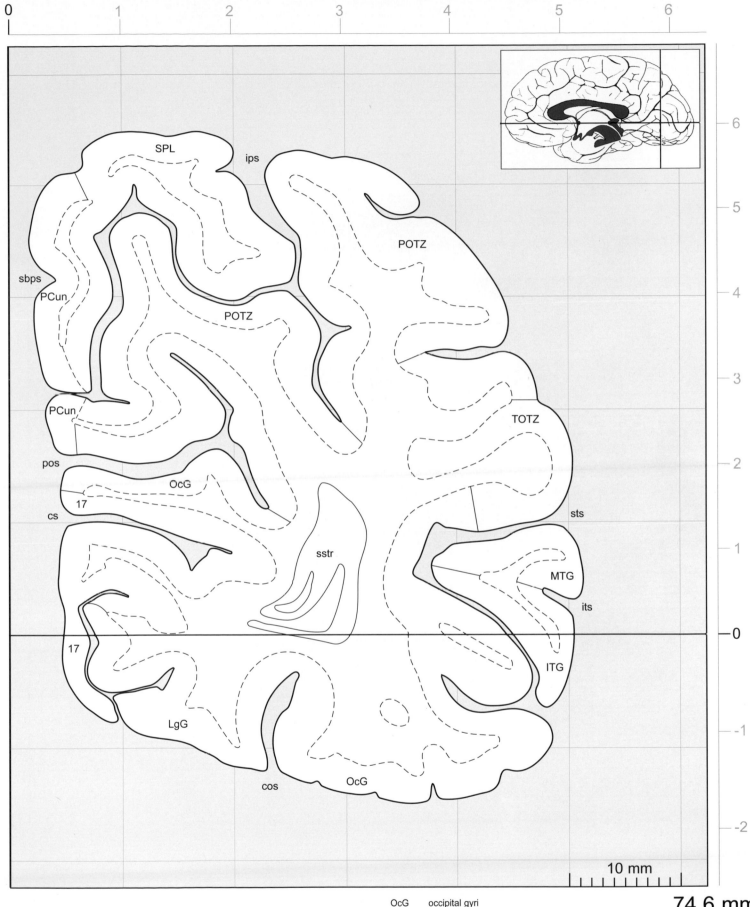

17	striate area
cos	collateral sulcus
cs	calcarine sulcus
ips	intraparietal sulcus
ITG	inferior temporal gyrus, T3
its	inferior temporal sulcus
LgG	lingual gyrus (O5)
MTG	medial temporal gyrus,T2

OcG	occipital gyri
PCun	precuneus
pos	parietooccipital sulcus
POTZ	parietooccipital transition zone
sbps	subparietal sulcus
SPL	superior parietal lobule
sstr	sagittal stratum
STG	superior temporal gyrus,T1
sts	superior temporal sulcus
TOTZ	temporooccipital transition zone

74,6 mm

64

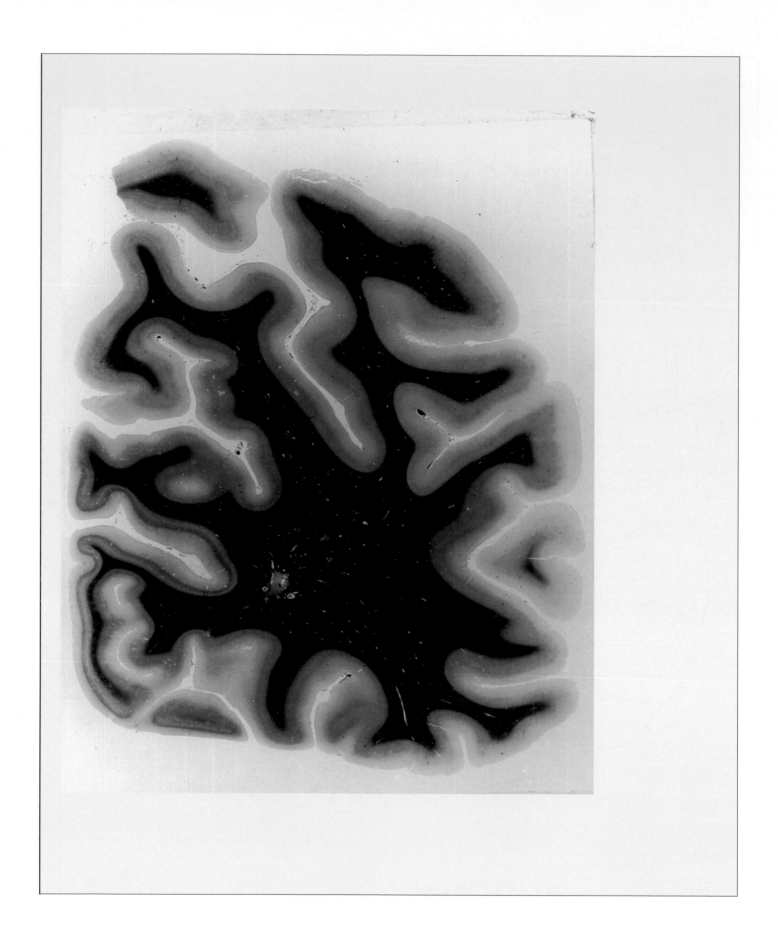

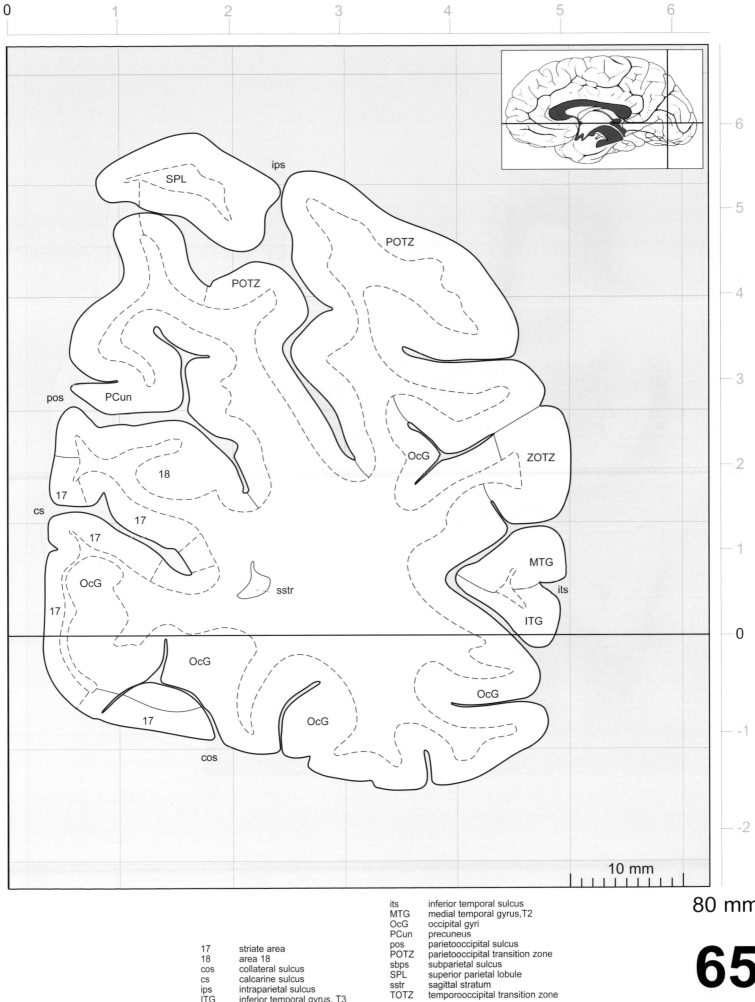

0	
1	
2	
3	
4	
5	
6	

SPL   ips

POTZ

POTZ

pos   PCun

18

17

cs

17

17

OcG

17

OcG

17

cos

POTZ

OcG   ZOTZ

sstr

MTG

ils

ITG

OcG

OcG

10 mm

80 mm

65

		its	inferior temporal sulcus
		MTG	medial temporal gyrus, T2
		OcG	occipital gyri
		PCun	precuneus
17	striate area	pos	parietooccipital sulcus
18	area 18	POTZ	parietooccipital transition zone
cos	collateral sulcus	sbps	subparietal sulcus
cs	calcarine sulcus	SPL	superior parietal lobule
ips	intraparietal sulcus	sstr	sagittal stratum
ITG	inferior temporal gyrus, T3	TOTZ	temporooccipital transition zone

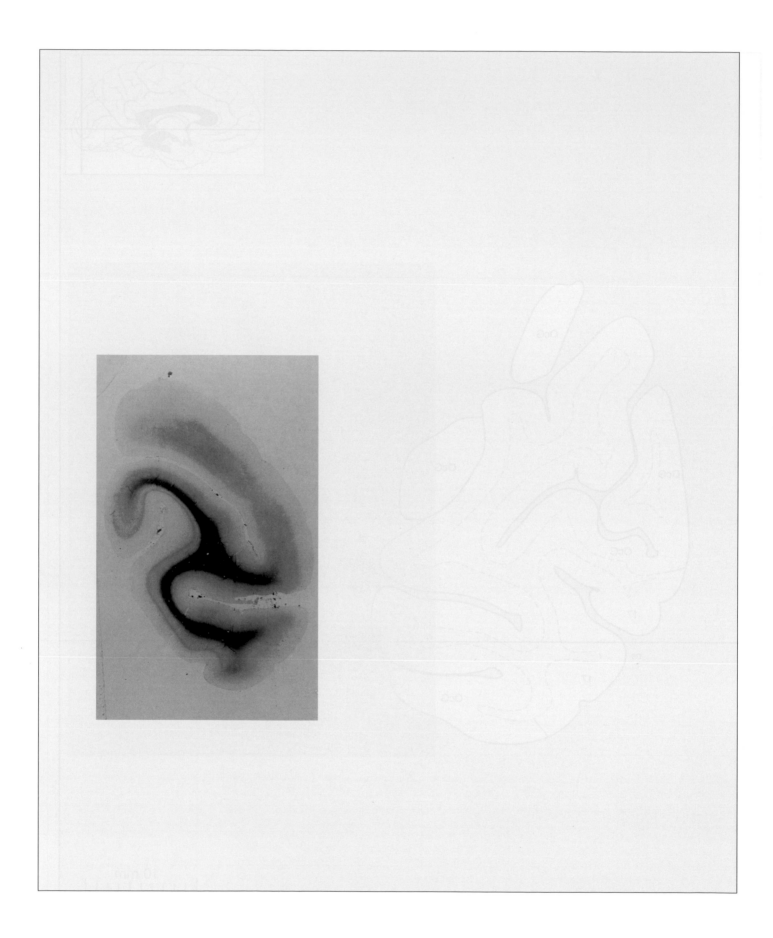

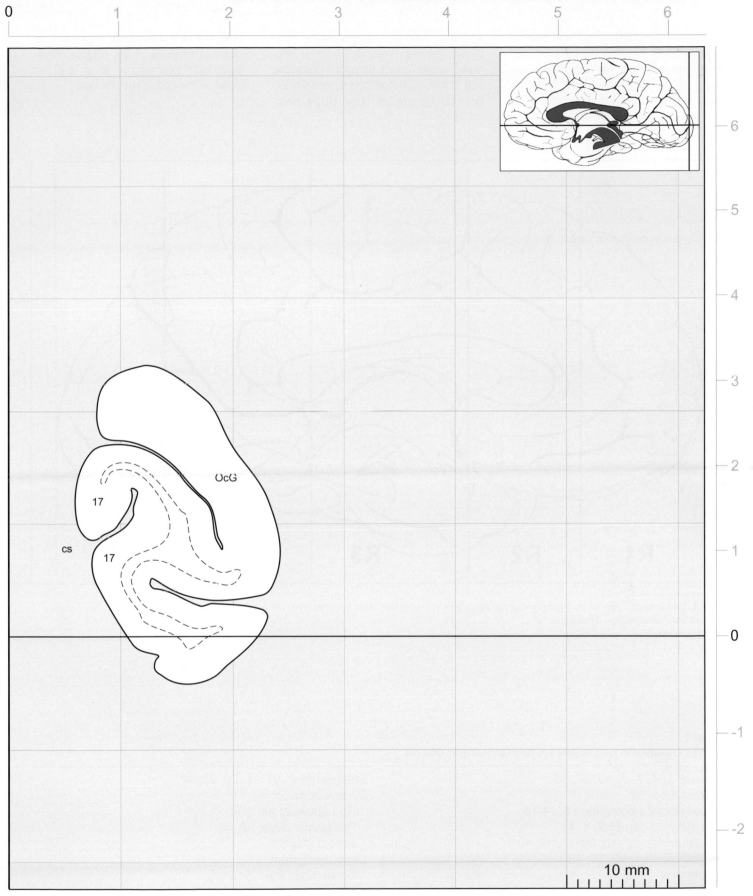

| 0 | 1 | 2 | 3 | 4 | 5 | 6 |

OcG

17

cs

17

6

5

4

3

2

1

0

-1

-2

10 mm

100 mm

69

17	striate area
cs	calcarine sulcus
OcG	occipital gyri

4.4 Past Histological, Morphometric, and Histochemical Studies of the Brain

Numerous descriptive and quantitative studies have been performed on the brain presented in the myeloarchitectonic atlas. Regions where analyses were perfomed are listed in Table 1. In addition, relevant morphometric data (fresh volume, volume of serial sections, numeric cell density, volumetric cell density, absolute cell numbers, etc.) have been compiled. If not stated otherwise, the designations of structures are identical to those of the original work. References pertinent to these data are found at the end of this section.

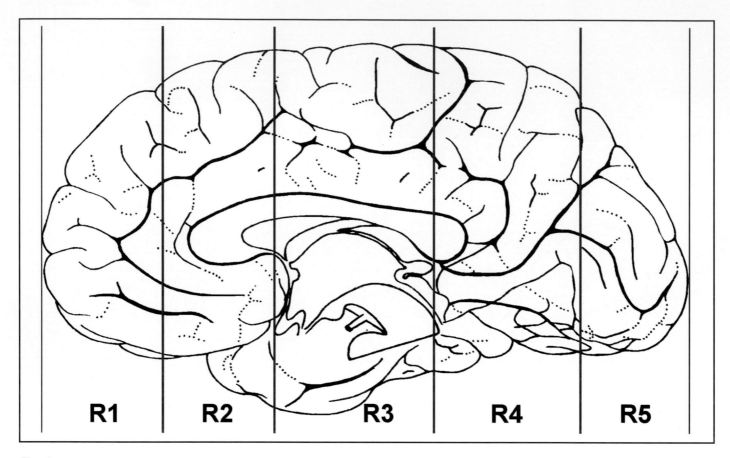

Fig. 1 Mediansagittal view of the brain (right hemisphere) from which all data listed below derived. The baseline shows the position where this hemisphere was cut into blocks before embedding.

Table 1
Previous Evaluations of Brain Regions and Their Corresponding Citations

Cortex: 1, 4, 7, 9, 13, 27, 43
Septal area: 12
Basal nuclear complex: 11, 14-16
Amygdaloid complex: 8, 41
Striatum: 12, 17, 18, 28-32, 36, 40
Hypothalamus: 10, 14, 48
Thalamus
  anterior ncl.: 19, 20
  mediodorsal ncl.: 2, 37
  mediolateral ncl.: 2, 3, 18, 25

Subthalamus: 10, 21, 26, 28-32
Mesencephalon:
  Red nucleus: 24, 39
  Substantia nigra: 22, 45
  Area 9, 10: 6
Lower brainstem: 51
  Locus coeruleus: 5
  Superior olive: 51
Cell studies: 23, 26, 42, 46
Neuroactive substances: 33-35, 38, 49, 50

[a]It is not specified on which hemispheres the evaluations were made. (See list of references at the end of this section.)

Morphometric Data

Weight, volume and linear dimensions	R	L
Brain weight (in formalin)	1383	
Fresh volume (cm^3)	1316	
Length (L)*	171	170
Width (W)*	71	71
Height (H)*	97	96
Length +	120	122
Width +	63	64
Height +	82	82

R: right hemisphere, L: left hemisphere

Shrinkage factors (SF)	R	L
SFw Lange, Thörner (1974)	2.13	2.22
SFl Lange, Thörner (1974)	1.89	1.81
SFl Sievert (1992)	1.74	1.82

Shrinkage factors (SF) describing the loss of volume from the fixed autopsy brains to the histological material. SFl : Linear calculated volume shrinkage factor = [L * W * H (autopsy brain in formaline)] / [L * W * H (serial paraffin sections)], where L = length of hemisphere; W = width of hemisphere; H = height of hemisphere). SFw : Weight related shrinkage factor (SFg) = [(Bw * 0,88 / 1,0365) / serial section volume of hemisphere], where Bw = brain weight, Factor 0,88 = [weight of hemisphere] / [brain weight], Factor 1.0365 = mean specific brain weight.

PROSENCEPHALON [1,27,28]	R	L
Fresh volume (cm^3)	549	527
Volume of serial sections (cm^3)	267	262

CORTEX [1,27,28]	R	L
Fresh volume (cm^3)	297	303
Volume of serial sections (cm^3)	144	139

CORTEX (fresh volume of cortical regions, (cm^3) [1]	R	L
socortex (ICx)	261	277
ICx.frontalis (ICx.f.)	101	103
ICx.f.convexitatis	63	64
ICx.f.medialis	22	22
ICx.f.opercularis dorsalis	3.6	3.2
ICx.f. opercularis basalis	0.8	1.2
ICx.f. basalis	11	12
Area (A.) gigantocellularis (gc)	5.1	5.5
A.gc. convexitatis	3.8	4.0
A.gc. medialis	1.3	1.5
ICx.parietalis (ICx.pa)	44	42
ICx.pa. convexitatis	24	22
ICx.pa. medialis	16	15
ICx.pa.opercularis	4.9	5.1
R.postcentralis.	13	15
R.p. convexitatis	11	12
R.p. medialis	2.1	2.5
ICx.temporalis (ICx.t)	41	49
ICx.t.dorsalis	7.7	7.8
R.temporalis transversalis (R.tv)	2.6	2.2
R.tv.1	1.9	1.6
R.tv.2	0.7	0.6
Parieto-temporal convexity	38	38
ICx. occipitalis	37	43
A18 + A19	30	35
A17	7.6	7.9
Allocortex (with Proisocortex): Claustro-Cx. temporalis	1.2	0.7
Claustro-Cx. insularis	7.4	7.3
Tbc. olfactorium, R. praepiri-formis frontalis, Peri-Palaeo-Cx. frontalis	0.9	0.5
Paleo-Cx. temporalis	0.5	0.4
Archi-Cx. frontalis	7.3	7.0
Archi-Cx.parietalis	5.6	4.4
Archi-Cx.temporalis	7.3	6.2

STRIATUM [1,27,28]	R	L
Volume of serial sections (10 mm^3)		
Caudate nucleus	298	269
Putamen	360	343
Numeric cell density (number / mm^3)		
Small neurons (x10)	2029	2248
Large neurons	156	156
Glial cells (x10)	7360	7835
Volumetric neuronal density (10^{-2} %)	454	393
Nuclear diameter (small neurons, 10^{-2} μm)	859	891

CAUDATE NUCLEUS [17,18]

Numeric cell density (number/mm^3)

Macroneurons (L)	270
Microneurons (S)	22,663
L/S	1/83
Average diameter in µm	10.78

PUTAMEN [17,18]

Numeric cell density (number/mm^3)

Macroneurons (L)	163
Microneurons (S)	19,953
L/S	1/119
Average diameter in µm	9.47

GLOBUS PALLIDUS [27]

		R	L
Volume of serial sections (mm^3)			
External globus pallidus	EGP	656	560
Internal globus pallidus	IGP	289	238
Numeric cell density (number/mm^3)			
Neurons	EGP	763	994
	IGP	625	588
Glial cells (*10^3)	EGP	124	132
	IGP	118	120
Volumetric cell density (10^{-3} %)			
Neurons	EGP	290	380
	IGP	210	270
Glial cells	EGP	450	620
	IGP	510	580

SUBTHALAMIC NUCLEUS [21]

		R	L
Fresh volume (cm^3)		0.139	0.119
Volumes of serial sections (mm^3)^a			
Subthalamic ncl., med. part	SThM	31.7	31.2
	SThL	35.7	26.6
	total	67.4	57.9
Numeric cell density (number / mm^3)			
Neurons (*10)	SThL	375	357
	SThM	591	516
Volumetric cell density			
Neurons (10-2%)	SThL	142	199
	SThM	162	223
Volumetric cell density (%)			
Neurons:	SThL	2.48	
	SThM	1.87	
Glia	SThL	0.99	
	SThM	0.923	
Numeric cell density (number / mm^3)			
	SThL	7,417	
	SThM	8,046	
Absolute cell numbers			
		232	700
		287	600

^{a} Without shrinkage factor correction.

THALAMUS [17,18]

Numeric cell density (number / mm^3)

Small neurons	anterior thalamus	3,522
	medial thalamus	4,544
	lateral thalamus	1,012
	posterior thalamus	4,686
Large neurons	anterior thalamus	6,177
	medial thalamus	5,538
	lateral thalamus	3,248
	posterior thalamus	7,618

RED NUCLEUS [24, 39]

		R	L
Volume of serial sections (mm^3)			
Dorsomedial quadrant	r1		26.6
Dorsolateral quadrant	r2		35.9
ventrolateral quadrant	r3		35.8
ventromedial quadrant	r4		35.2
Numeric cell density (number / mm^3)			
Neurons	r1	171	172
	r2	124	95
	r3	104	103
	r4	104	104
Glial cells	r1	446	421
	r2	384	336
	r3	320	402
	r4	309	308
Volumetric density (%)			
Neurons	r1	57	51
	r2	28	24
	r3	25	27
	r4	21	23
Glial cells	r1	78	69
	r2	74	58
	r3	74	60
	r4	72	56

References:

1. Albring, K.M. (1983). *Quantitative Untersuchungen an 33 Rindenregionen des menschlichen Gehirns*. Thesis, Düsseldorf.
2. Bäumer, H. (1952). Untersuchungen am Ncl. medialis und lateralis thalami bei Schizophrenie. *Proc. Ist Intl. Congr. Neuropathol. Rom*. Rosenberg & Sellier, Torino. Vol. 3, pp. 636-647.
3. Bäumer, H. (1954). Veränderungen des Thalamus bei Schizophrenie. *J. Hirnforsch*. 1, 156-172.
4. Beheim-Schwarzbach, D. (1952). Anatomische Veränderungen im Schläfenlappen bei "funktionellen" Psychosen. *Proc. Ist. Intl. Congr. 6. Neuropathol. Rom*. Rosenberg & Sellier, Torino. Vol. 3, pp. 609-620.
5. Beheim-Schwarzbach, D. (1955). Lebensgeschichte der melaninhaltigen Nervenzellen des Ncl. coeruleus unter normalen und pathogenen Bedingungen. *J. Hirnforsch*. 2, 62-95.
6. Bogerts, B., Häntsch, J., & Herzer, M. (1982). *A morphometric study of the dopamine-containing cell groups in the mesencephalon of normals, Parkinson patients and schizophrenics*. Thesis, Düsseldorf.
7. Braitenberg, G. V. (1952). Ricerche istopatologiche sulla corteccia frontale di schizofrenici. *Proc. Ist. Intl. Cong. Neuropathol. Rom*. Rosenberg & Sellier, Torino. Vol. 3, pp. 621-626.
8. Brockhaus, H. (1938). Zur normalen und pathologischen Anatomie des Mandelkerngebietes. *J. Psychol. Neurol*. 49, 1-136.
9. Brockhaus, H. (1940). Die Cyto- und Myeloarchitektonik des Cortex claustralis und des Claustrum beim Menschen. *J. Psychol. Neurol*. 49, 249-348.
10. Brockhaus, H. (1942). Beitrag zur normalen Anatomie des Hypothalamus und der Zona incerta beim Menschen. *J. Psychol. Neurol*. 51, 96-195.
11. Brockhaus, H. (1942). Vergleichend-anatomische Untersuchungen über den Basalkernkomplex. *J. Psychol. Neurol*. 51, 57-95.
12. Brockhaus, H. (1942). Zur feinen Anatomie des Septum und des Striatum. *J. Psychol. Neurol*. 51, 1-56. *Translated in:* "Human Brain Dissection, (Pope, A., ed.). U.S. Government Printing Office Publ. 381-132: 3096. (1983).
13. Busch, K.-T. (1960). Individuelle architektonische Differenzen der Area striata. *J. Hirnforsch*. 4, 535-552.
14. Buttlar-Brentano, K.v. (1954). Zur Lebensgeschichte des Ncl. basalis, tuberomammillaris, supraopticus und para ventricularis unter normalen und pathogenen Bedingungen. *J. Hirnforsch*. 1, 337-419.
15. Buttlar-Brentano, K.v. (1955). Das Parkinsonsyndrom im Lichte der lebensgeschichtlichen Veränderungen des Nucleus basalis. *J. Hirnforsch*. 2, 55-76.
16. Buttlar-Brentano, K.v. (1956) Zur weiteren Kenntnis der Veränderung des Basalkerns bei Schizophrenen. *J. Hirnforsch*. 2, 271-291.
17. Dom, R., De Saedeleer, J., Bogerts, B., & Hopf, A. (1981). Quantitative cytometric analysis of basal ganglia in catatonic schizophrenics. *In:* "Biological Psychiatry," (Perris, C, Struwe, G & Jansson B. eds.), Elsevier, North-Holland, pp. 723-726.
18. Dom, R. (1976). *Neostriatal and Thalamic Interneurons. Their role in the pathophys-iology of Huntington's chorea, Parkinson's disease, and catatonic schizophrenia*. Thesis, Leuven.
19. Fünfgeld, E.W. (1952). Pathologisch-anatomische Untersuchungen im Nucleus anterior thalami bei Schizophrenie. *Proc. Ist. Intl. Cong. Neuropathol. Rom*. Rosenberg & Sellier, Torino. Vol. 3, pp. 648-659.
20. Fünfgeld, E.W. (1954). Der Nucleus anterior thalami bei Schizophrenie. *J. Hirnforsch*. 1, 146-155.
21. Füssenich, M.S.U. (1967). *Vergleichend anatomische Studien über den Nucleus subthalamicus (Corpus Luysi) bei Primaten*. Thesis, Freiburg.
22. Hassler (1937). Zur Normalanatomie der Substantia nigra. Versuch einer architektonischen Gliederung. *J. Psychol. Neurol*. 48, 1-55.
23. Hempel, K.-J., & Treff, W.M. (1959). Die Gliazelldichte bei klinisch Gesunden und Schizophrenen. *J. Hirnforsch*. 4, 371-411.
24. Herbel, W. (1979). *Zur Neuroanatomie und Neuropathologie des Nucleus ruber beim Menschen*. Thesis, Düsseldorf.
25. Hopf, A., Gihr, M., & Kraus, C. (1967). Vergleichende Architektonik des Primatenthalamus. *Progr. Primatol. I. Congress of the International Primatological Society*, Frankfurt, pp.120-127.
26. Klatzo, I. (1954). Über das Verhalten des Nukleolarapparates in den menschlichen Pallidumzellen. *J. Hirnforsch*. 1, 47-60.
27. Lange, H., & Albring, K.M. (1979). Quantitative Untersuchungen an 33 Rindenregionen des menschlichen Gehirns. *Verh. Anat. Ges*. 73, 107-109.
28. Lange, H., & Thörner, G. (1974). *Zur Neuroanatomie und Neuropathologie des Corpus striatum, Globus pallidus und Nucleus subthalamicus beim Menschen*, Thesis, Düsseldorf.
29. Lange, H., Thörner G., & Hopf, A. (1975).Morphometrisch-statistische Strukturanalysen des Striatum, Pallidum und Nucleus subthalamicus beim Menschen, Teil 1, *J. Hirnforsch*. 16, 333-350.
30. Lange, H., Thörner G., & Hopf, A. (1975). Morphometrisch-statistische Struktur-analysen des Striatum, Pallidum und Nucleus subthalamicus beim Menschen, Teil 2, *J. Hirnforsch*. 16, 401-413.
31. Lange, H., Thörner, G., & Hopf, A. (1976). Morphometrisch-statistische Strukturanalysen des Striatum, Pallidum und Nucleus subthalamicus beim Menschen, Teil 3, *J. Hirnforsch*. 17.
32. Lange, H., Thörner, G., Hopf, A. & Schröder, K.F. (1976). Morphometric studies of the neuropathological changes in choreatic diseases. *J. Neurol. Sci*. 28, 401-425.
33. Mai, J. K., Kedziora, O., Teckhaus, L., & Sofroniew, M.V.(1991). Evidence for subdivisions in the human suprachiasmatic nucleus. *J. Comp. Neurol*. 305, 508-525.
34. Mai, J. K., Stephens, P., Hopf, A. & A.C. Cuello, (1986). Substance P in the human brain. *Neuroscience* 17, 709-739.
35. Mai, J. K., & Reifenberger, G. (1988). Distribution of the carbohydrate epitope 3-fucosyl-*N*-acetyl-lactosamine (FAL) in the adult human brain. *J. Chem. Anat*. 1, 255-285.
36. Namba, M. (1957). Cytoarchitektonische Untersuchung am Striatum. *J. Hirnforsch*. 3, 24-48.
37. Namba, M. (1958). Über die feineren Strukturen des medio-dorsalen Supranucleus und der Lamella medialis des Thalamus beim Menschen. *J. Hirnforsch*. 4, 1-41.
38. Pioro, E. P., Mai, J. K. & Cuello, A. C. (1990). Distribution of substance P- and enkephalin-immunoreactive neurons and fibers. *In:* "The Human Nervous System," G. Paxinos (ed.). Academic Press, 1051-1094.
39. Sander, H.A. (1981). *Morphometrische Analyse der neuropathologischen Veränderungen im Nucleus ruber bei Parkinson'scher Krankheit*. Thesis, Düsseldorf.
40. Sanides, F. (1957). Die Insulae terminales des Erwachsenengehirns des Menschen. *J. Hirnforsch*. 3, 243-273.
41. Sanides, F. (1957). Untersuchungen über die histologische Struktur des Mandelkerngebietes. *J. Hirnforsch*. 2, 354-390.
42. Schiffer, D.(1954) Sur l'action reparatrice dunoyau des cellules nerveuses. *J. Hirnforsch*. 1, 326-336.
43. Schulze, H.A.(1960). Zur individuellen cytoarchitektonischen Gestaltung der linken und echten Hemisphäre des Lobulus parietalis inferior. *J. Hirnforsch*. 4, 486-534
44. Schröder, K. F. (1970). *Quantitativ-mor-*

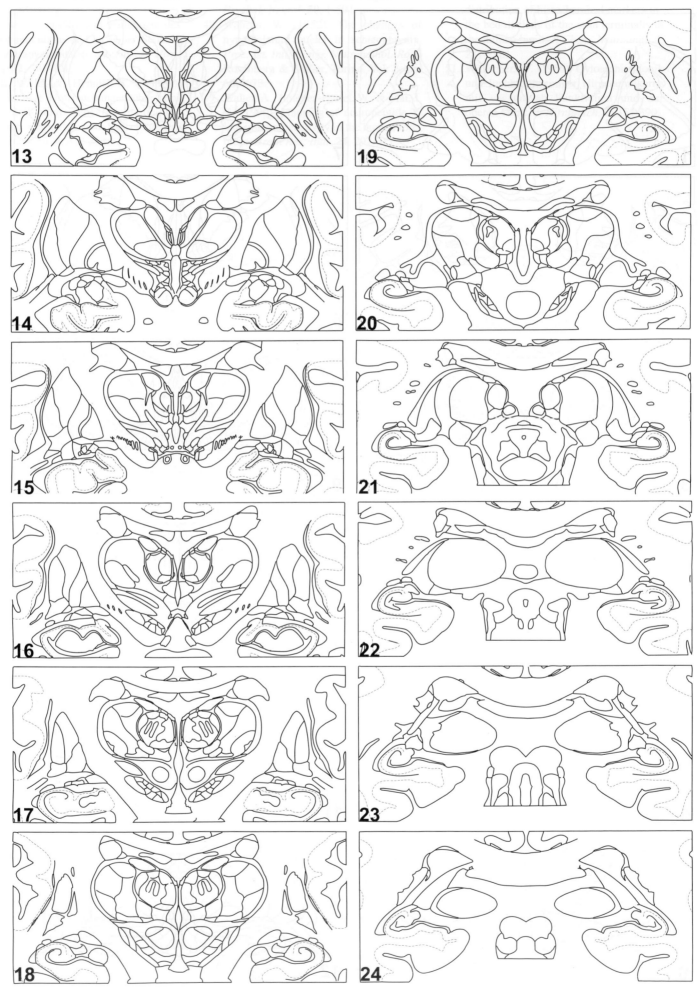

4.6 Template Diagrams (Schematized "Model Brain")

The following pages show diagrams transformed to the dimensions of the mean Talairach space (see Section 2.2.8). Details are suppressed so that the diagrams can function as templates for the supreme position of structural and functional data. The section diagrams show the same levels as those shown in Section 4.1. The surface drawings are derived from the diagrams in Section 3.2.

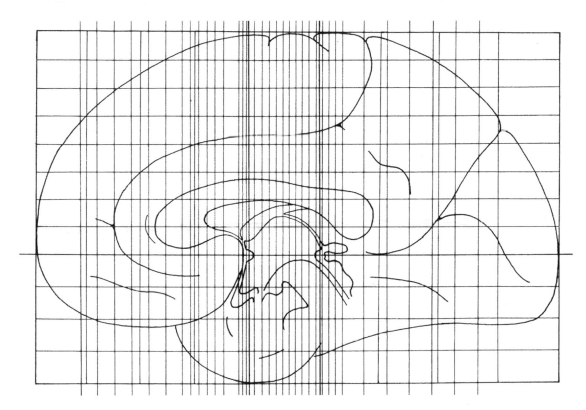

Location of the following 36 diagrams of suppressed details.

Amygdaloid Complex [1]

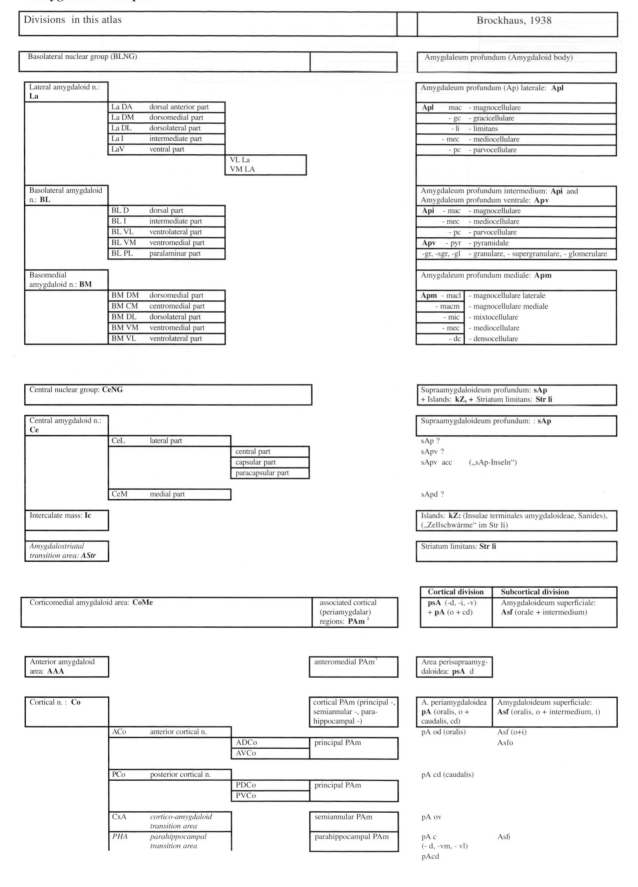

Divisions in this atlas		Brockhaus, 1938

Basolateral nuclear group (BLNG) — Amygdaleum profundum (Amygdaloid body)

Lateral amygdaloid n.: **La**

La DA	dorsal anterior part
La DM	dorsomedial part
La DL	dorsolateral part
La I	intermediate part
La V	ventral part

VL La
VM LA

Amygdaleum profundum (Ap) laterale: **Apl**

Apl mac - magnocellulare
- gc - gracilicellulare
- li - limitans
- mec - mediocellulare
- pc - parvocellulare

Basolateral amygdaloid n.: **BL**

BL D	dorsal part
BL I	intermediate part
BL VL	ventrolateral part
BL VM	ventromedial part
BL PL	paralaminar part

Amygdaleum profundum intermedium: **Api** and
Amygdaleum profundum ventrale: **Apv**

Api - mac - magnocellulare
- mec - mediocellulare
- pc - parvocellulare
Apv - pyr - pyramidale
-gr, -sgr, -gl - granulare, - supergranulare, - glomerulare

Basomedial amygdaloid n.: **BM**

BM DM	dorsomedial part
BM CM	centromedial part
BM DL	dorsolateral part
BM VM	ventromedial part
BM VL	ventrolateral part

Amygdaleum profundum mediale: **Apm**

Apm - macl - magnocellulare laterale
- macm - magnocellulare mediale
- mic - mixtocellulare
- mec - mediocellulare
- dc - densocellulare

Central nuclear group: CeNG — Supraamygdaloideum profundum: **sAp**
+ Islands: **kZ**, + Striatum limitans: **Str li**

Central amygdaloid n.: **Ce**

CeL	lateral part
	central part
	capsular part
	paracapsular part
CeM	medial part

Supraamygdaloideum profundum: : **sAp**

sAp ?
sApv ?
sApv acc („sAp-Inseln")

sApd ?

Intercalate mass: **Ic** — Islands: **kZ:** (Insulae terminales amygdaloideae, Sanides), („Zellschwärme" im Str li)

Amygdalostriatal transition area: AStr — Striatum limitans: **Str li**

	Cortical division	Subcortical division

Corticomedial amygdaloid area: **CoMe** — associated cortical (periamygdalar) regions: **PAm** [2] — **psA** (-d, -i, -v) + **pA** (o + cd) — Amygdaloideum superficiale: **Asf** (orale + intermedium)

Anterior amygdaloid area: **AAA** — anteromedial PAm [3] — Area perisupraamyg-daloidea: **psA** d

Cortical n. : **Co** — cortical PAm (principal -, semiannular -, para-hippocampal -) — A. periamygdaloidea **pA** (oralis, o + caudalis, cd) — Amygdaloideum superficiale: **Asf** (oralis, o + intermedium, i)

ACo	anterior cortical n.			pA od (oralis)	Asf (o+i)
		ADCo	principal PAm		Asfo
		AVCo			
PCo	posterior cortical n.			pA cd (caudalis)	
		PDCo	principal PAm		
		PVCo			
CxA	*cortico-amygdaloid transition area*		semiannular PAm	pA ov	
PHA	*parahippocampal transition area*		parahippocampal PAm	pA c (- d, -vm, - vl) pAcd	Asfi

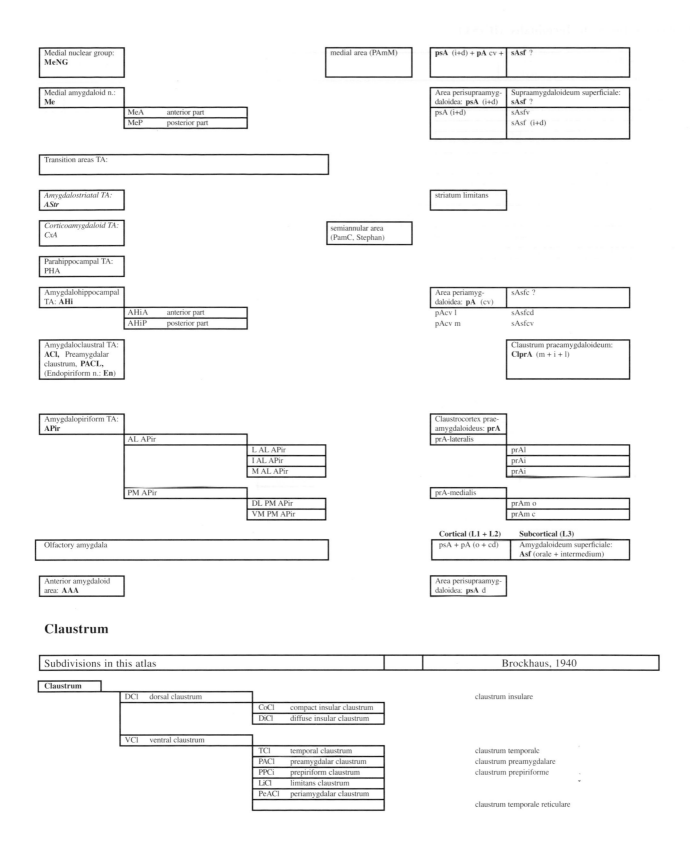

Medial nuclear group: **MeNG**

medial area (PAmM)

psA (i+d) + **pA** cv + **sAsf** ?

Medial amygdaloid n.: **Me**

| MeA | anterior part |
| MeP | posterior part |

Area perisupraamyg-daloidea: **psA** (i+d)	Supraamygdaloideum superficiale: **sAsf** ?
psA (i+d)	sAsfv
	sAsf (i+d)

Transition areas TA:

Amygdalostriatal TA: ***AStr***

striatum limitans

Corticoamygdaloid TA: *CxA*

semiannular area (PamC, Stephan)

Parahippocampal TA: PHA

Amygdalohippocampal TA: **AHi**

| AHiA | anterior part |
| AHiP | posterior part |

Area periamyg-daloidea: **pA** (cv)	sAsfc ?
pAcv l	sAsfcd
pAcv m	sAsfcv

Amygdaloclaustral TA: **ACl,** Preamygdalar claustrum, **PACL,** (Endopiriform n.: **En**)

Claustrum praeamygdaloideum: **ClprA** (m + i + l)

Amygdalopiriform TA: **APir**

AL APir	
	L AL APir
	I AL APir
	M AL APir

Claustrocortex prae-amygdaloideus: prA	
prA-lateralis	
	prAl
	prAi
	prAi

PM APir	
	DL PM APir
	VM PM APir

prA-medialis	
	prAm o
	prAm c

Cortical (L1 + L2) **Subcortical (L3)**

psA + pA (o + cd)	Amygdaloideum superficiale: **Asf** (orale + intermedium)

Olfactory amygdala

Anterior amygdaloid area: **AAA**

Area perisupraamyg-daloidea: **psA** d

Claustrum

Subdivisions in this atlas		Brockhaus, 1940

Claustrum

DCl	dorsal claustrum		claustrum insulare
		CoCl compact insular claustrum	
		DiCl diffuse insular claustrum	

VCl	ventral claustrum		
		TCl temporal claustrum	claustrum temporalc
		PACl preamygdalar claustrum	claustrum preamygdalare
		PPCi prepiriform claustrum	claustrum prepiriforme
		LiCl limitans claustrum	
		PeACl periamygdalar claustrum	
			claustrum temporale reticulare

---

[1] This division is based on the schema proposed by De Olmos (1990).

Globus pallidus and Substantia nigra

Subdivisions in this atlas	Hassler, 1937

Globus pallidus (GP)

DP	dorsal pallidum

IGP*	internal globus pallidus
EGP*	external globus pallidus

	medial part
	lateral part

SCGP	supracapsular part

VP	ventral pallidum

Substantia nigra (SN)

SNC	Pars compacta

SNR	Pars reticulata

SNL	Pars lateralis

SNCA	Sam, Sai, Sal
SNCP	Spv, Spe, Spd
SNRA	rab, rad, raf
SNRP	rKu

*Lamina pallidi externa, interna, incompleta (accessoria), limitans (lateral medullary lamina, lml; medial medullary lamina, mml; incomplete medullary lamina, icml; limiting medullary lamina, liml).

Thalamus

Subdivisions in this atlas			Hirai/Jones1989	Hassler, 1959, 1977	
Anterior nuclear group (anterior thalamus, ATh):				**A**	**n. anterior**
	AD	anterodorsal thalamic n.	AD	A.d	n. anterodorsalis
	APr	anteroprincipal thalamic n.	AV	A.pr	n. anteroprincipalis
	AM	anteromedial thalamic n.	AM	A.m	n. anteromedialis
		anteroinferior	part of AM	A. if	n. anteroinferior
		(antero-) reuniens	part of AM	A.r	n. (antero-) reuniens
Medial nuclear region					
	MD	mediodorsal thalamic n.	MD	**M**	**n. medialis dorsalis**
		MDFi pars fibrosa	- mc	M. fi	n..fibrosus
		MDFa pars fasciculosa	- l	M. fa	n. fasciculosus (p,f)
		MDV pars dorsalis	- v	M. c	n. magnocellularis (i,e)
		MDMC pars magnocellularis	part of CL		n. paralamellaris
		MDV pars ventralis			
Central nuclei (gray), (Midline nuclei)					
	Re	reuniens n.	MV (Re)	Edy	n. endymalis
	PV	paraventricular n.	Pv	Pm	n. paramedianus (o, pr, c)
	SubH	subhabenular n.		sHb	n. subhabenularis
Envelope (Nuclei of the internal medullary lamina)					
	PF	parafascicular n.	t.pf	Pf	n. parafascicularis
	CM	centromedian n.	CM	Ce	n. centralis
		CMPC parvocellular part			- . pc
		CMMC magnocellular part			- . mc
		CMV ventral part			
	Lim	limitans n.	t.li , part of CL.p to MD	Li	n. limitans (m,opticus portae)
	Cuc	cucullaris n.	dorsomedial CL	Cu	n. cucullaris
	Com	commissuralis n.	t.com	Co	n. commissuralis
	PT	paratenialis n.	t.pt	Pt	n. paratenialis
	ILa	intralamellaris	Cl and Pc	iLa	(o,v,interpol.c)
		CIL central part			
		PCIL paracentral part			
	Fa	fasciculosus n.	part of MV	Fa	n. fasciculosus
	SGe	suprageniculate n.			
Lateral nuclear region: Ventral (group) nuclei					
Lateropolar region					
	VA	ventroanterior n.	VA	**Lpo**	**n. lateropolaris**
		VAMC magnocellular part		Lpo.mc	
		Fas fasciculosus n.			
Ventral nuclei					
	VL	ventrolateral n.			
		VLA ventrolateral anterior n. (internal part, external part)	VLa, am part of VLp	**V.o** V.oa	**n. ventro-oralis** (- i ,m)
		VLP ventrolateral posterior n. (internal part, external part)		V.op	(- i ,m)
		VIM ventrointermedius n.		**V. im**	**n. ventro-intermedius**
	VP	ventroposterior n.		**V.c**	**n. ventro-caudalis**
		VPL ventroposterior lateralis (anterior part, posterior part)	VPLa	**V.c.e** V.c. e. a. V.c. e. p.	**n. ventro-caudalis externus** n. ventro-caudalis anterior ext. n. ventro-caudalis post. ext.
		VPI ventroposterior inferior (internus)	VPI	**V.c.pc.e**	**n. ventro-caudalis parvocellularis externus**
		VPM ventroposterior medialis	VPM VMb (+ n. submedius)	**V.c.(a).i** **V.c.pc.i**	**n. ventro-caudalis internus** **n. ventro-caudalis parvocellularis internus**
		PLa ventroposterior portae	PLa	.po	- portae
Dorsal nuclei					
	LD	laterodorsal n.	LD	**D.**	**n. dorsalis**
		LDSF superficial part		d.sf	n. dorsalis sf.
		LDO oral part	parts of VA	d.o	n. dorso-oralis (e,i)
		LDI intermediate part	dorsal parts of VLp	d.im	n. dorso-intermedius (e,i,s)
		LDC caudal part	LP	d.c	n. dorso-caudalis

Latin	English	Abbreviation
Bulbus olfactorius	olfactory bulb	OB
Bulla ethmoidalis	ethmoidal bulla	EthBu
Bulla tympanica	tympanic bulla	TyBu
Calcar avis	calcar avis	cal
Canalis	facial canal *see* facial nerve canal	
Canalis caroticus	carotid canal	CtdC
Canalis centralis	central canal	CC
Canalis facialis	facial canal *see* facial nerve canal	
Canalis hypoglossi	hypoglossal	12C
Canalis incisivus	incisive canal	IncC
Canalis infraorbitalis	infraorbital canal	IOC
Canalis mandibulae	mandibular canal	ManC
Canalis nervi facialis	facial nerve canal	7C
Canalis pterygoideus	pterygoid canal	PtgC
Canalis semicircularis	semicircular canals	SCC
Capsula corporis geniculati mediale	capsule of medial geniculate nucleus	cmg
Capsula externa	external capsule	ec
Capsula extrema	extreme capsule	ex
Capsula interna	internal capsule	ic
Capsula interna, genu	genu of the internal capsule	gic
Capsula interna, pars anterior	anterior limb of internal capsule	aic
Capsula interna, pars lenticularis	lenticulothalamic part of the internal capsule	ltic
Capsula interna, pars posterior	posterior limb of the internal capsule	pic
Capsula interna, pars retrolenticularis	retrolenticular part of the internal capsule	rlic
Capsula interna, pars sublenticularis	sublenticular part of the internal capsule	slic
Caput nuclei caudati	head of caudate nucleus	HCd
Cartilago arytenoidea	arytenoid cartilage of the larynx	Ary
Cartilago nasi	greater nasal cartilage	GNaC
Cartilago nasi	nasal cartilage	NaCa
Cartilago septi nasi	septal (nasal) cartilage	SeC
Cartilago thyroidea	thyroid cartilage	ThC
Cartilago tubae auditivae	auditory tube cartilage	AudC
Cauda ncl. caudati	tail of caudate nucleus	TCd
Caudato-Putamen	caudate putamen *see* striatum	CPu
Cavitas orbitae	orbital cavity	Orbit
Cavum nasi	nasal cavity	Nasal
Cavum oris	oral cavity	Oral
Cavum tympani	tympanic cavity	TyC
Cellulae mastoideae	mastoid cells	mstc
Centrum medianum *see* Ncl.centromedianus	centromedian thalamic nucleus	CM
Centrum semiovale	semioval center	sovc
Cerebellum	cerebellum	Cb
Chiasma opticum	optic chiasm	ox
Chorda tympani	chorda tympani nerve	cty
Cingulum	cingulum	cg
Cisterna	cistern	Ci
Cisterna basalis	basal cistern	BslCi
Cisterna basilaris	basilar cistern	BasCi
Cisterna cerebello-medullaris	cerebello-medullary cistern	CMCi
Cisterna interpeduncularis	interpeduncular cistern	IPCi
Cisterna magna (cerebello-medullaris)	great cistern	GrCi
Cisterna pontis	pontine cistern	PoCi
Claustrum	claustrum	Cl
Claustrum compactum	dorsal (compact) insular claustrum	DCl
Claustrum diffusum	diffuse insular claustrum	DiCl
Claustrum dorsale	(compact) insular claustrum	CoCl
Claustrum insulare (*see* dorsale)	insular claustrum *see* dorsal claustrum	
Claustrum temporale	temporal claustrum	TCl
Claustrum temporale, subregio praeamygdaleum	preamygdalar claustrum	PACl
Claustrum temporale, subregio praepiriformis	prepiriform claustrum	PPCl
Claustrum ventrale	ventral claustrum	VCl
Clavicula	clavicle	Clav
Cochlea	cochlea	Co
Colliculus facialis	facial colliculus	7c
Colliculus inferior	inferior colliculus	IC
Colliculus superior	superior colliculus	SC
Columna anterior, cornu anterius	ventral horn of spinal cord	VH
Columna fornicis, *see* fornix	column of fornix *see* anterior column	
Columna intermediolateralis	intermediolateral cell column	IML
Columna lateralis, cornu laterale	lateral horn of spinal cord	LH
Columna posterior, cornu posterius	dorsal horn of spinal cord	DH
Commissura anterior	anterior commissure	ac
Commissura anterior, pars anterior	anterior commissure, anterior part	aca
Commissura anterior, pars olfactoria	anterior commissure, olfactory limb	aco
Commissura anterior, pars posterior	anterior commissure, posterior part	acp
Commissura colliculi inferioris	commissure of the inferior colliculi	cic
Commissura colliculi superioris	commissure of the superior colliculi	csc
Commissura fornicis	commissure of fornix	cfx
Commissura habenularum	habenular commissure	hbc
Commissura hippocampalis dorsalis	dorsal hippocampal commissure	dhc
Commissura posterior	posterior commissure	pc
Commissura supramamillaris *see* decussatio	supramammillary commissure *see* decussation	
Commissura ventralis hippocampi	ventral hippocampal commissure	vhc
Concha nasalis inferior	inferior nasal concha (turbinate)	INaC
Concha nasalis media	middle nasal concha	MNaC
Concha nasalis superior	superior nasal concha	SNaC
Confluens sinuum	confluence of sinuses	cosi
Cornu Ammonis	Ammon's horn	CA
Cornu majus ossis hyoidei	greater horn of hyoid bone	GHHy
Cornu superius cartilaginis thyroideae	superior horn of thyroid cartilage	SHThC
Corona radiata	thalamic radiation	tra

Corpus adiposum buccae	buccal fat pad	buf
Corpus adiposum orbitae	orbital fat pad	off
Corpus amygdaloideum	amygdaloid body *see* amygdala	Amg
Corpus callosum	corpus callosum	cc
Corpus callosum, corpus	body of the corpus callosum	bcc
Corpus callosum, forceps major	forceps major of the corpus callosum	fmj
Corpus callosum, forceps minor	forceps minor of the corpus callosum	fmi
Corpus callosum, genu	genu of the corpus callosum	gcc
Corpus callosum, rostrum	rostrum of the corpus callosum	rcc
Corpus callosum, splenium	splenium of the corpus callosum	scc
Corpus fornicis	body of fornix	bfx
Corpus geniculatum laterale	lateral geniculate nucleus	LG
Corpus geniculatum laterale, pars magnocellularis	ventral lateral geniculate nucleus, magnocellular part	LGMC
Corpus geniculatum laterale, pars parvocellularis	ventral lateral geniculate nucleus, parvocellular part	LGPC
Corpus geniculatum mediale	medial geniculate nucleus	MG
Corpus geniculatum mediale, pars fibrosa	ventral lateral geniculate nucleus, fibrosal part	MGFi
Corpus geniculatum mediale, pars limitans	ventral lateral geniculate nucleus, limitans part	MGLi
Corpus geniculatum mediale, pars magnocellularis	ventral lateral geniculate nucleus, magnocellular part	MGMC
Corpus geniculatum mediale, pars parvocellularis	ventral lateral geniculate nucleus, parvocellular part	MGPC
Corpus mamillare	mammillary body	MB
Corpus nuclei caudati	body of caudate nucleus	BCd
Corpus ossis hyoidei	body of hyoid bone	BHy
Corpus pineale	pineal gland	Pi
Corpus pontobulbare (Substantia -)	pontobulbar substance	PBS
Corpus trapezoideum	trapezoid body	tz
Corpus vitreum	vitreous of the eye	Vitr
Crista ampullaris	crista of anterior ampulla	CrAnt
Crista galli	crista galli	CGal
Crus fornicis, *see* fornix	crus of fornix, *see* posterior crus	pfx
Cuneus	cuneus	Cun
Cx. cerebri	cerebral cortex	Cx
Cx. entorhinalis	entorhinal cortex	Ent
Cx. frontalis	frontal cortex	Fr
Cx. infralimbicus	infralimbic cortex	IL
Cx. insularis agranularis	agranular insular cortex	AIn
Cx. occipitalis	occipital cortex	Oc
Cx. orbitalis	orbital cortex	Orb
Cx. parietalis	parietal cortex	Par
Cx. periamygdaloideus	periamygdaloid cortex	PAC
Cx. perirhinalis	perirhinal cortex	PRC
Cx. piriformis	piriform cortex	Pir
Cx. praeamygdaloideus	preamygdaloid cortex	PrAC
Cx. retrosplenialis agranularis	retrosplenial agranular cortex	RSA
Cx. retrosplenialis granularis	retrosplenial granular cortex	RSG
Cx. temporalis	temporal cortex, area 2	Te
Cx. temporalis, area 1	temporal cortex, area 1 (primary auditory cortex)	Te1
Decussatio lemniscorum med.	decussation of medial lemniscus	xml
Decussatio n. trochlearis	decussation of trochlear nerve	x4n
Decussatio pedunculorum cerebellarium inf.	decussation of inferior cerebellar peduncle	xicp
Decussatio pedunculorum cerebellarium sup.	decussation of the superior cerebellar peduncle	xscp
Decussatio pyramidum	pyramidal decussation	pyx
Decussatio supramamillaris	supramammillary decussation	sumx
Decussatio supraoptica	supraoptic decussation	sox
Decussatio supraoptica ventralis	ventral supraoptic decussation	vsox
Decussatio tegmenti dorsalis	dorsal tegmental decussation	dtgx
Decussatio tegmenti ventralis (=Forel)	ventral tegmental decussation	vtgx
Dens axis	dens axis	DAx
Diaphragma sellae	diaphragma sellae	DS
Diencephalon	diencephalon	Dien
Discus articularis	temporomandibular disc	TMD
Discus articularis mandibulae	articular disc of temporo-mandibular joint, *see also* temporomandibular disc	Disc
Discus intervertebralis	intervertebral disc	Disc
Diverticulum unci *see* sulcus unci		
dopaminergic cell group	dopaminergic cell group	DA#
Dorsum sellae	dorsum sellae	DSel
Ductus cochlearis	cochlear duct	CD
Ductus nasolacrimalis	nasolacrimal duct	nlac
Ductus parotideus	parotid duct	ptdd
Ductus semicircularis (ampulla)	ampulla of anterior semicircular duct	AntA
Ductus semicircularis (ampulla)	ampulla of horizontal semicircular duct	HorA
Ductus semicircularis (ampulla)	ampulla of posterior semicircular duct	PostA
Ductus semicircularis anterior	anterior semicircular duct	Ant
Ductus semicircularis horizontalis	horizontal semicircular duct	Hor
Ductus semicircularis posterior	posterior semicircular duct	Post
Ductus semicircularis, crus commune	common crus of anterior and posterior semicircular ducts	CCrus
Ductus sublingualis	sublingual duct	sld
Ductus submandibularis	submandibular duct	smd
Dura mater	dura	Dura
Eminentia arcuata	arcuate eminence of the petrosal part of the temporal bone	ArcE
Eminentia collateralis	collateral eminence	coe
Eminentia mediana	median eminence	ME
Eminentia mediana rhombencephali	medial eminence of fourth ventricle	me4V
Ependyma	ependyma/subependymal layer	EpL
Epiglottis	epiglottis	EGl

Epithelium	respiratory epithelium	respepith
Falx cerebelli	falx cerebelli	FxCb
Falx cerebri	falx cerebri	FxC
Fascia dentata	fascia dentata *see* dentate gyrus	FD
Fascia nuchae	nuchal fascia	nuf
Fascia parotidea	parotid fascia	ptdf
Fascia praevertebralis	prevertebral fascia	pvf
Fascia superficialis	superficial fascia	sff
Fascia temporalis	temporal fascia	tf
Fasciculus thalamicus	thalamic fasciculus	thf
Fasciola cinerea	fasciola cinerea	FC
Fc. cuneatus	cuneate fasciculus	cu
Fc. dorsolateralis	dorsolateral fasciculus of spinal cord	dl
Fc. fronto-occipitalis inferior	inferior longitudinal fasciculus	ilf
Fc. fronto-occipitalis superior (Fc. occipito-frontalis sup.)	superior longitudinal fasciculus *see* fc. subcallosus	
Fc. gracilis	gracile fasciculus	gr
Fc. lenticularis (FOREL's field H2)	lenticular fasciculus	lenf (H2)
Fc. longitudinalis dorsalis	dorsal longitudinal fasciculus	dlf
Fc. longitudinalis inferior, *see* Fc. fronto-occipitalis inf.	inferior longitudinal fasciculus	ilf
Fc. longitudinalis medialis	medial longitudinal fasciculus	mlf
Fc. longitudinalis pontis	longitudinal fasciculus of the pons	lfp
Fc. longitudinalis superior	superior longitudinal fasciculus *see* subcallosal fasciculus	
Fc. longitudinalis telencephali medialis	medial forebrain bundle	mfb
Fc. mamillaris	principal mammillary fasciculus	pm
Fc. mamillo peduncularis = Ped. mamillaris	mammillary peduncle	mp
Fc. occipito-frontalis sup. *see* fronto-occ. fc.	superior occipito-frontal fascicle *see* subcallosal fasciculus	
Fc. pallido-habenularis	pallido-habenular bundle	phb
Fc. pallido-tegmentalis	pallido-tegmental fasciculus	ptf
Fc. princeps	Fc. princeps *see* Fc. mammillothalamicus	
Fc. pyramidalis	pyramidal fibers	pyr
Fc. retroflexus	fasciculus retroflexus	fr
Fc. subcallosus	subcallosal bundle (sup. fronto-occipital bundle)	scal
Fc. subthalamicus	subthalamic fasciculus	sth
Fc. thalamicus (FOREL's field H1)	thalamic fasciculus	th/H2
Fc. uncinatus	uncinate fasciculus	unc
Fibrae arcuatae	arcuate fasciculus	ar
Fibrae arcuatae int.	internal arcuate fibers	ia
Fibrae corticopontinae	corticopontine fibers	cpo
Fibrae dentatorubrales	dentatorubral fibers	dr
Fibrae frontopontinae	frontopontine fibers	fpo
Fibrae pallidohypothalamicae	pallidohypothalamic fibers (X-bundle)	phy
Fibrae parietotemporopontinae	parietotemporopontine fibers	patepo
Fibrae perforantes penduculi	comb system	comb
Fibrae pericommissurales	pericommissural fibers	pcom
Fibrae periventriculares thalami	periventricular thalamic fibers	pvth
Fibrae pontis longitudinales	longitudinal fibers of the pons	lfp
Fibrae pontis transversae	transverse fibers of the pons	tfp
Fimbria hippocampi	fimbria of the hippocampus	fi
Fissura amygdaloidea	amygdaloid fissure	af
Fissura cerebro-cerebellaris	cerebro-cerebellar fissure	ccbf
Fissura choroidea	choroidal fissure	chf
Fissura hippocampi	hippocampal fissure	hif
Fissura lateralis	lateral fissure	lf
Fissura longitudinalis cerebri	longitudinal fissure of hemisphere	lfh
Fissura medialis anterior	ventral median fissure of the spinal cord	vmnf
Fissura mediana anterior	anterior median fissure	amf
Fissura orbitalis superior	superior orbital fissure	sorf
Fissura telo-diencephalica	telo-diencephalic fissure	tdf
Flocculus	flocculus	Fl
For. infratemporale	infratemporal foramen	ITF
For. interventriculare	interventricular foramen	IVF
For. jugulare	jugular foramen	JugF
For. lacerum	lacerated foramen	LF
For. mentale	mental foramen	MF
For. opticum	optic foramen	OptF
For. ovale	oval foramen	Oval
For. palatinum majus	greater palatine foramen	GPalF
For. rotundum	foramen rotundum (round window)	FOR/ RW
For. stylomastoideum	stylomastoid foramen	StyMF
Forceps major	posterior forceps *see* forceps major	
Forceps minor	anterior forceps *see* forceps minor	
Formatio	medullary reticular formation	MeRF
Fornix	fornix	fx
Fornix praecommissuralis (longus)	precommissural fornix	pcfx
Fornix, commissura	commissure of fornix	cfx
Fornix, corpus	body of fornix	bfx
Fornix, crus anterius (pars libera, pars tecta)	anterior column of fornix	afx
Fornix, crus posterius	posterior crus of fornix	pfx
Fossa interpeduncularis	interpeduncular fossa	ipf
Fossa mandibularis	mandibular fossa (of TMJ)	ManF
Fossa pterygopalatina	pterygopalatine fossa	PtPf
Fossa rhomboidea	rhomboid fossa	RhF
Fossa subarcuata	subarcuate fossa	SAF
Fundus	fundus	Fu
Fundus caudati	caudate fundus	FCd
Fundus putaminis	putaminal fundus	FPu
Fundus striati	fundus striati	FStr

Fundus subventricularis	subventricular fundus	FSV
Funiculus anterolateralis	anterolateral system	als
Funiculus dorsalis	dorsal funiculus of spinal cord	dfu
Funiculus lateralis medullae spinalis	lateral funiculus of the spinal cord	lfu
Funiculus ventralis medullae spinalis	ventral funiculus of the spinal cord	vfu
Galea aponeurotica	galea aponeurotica	gap
Gdl. adrenalis	adrenal gland	Adr
Gdl. lacrimalis	lacrimal gland	LacG
Gdl. lingualis ant.	lingual gland	LgGl
Gdl. maxillaris	maxillary gland	MxG
Gdl. nasalis	nasal glands	NasG
Gdl. parotidea	parotid gland	Par
Gdl. sublingualis	sublingual gland	SLGl
Gdl. submandibularis	submandibular gland	SMGl
Gdl. thyroidea	thyroid gland	Thyr
Gdll. buccales	buccal glands	BucG
Gdll. palatinae	palatine glands	PalG
Genu capsulae internae	genu of the internal capsule	gic
Genu nervi facialis	genu of the facial nerve	g7
Ggl. cervicale inferius	inferior cervical ganglion	ICGn
Ggl. cervicale superius	superior cervical ganglion	SCGn
Ggl. ciliare	ciliary ganglion	Cil
Ggl. geniculi	geniculate ganglion	Gen
Ggl. nervi glossopharyngei	glossopharyngeal ganglion	9Gn
Ggl. nervi glossopharyngei (inf.)	inferior glossopharyngeal (petrosal) ganglion	I9Gn
Ggl. nervi glossopharyngei (sup.)	superior glossopharyngeal ganglion	S9Gn
Ggl. nervi vagi	inferior vagal (nodose) ganglion	I10Gn
Ggl. nervi vagi (inf.)	superior vagal (jugular) ganglion	S10Gn
Ggl. nervi vagi (sup.)	vagal ganglion	10Gn
Ggl. oticum	otic ganglion	Otic
Ggl. pterygopalatinum	pterygopalatine ganglion, *see* spheno-palatine ganglion	
Ggl. sphenopalatinum	sphenopalatine ganglion	SphP
Ggl. spinale	dorsal root ganglion	DRG
Ggl. spirale cochleae	cochlear (spiral) ganglion	CGn
Ggl. stellatum	stellate ganglion	StGn
Ggl. trigeminale (Gasseri)	trigeminal ganglion	5Gn
Ggl. vestibulare	vestibular ganglion	VeGn
Ggl. vestibulocochleare	ganglion of vestibulocochlear nerve	8Gn
Glia glia	glia	
Globus pallidus	globus pallidus	GP
Globus pallidus externus	external globus pallidus	EGP
Globus pallidus internus	internal globus pallidus	IGP
Globus pallidus, pars supracapsularis	supracapsular part of the globus pallidus	SCGP
Glomus caroticum	carotid body	CtdB
Granulationes arachnoidales	arachnoid granulations	argr
Griseum centrale pontis	central gray of the pons	CGPn
Gyri breves insulae	short insular gyri	SIG
Gyri digitati unci	uncal gyrus	UnG
Gyri temporales transversi	transverse temporal gyrus/gyri	TTG
Gyrus ambiens	ambiens gyrus	AG
Gyrus Andreas Retzius	Andreas Retzius gyrus	ARG
Gyrus angularis	angular gyrus	AnG
Gyrus cinguli	cingulate gyrus	CG
Gyrus dentatus	dentate gyrus	DG
Gyrus diagonalis	diagonal gyrus *see* #	
Gyrus entorhinalis	entorhinal gyrus	EntG
Gyrus fasciolaris	fasciolar gyrus	FG
Gyrus fornicatus	gyrus fornicatus *see* isthmus of cingulate gyrus	
Gyrus frontalis inf.	inferior frontal gyrus	IFG
Gyrus frontalis inf., pars opercularis	inferior frontal gyrus, opercular part	IFGOp
Gyrus frontalis inf., pars orbitalis	inferior frontal gyrus, orbital part	IFGOr
Gyrus frontalis inf., pars triangularis	inferior frontal gyrus, triangular part	IFGTr
Gyrus frontalis medius	middle frontal gyrus	MFG
Gyrus frontalis sup	superior frontal gyrus	SFG
Gyrus frontomarginalis	frontomarginal gyrus	FMG
Gyrus frontoorbitalis	fronto-orbital gyrus	FOG
Gyrus frontopolaris	fronto-polar gyrus	FPG
Gyrus frontopolaris transversus	transverse frontopolar gyrus	TFPG
Gyrus frontopolaris transversus inferior	inferior transverse frontopolar gyrus	TFPGI
Gyrus frontopolaris transversus med.	medial transverse frontopolar gyrus	TFPGM
Gyrus frontopolaris transversus superior	superior transverse frontopolar gyrus	TFPGS
Gyrus fusiformis (occipito-temp.lat. =T4)	fusiform gyrus	FuG
Gyrus insulae/insularis	insular gyrus (gyri)	IG
Gyrus lingualis (part of G. occipito-temp.med., T5)	lingual gyrus	LgG
Gyrus occipitalis (primus, secundus, tertius)	occipital gyrus	OcG
Gyrus occipito-temporalis	occipito-temporal gyrus	OTG
Gyrus occipito-temporalis lateralis	lateral occipito-temporal gyrus *see* fusiform g.	
Gyrus occipito-temporalis medialis	medial occipito-temporal gyrus *see* lingual g.	
Gyrus olfactorius lateralis	lateral olfactory gyrus	LOG
Gyrus orbitalis	orbital gyrus (gyri)	OrG
Gyrus orbitalis lateralis	lateral orbital gyrus	LOrG
Gyrus orbitalis medius	medial orbital gyrus	MOrG
Gyrus orbitofrontalis	orbitofrontal gyrus (gyri) *see* orbital gyri	
Gyrus parahippocampalis	parahippocampal gyrus	PHG
Gyrus paraterminalis (*see* G. subcallosus)	paraterminal gyrus	PTG
Gyrus perirhinalis	perirhinal gyrus	PRhG
Gyrus postcentralis	postcentral gyrus	PoG
Gyrus praecentralis	precentral gyrus	PrG
Gyrus rectus	rectus gyrus *see* gyrus rectus	

Latin	English	Abbreviation
Gyrus rectus	gyrus rectus	GRe
Gyrus rostralis	rostral gyrus	RoG
Gyrus rostralis inferior	inferior rostral gyrus	IRoG
Gyrus rostralis superior	superior rostral gyrus	SRoG
Gyrus semilunaris	semilunar gyrus	SLG
Gyrus subcallosus (PNA)	subcallosal gyrus	SuCG
Gyrus subsplenialis	subsplenial gyrus	SSpG
Gyrus supracallosus *see* G. paraterminalis	supracallosal gyrus *see* paraterminal gyrus	
Gyrus supramarginalis	supramarginal gyrus	SMG
Gyrus temporalis (.if, .m., .s, .tv-a, tv-p)	temporal gyrus	TG
Gyrus temporalis inferior	inferior temporal gyrus	ITG
Gyrus temporalis medius	middle temporal gyrus	MTG
Gyrus temporalis superior	superior temporal gyrus	STG
Gyrus temporopolaris	temporopolar gyrus	TPG
Gyrus transversus (I,II,III, Heschl)	transverse gyrus	TrG
Gyrus uncinatus	uncinate gyrus	UG
Habenula	habenula	Hb
Haemisphaerium cerebelli	cerebellar hemisphere	CH
Hamulus ossis pterygoidei	hamulus of the pterygoid bone	HPtg
Hamulus pterygoideus	pterygoid hamulus *see* hamulus of the pterygoid bone	
Hemisphaerium cerebelli	hemisphere of cerebellum *see* cerebellar hemisphere	
Hilum	hilum of dentate nucleus	HDt
Hilum	hilum of inferior olive	HIO
Hippocampus	CA2 field of the hippocampus	CA2
Hippocampus	CA3 field of the hippocampus	CA3
Hippocampus	hippocampus	Hi
Hippocampus (Cornu Ammonis)	CA1 field of the hippocampus	CA1
Hippocampus (praecommissuralis)	hippocampus, praecommissural part	HiP
Hippocampus (retrocommissuralis)	hippocampus, retrocommissural	HiR
Hippocampus (supracommissuralis)	hippocampus, supracommissural part	HiS
Hippocampus, caput	hippocampal head	HiH
Hippocampus, cauda	hippocampal tail	HiT
Hippocampus, corpus	hippocampal body	HiB
Hippocampus, digitationes	hippocampal digitations	HiD
Hypophysis cerebri	pituitary gland *see* hypophysis	
Hypophysis cerebri	hypophysis	Hp
Hypophysis, lobus anterior	anterior lobe of the pituitary	APit
Hypophysis, pars intermedia	intermediate lobe of the pituitary	IPit
Hypothalamus	hypothalamus	Hy
Incisura	incision	inc
Incisura tentorii cerebelli	tentorial edge (free edge of tentorium cerebelli)	TeE
Incisura unci (impressio unci)	uncal notch	unn
Incus incus (ossicle)	Incus	
Indusium griseum	indusium griseum	IGr
Infundibulum	infundibular stalk	InfS
Insertio: M. levator scapulae	levator scapulae muscle insertion	LScI
Insula amygdaloidea	amygdaloid island(s), extended amygdala	AI
Insula terminalis	terminal island(s)	TI
Insula terminalis amygdalaris,	amygdalar terminal island(s)	ATI
Insula terminalis magna (Insula Calleja)	islands of Calleja *see* striatal terminal islands, major island	ICjM
Insula terminalis magna,	great magna terminal island	GTI
Insula terminalis praeputaminalis	preputaminal terminal island	PPuTI
Insula terminalis subcaudata	subcaudate terminal island	SCTI
Insula terminalis substriatalis	substriatal terminal island	SSTI
Insula terminalis subventricularis	subventricular terminal island	SVTI
Insula terminalis tubercularis	tubercular terminal island(s)	TuTI
Insula, Cx. insularis	insula, insular cortex	Ins
Insulae striatales	striatal terminal islands	StrTI
Involucrum thalami/ internal medullary lamina	envelope of thalamus	EnvT
Isthmus cinguli	isthmus of cingulate gyrus	ICG
Jugum sphenoidale	jugum of sphenoid bone	JSph
Lamina (lamella) pallidi interna	medial medullary lamina of the globus pallidus	mml
Lamina (lamella) pallidi externa	lateral medullary lamina of the globus pallidus	lml
Lamina (lamella) pallidi incompleta (accessoria) (Hassler)	incomplete medullary lamina of the globus pallidus	icml
Lamina (lamella) pallidi limitans (Hassler)	limiting medullary lamina of the globus pallidus	liml
Lamina corticalis I-VI	cortical layer I-VI	I-VI
Lamina lateralis processus pterygoidei	lateral pterygoid plate of sphenoid bone	LPSph
Lamina medialis processus pterygoidei	medial pterygoid plate of sphenoid bone	MPSph
Lamina medullaris externa (thalami)	external medullary lamina of the thalamus	eml
Lamina medullaris interna (thalami)	internal medullary lamina of the thalamus	iml
Lamina quadrigemina	quadrigeminal plate (*see* Carpenter)	QuPl
Lamina subependymalis	subependymal layer	SEL
Lamina terminalis	lamina terminalis	LT
Larynx	larynx	Lx
Lemniscus	lemniscal system	Lem
Lemniscus lateralis	lateral lemniscus	ll
Lemniscus medialis	medial lemniscus	ml
Lens	lens	Lens
Lig. apicis dentis	apical ligament of dens	ald
Lig. longitudinale ant.	anterior longitudinal ligament	all
Lig. nuchae	nuchal ligament	nl
Lig. sphenomandibulare	sphenomandibular ligament	sphml
Lig. stylohyoideum	stylohyoid ligament	shl
Lig. stylomandibulare	stylomandibular ligament	sml
Lig. thyrohyoideum medianum	median thyrohyoid ligament	thh
Lig. transversum atlantis	transverse ligament of atlas	tla
Lig. vocale	vocal ligament	vl

Latin	English	Abbreviation
Ligg. alaria	alar ligament of dens	alaI
Limen insulae (angulus gyri olfactorii lat.)	limen insulae	Li
Linea intercommissuralis	intercommissural line	ICL
Lingua	tongue	Tongue
Lingula cerebelli	lingula cerebelli	Lg
Lobulus	lobule	Lbl
Lobulus paracentralis	paracentral lobule	PCL
Lobulus parietalis inferior	inferior parietal lobule	IPL
Lobulus parietalis superior	superior parietal lobule	SPL
Lobus	lobe	Lb
Lobus flocculo-nodularis	flocculo-nodular lobe	FNL
Lobus frontalis	frontal lobe	FL
Lobus occipitalis	occipital lobe	OL
lobus parietalis	parietal lobe	PL
Lobus temporalis	temporal lobe	TL
Locus coeruleus	locus coeruleus	LC
M. aryepiglotticus	aryepiglotticus muscle	AryE
M. arytenoideus	arytenoid muscle	AryM
M. auricularis posterior	posterior auricular muscle	PAu
M. buccinator	buccinator muscle	BucM
M. cervicalis anterior	anterior cervical muscle	ACeM
M. ciliaris	ciliary muscle	CilM
M. constrictor nasi sup.	superior nasal constrictor muscle	SNaCM
M. constrictor pharyngis	constrictor of pharynx	PhC
M. constrictor pharyngis inferior	inferior constrictor muscle of pharynx	ICM
M. constrictor pharyngis medius	medial constrictor muscle of pharynx	MCM
M. constrictor pharyngis superior	superior constrictor muscle	SCM
M. corrugator cilii	corrugator cilii muscle	CCil
M. corrugator supercilii	corrugator supercilii muscle	CSCil
M. cricoarytenoideus	cricoarytenoid (lat., post.) muscle	CrAr
M. cricothyroideus	cricothyroid muscle	CrTh
M. deltoideus	deltoid muscle	DetM
M. depressor anguli oris	depressor anguli oris muscle	DpAO
M. depressor cilii	depressor cilii muscle	DPCil
M. depressor labii inferior	depressor labii inferioris muscle	DpLb
M. depressor supercilii	depressor supercilii muscle	DpSCil
M. digastricus	digastric muscle (ant. belly, post belly)	DiM
M. digastricus (tendo)	digastric muscle	DiT
M. epicranius	epicranius muscle	EpCr
M. erector spinae	erector spinae muscle	ESp
M. frontalis	frontalis muscle	FrM
M. genioglossus	genioglossus muscle	GGM
M. genohyoideus	geniohyoid muscle	GeHy
M. hyoglossus	hyoglossus muscle	HyGl
M. iliocostalis cervicis	iliocostalis cervicis muscle	ICCe
M. infraspinatus	infraspinatus muscle	InfSM
M. interspinalis	interspinalis muscle	ISM
M. interspinalis cervicis	cervical interspinal muscle	CISM
M. interspinalis, tendo	interspinalis muscle, tendon	ISMT
M. intertransversarius	anterior cervical intertransversarii muscle	ACeIT
M. levator anguli oris	levator anguli oris muscle	LAng
M. levator anguli oris alaequae nasi	levator anguli oris alaequae nasi muscle	LAngO
M. levator labii sup. alaequae nasi (M. nasalis)	levator labii sup. alaequae nasi muscle	LLbAN
M. levator labii superior	levator labii sup. muscle	LLb
M. levator palati	levator palati muscle	LPM
M. levator palpebrae superioris	levator palpebrae superioris muscle	LPal
M. levator scapulae	levator scapulae muscle	LScM
M. levator veli palatini	levator veli palatini muscle	LVePa
M. longissimus	longissimus muscle	LgsM
M. longissimus capitis	longissimus capitis muscle	LgsCa
M. longissimus cervicis	longissimus cervicis muscle	LgsCe
M. longissimus cervicis, tendo	longissimus cervicis muscle, tendon	LgsCeT
M. longus capitis	longus capitis muscle	LgCa
M. longus colli	longus colli muscle	LgCo
M. longus colli et capitis	longus colli and capitis muscles	LgC
M. masseter	masseter muscle	MasM
M. masseter (pars profunda)	deep masseter muscle	DpMasM
M. masseter (pars superficialis)	superficial masseter muscle	SuMas
M. mentalis	mentalis muscle	MentM
M. multifidus	multifidus muscle	Mult
M. mylohyoideus	mylohyoid muscle	MyHy
M. nasalis	nasalis muscle	NaM
M. obliquus capitis inf.	inferior oblique capitis muscle	IObCa
M. obliquus capitis sup.	superior oblique capitis muscle	SObCa
M. obliquus inferior	inferior oblique muscle	IOb
M. obliquus superior	superior oblique muscle	SOb
M. occipitalis	occipitalis muscle	OcM
M. occipito-frontalis	occipito-frontal muscle	OcFr
M. occipito-frontalis, venter ant.	occipito-frontal muscle, frontal belly	OcFrF
M. occipito-frontalis, venter posterior	occipito-frontal muscle, occipital belly	OcFrO
M. omohyoideus	omohyoid muscle	OmHy
M. orbicularis oculi	orbicularis oculi muscle	OOM
M. orbicularis oris	orbicularis oris muscle	OOrM
M. orbicularis posterior	posterior orbicular muscle	POrbM
M. palatoglossus	palatoglossus muscle	PlGl
M. palatopharyngeus	palatopharyngeus muscle	PlPh
M. proccrus	procerus muscle	Prc
M. pterygoideus lat., venter inferior	lateral pterygoid muscle, inferior part	LPtgI
M. pterygoideus lateralis, venter superior	lateral pterygoid muscle, superior part	LPtgS
M. pterygoideus medialis	medial pterygoid muscle	MPtg
M. rectus capitis ant.	anterior rectus capitis muscle	AReCa

M. rectus capitis lat.	lateral rectus capitis muscle	LReCa
M. rectus capitis posterior major	posterior major rectus capitis muscle	PMjRe
M. rectus capitis posterior minor	posterior minor rectus capitis muscle	PMiRe
M. rectus inferior	inferior rectus muscle	IRec
M. rectus lateralis	lateral rectus muscle	LRec
M. rectus medialis	medial rectus muscle	MRec
M. rectus superior	superior rectus muscle	SRec
M. risorius	risorius muscle	Ris
M. salpingopharyngeus	salpingopharyngeus muscle	SalPh
M. scalenus	scalenus muscle	ScalM
M. scalenus ant.	anterior scalenus muscle	AScal
M. scalenus medius	medial scalenus muscle	MScal
M. scalenus posterior	posterior scalenus muscle	PScal
M. semispinalis	semispinalis muscle	SSpM
M. semispinalis capitis	semispinal capitis muscle	SSpCa
M. semispinalis cervicis	semispinal cervicis muscle	SSpCe
M. sphincter et dilatator pupillae	pupillary muscle	PupM
M. spinalis	spinalis muscle	SpM
M. splenius capitis	splenius capitis muscle	SpCa
M. splenius cervicis	splenius cervicis muscle	SpCe
M. stapedius	stapedius muscle	StpM
M. sternocleidomastoideus	sternomastoid muscle	StM
M. sternocleidomastoideus, tendo	sternomastoid muscle, tendon	StT
M. sternohyoideus	sternohyoid muscle	StHy
M. sternothyroideus	sternothyroid muscle	StTh
M. sternothyroideus, tendo	sternothyroid muscle, tendon	StThT
M. styloglossus	styloglossus muscle	StyGl
M. stylohyoideus	stylohyoid muscle	StyHy
M. stylopharyngeus	stylopharyngeus muscle	StyPh
M. subclavius	subclavius muscle	SClv
M. subscapularis	subscapularis muscle	SSc
M. supraspinatus	supraspinatus muscle	SSpM
M. temporalis	temporalis muscle	TempM
M. temporalis, tendo	temporalis muscle, tendon	TempT
M. tensor et levator palati	tensor et levator palati muscle	TeLePa
M. tensor tympani	tensor tympani muscle	TenT
M. tensor veli palatini	tensor palatini muscle	TeVePa
M. thyroarytenoideus	thyroarytenoid muscle	ThArTe
M. thyroepiglotticus	thyroepiglotticus muscle	ThyE
M. thyrohyoideus	thyrohyoid muscle	ThHy
M. trapezius	trapezius muscle	TzM
M. uvulae	uvula muscle	UvM
M. vocalis	vocalis muscle	Voc
M. zygomaticus major	greater zygomatic muscle	GZgM
M. zygomaticus minor	minor zygomaticus muscle	MiZyM
Macula sacculi	saccular macula	SMac
Macula utriculi	utricular macula	UMac
Malleus	malleus (ossicle)	Mal
Malleus, -	handle of Malleus	HandleM
Massa intercalata	intercalated masses *see* intercalated nuclei of amygdala	
Maxilla	maxilla	Mx
Meatus acusticus ext.	external auditory meatus	EAM
Meatus acusticus int.	internal auditory meatus	IAud
Meatus nasi	nasal meatus	Nas
Meatus nasi inferior	inferior meatus of nasal cavity	InfMe
Meatus nasi med.	middle meatus of nasal cavity	MidM
Medulla oblongata	medulla oblongata	Md
Medulla spinalis	spinal cord	Spinal
Membrana atlanto-occipitalis	atlanto occipital membrane	AtOcM
Membrana tectoria	tectorial membrane	TecMe
Membrana thyrohyoidea	thyrohyoid membrane	ThHyMe
Membrana tympanica	tympanic membrane	TyMe
Mesencephalon	mesencephalon, midbrain	Mes
Mm. intertransversarii	intertransversarii muscle	InTrM
N. abducens	abducens nerve or its root	6n
N. accessorius, pars spinalis	spinal accessory nerve	11n
N. alveolaris inferior	inferior alveolar nerve	ialvn
N. alveolaris superior ant.	anterior superior alveolar nerve	asan
N. alveolaris superior posterior	posterior superior alveolar nerve	psan
N. auriculotemporalis	auriculotemporal nerve	aute
N. buccalis	buccal nerve	bucn
N. canalis pterygoidei	nerve of the pterygoid canal	ptgcn
N. cervicalis	cervical nerve	cern
N. facialis	facial nerve or its root	7n
N. facialis, -	descending fibers of facial nerve	7dsc
N. frontalis	frontal nerve of V	5fr
N. glossopharyngeaus, ramus tympanicus	tympanic branch of glossopharyngeal nerve	9ty
N. glossopharyngeus	glossopharyngeal nerve	9n
N. hypoglossus	hypoglossal nerve or its root	12n
N. infraorbitalis	infraorbital nerve	5inf
N. intercostalis	intercostal nerve	icn
N. lacrimalis	lacrimal nerve of trigeminus	5lac
N. laryngeus externus	external laryngeal nerve	eln
N. laryngeus internus	internal laryngeal nerve	ilxn
N. laryngeus recurrens	recurrent laryngeal nerve	rln
N. laryngeus sup.	superior laryngeal nerve	sln
N. lingualis	lingual nerve	5lgn
N. mandibularis	mandibular nerve	5mand
N. massetericus	masseteric nerve	masn
N. maxillaris	maxillary nerve of the trigeminal	mx5

Latin	English	Abbr.
N. mylohyoideus	mylohyoid nerve	myhy
N. nasociliaris	nasociliar nerve	5nc
N. nasopalatinus	nasopalatine nerve	npal
N. occipitalis	occipital nerve	occn
N. occipitalis major	greater occipital nerve	gocn
N. oculomotorius	oculomotor nerve or its root	3n
N. oculomotorius, pars communicans	oculomotor nerve, branches to inf. oblique muscle	3iob
N. oculomotorius, radix inf.	inferior division of oculomotor nerve	3n
N. oculomotorius, ramus inferior	oculomotor nerve, inferior ramus	3ni
N. olfactorius	olfactory nerve	1n
N. ophthalmicus	ophthalmic nerve of trigeminal	oph5
N. opticus	optic nerve	2n
N. palatinus	palatine nerve (s)	paln
N. palatinus major	greater palatine nerve	gpaln
N. palatinus minor	lesser palatine nerve	lpaln
N. petrosus (superficialis) major	greater petrosal nerve	7gp
N. petrosus minor	lesser petrosal nerve	lpet
N. petrosus profundus	deep petrosal nerve	dpetn
N. pharyngeus sup.	superior pharyngeal nerve	sphn
N. phrenicus	phrenic nerve	phrn
N. pterygoid medialis	medial pterygoid nerve	mptg
N. sublingualis	sublingual nerve	slin
N. supraorbitalis	supraorbital nerve	suorbn
N. supratrochlearis	supratrochlear nerve	sutrn
N. temporalis profundus	deep temporal nerve	dtn
N. trigeminalis	trigeminal nerve	5n
N. trigeminus, radix motoria	motor branch of trigeminal nerve	m5
N. trochlearis	trochlear nerve or its root	4n
N. vagus	vagus nerve	10n
N. vestibulocochlearis	vestibulocochlear nerve	8n
N. vestibulocochlearis(stato-acusticus)	cochlear root of the vestibulocochlear nerve	8cn
N. vestibulocochlearis, pars vestibularis	vestibular root of the vestibulocochlear nerve	8vn
N. vomeronasalis	nerve of vomeronasal organ	vno
N. zygomaticus	zygomatic nerve	5zg
Ncl. (nervi) abducentis	abducens nucleus	6
Ncl. abducens accessorius	accessory abducens nucleus	Acs6
Ncl. accumbens	accumbens nucleus	Acb
Ncl. accumbens, pars centrolateralis	accumbens nucleus, centrolateral part	AcCL
Ncl. accumbens, pars centromedialis	accumbens nucleus, centromedial part	AcCM
Ncl. accumbens, pars subcaudata	accumbens n., caudate fundus region, *see* fundus	
Ncl. accumbens, pars subputaminalis	accumbens n., putaminal fundus region *see* fundus	
Ncl. accumbens, pars ventricularis	accumbens nucleus, subventricular part	AcSV
Ncl. ambiguus	ambiguus nucleus	Amb
Ncl. amygdaloideus	amygdaloid nucleus	A
Ncl. amygdaloideus anterior	anterior amygdaloid nucleus	AA
Ncl. amygdaloideus basalis	basal amygdaloid nucleus	BA
Ncl. amygdaloideus basalis accessorius	accessory basal amygdaloid nucleus	AB
Ncl. amygdaloideus basolateralis	basolateral amygdaloid nucleus	BL
Ncl. amygdaloideus basolateralis, p.dorsalis	basolateral amygdaloid nucleus, dorsal part	BLD
Ncl. amygdaloideus basolateralis, pars intermedius	basolateral amygdaloid nucleus, ventromedial part	BLI
Ncl. amygdaloideus basolateralis, pars paralaminaris	basolateral amygdaloid nucleus, ventromedial part	BLPL
Ncl. amygdaloideus basolateralis, pars ventrolateralis	basolateral amygdaloid nucleus, ventrolateral part	BLVL
Ncl. amygdaloideus basolateralis, pars ventromedialis	basolateral amygdaloid nucleus, ventromedial part	BLVM
Ncl. amygdaloideus basomedialis	basomedial amygdaloid nucleus	BM
Ncl. amygdaloideus basomedialis, pars anterior	basomedial amygdaloid nucleus, anterior part	BMA
Ncl. amygdaloideus centralis	central amygdaloid nucleus	Ce
Ncl. amygdaloideus corticalis	cortical amygdaloid nucleus	CoA
Ncl. amygdaloideus corticalis anterior	anterior cortical amygdaloid nucleus	ACo
Ncl. amygdaloideus corticalis anterior, pars dorsalis	anterior cortical amygdaloid nucleus, dorsal part	ACoD
Ncl. amygdaloideus corticalis anterior, pars ventralis	anterior cortical amygdaloid nucleus, ventral part	ACoV
Ncl. amygdaloideus corticalis posterior	posterior cortical amygdaloid nucleus	PCo
Ncl. amygdaloideus intercalatus	intercalated nuclei of the amygdala	I
Ncl. amygdaloideus lat. pars dorsomedialis	lateral amygdaloid nucleus, dorsomedial part	LaDM
Ncl. amygdaloideus lat. pars ventralis	lateral amygdaloid nucleus, ventral part	LaV
Ncl. amygdaloideus lat., pars dorsolateralis	lateral amygdaloid nucleus, dorsolateral part	LaDL
Ncl. amygdaloideus lat., pars intermedia	lateral amygdaloid nucleus, intermediate part	LaI
Ncl. amygdaloideus lat., pars magnocellul.	lateral amygdaloid nucleus, magnocellular part	LaMC
Ncl. amygdaloideus medialis	medial amygdaloid nucleus	Me
Ncl. amygdaloideus medialis, pars anteroventralis	medial amygdaloid nucleus, anteroventral part	MeAV
Ncl. amygdaloideus medialis, pars posterodorsalis	medial amygdaloid nucleus, posterodorsal part	MePD
Ncl. amygdaloideus medialis, pars posteroventralis	medial amygdaloid nucleus, posteroventral part	MePV
Ncl. ansae lenticularis	nucleus of the ansa lenticularis	AL
Ncl. ansae peduncularis	nucleus of the ansa peduncularis	APd
Ncl. anterior hypothalami *see* Ncl. hypothalamicus -	anterior hypothalamic nucleus	
Ncl. anterior hypothalami *see* Ncl. hypothalamicus -	anterior hypothalamic nucleus, dorsal part	
Ncl. anterior thalami, *see* Ncl. thalamicus -	anterior thalamus	
Ncl. anterodorsalis thalami *see* Ncl. thalamicus -	anterodorsal thalamic nucleus	
Ncl. anteromedialis thalami, *see* Ncl. thalamicus -	anteromedial thalamic nucleus	
Ncl. anteroventralis thalami, *see* Ncl. thalamicus -	anteroprincipal thalamic nucleus	
Ncl. arcuatus hypothalami	arcuate hypothalamic nucleus	Arc

Ncl. rotundus (ncl. tractus solitarius, subnucleus rotundus)	rotund nucleus	Ro
Ncl. ruber	red nucleus	R
Ncl. ruber, capsula	capsule of red nucleus	cr
Ncl. ruber, pars magnocellularis	red nucleus, magnocellular part	RMC
Ncl. ruber, pars parvocellularis	red nucleus, parvocellular part	RPC
Ncl. sagulum	sagulum nucleus	Sag
Ncl. septi lateralis	lateral septal nucleus	LS
Ncl. septi lateralis, pars dorsalis	lateral septal nucleus, dorsal part	LSD
Ncl. septi lateralis, pars intermedia	lateral septal nucleus, intermediate part	LSI
Ncl. septi lateralis, pars ventralis	lateral septal nucleus, ventral part	LSV
Ncl. septi medialis	medial septal nucleus	MS
Ncl. septi posterior	posterior septal nucleus	PS
Ncl. septi triangularis	triangular septal nucleus	TS
Ncl. septi ventralis	ventral septal nucleus	VS
Ncl. septodiagonalis	septodiagonal nucleus	SD
Ncl. septofimbrialis	septofimbrial nucleus	SFi
Ncl. septohippocampalis	septohippocampal nucleus	SHi
Ncl. septohypothalamicus	septohypothalamic nucleus	SHy
Ncl. solitarius, pars commissuralis	solitary nucleus, commissural part	SolC
Ncl. spinalis lateralis	lateral spinal nucleus	LSp
Ncl. spinalis nervi trigemini	spinal trigeminal nucleus	Sp5
Ncl. striae medullaris	nucleus of the stria medullaris	SM
Ncl. subcoeruleus	subcoeruleus nucleus/ A7 noradrenaline cells	SubC/ A7
Ncl. subhabenularis	subhabenular nucleus	SubH
Ncl. subincertus	subincertal nucleus	SubI
Ncl. sublentiformis	sublentiform nucleus	SLn
Ncl. subparafascicularis thalami	subparafascicular thalamic nucleus	SPF
Ncl. subthalamicus	subthalamic nucleus	STh
Ncl. subthalamicus, capsula	capsule of subthalamic nucleus	csth
Ncl. suprachiasmaticus	suprachiasmatic nucleus	SCh
Ncl. suprageniculatus	suprageniculate nucleus	SGe
Ncl. supramamillaris	supramammillary nucleus	SuM
Ncl. supraopticus	supraoptic nucleus	SO
Ncl. supraopticus, pars dorsolateralis	supraoptic nucleus, dorsolateral part	SODL
Ncl. supraopticus, pars posterior	supraoptic nucleus, posterior part	SOP
Ncl. supraopticus, pars retrochiasmaticus	supraoptic nucleus, retrochiasmatic part	SOR
Ncl. supraopticus, pars tuberalis	supraoptic nucleus, tuberal part	SOT
Ncl. supraopticus, pars ventromedialis	supraoptic nucleus, ventromedial part	SOVM
Ncl. tegmentalis laterodorsalis	laterodorsal tegmental nucleus	LDTg
Ncl. tegmentalis pedunculopontinus	pedunculopontine tegmental nucleus	PPTg
Ncl. tegmentalis ventralis (Gudden)	ventral tegmental nucleus (Gudden)	VTg
Ncl. tegmenti dorsalis	dorsal tegmental nucleus	DTg
Ncl. terminalis dorsalis	dorsal terminal ncl. of the accessory optic system	DT
Ncl. terminalis lateralis	lateral terminal ncl. of the AOS	LTe
Ncl. thalamicus anterior	anterior thalamic nucleus	ATh
Ncl. thalamicus anterodorsalis	anterodorsal thalamic nucleus	AD
Ncl. thalamicus anteromedialis	anteromedial thalamic nucleus	AM
Ncl. thalamicus anteroprincipalis	anteroprincipal thalamic nucleus	APr
Ncl. thalamicus centralis medialis	centromedian thalamic nucleus	CM
Ncl. thalamicus centralis medialis, pars magnocellularis	centromedian thalamic nucleus, magnocellular	CMMC
Ncl. thalamicus centralis medialis, pars parvocellularis	centromedian thalamic nucleus, parvocellular part part	CMPC
Ncl. thalamicus centralis medialis, pars ventralis	centromedian thalamic nucleus, ventral part	CMV
Ncl. thalamicus fasciculosus	fasciculosus thalamic nucleus	Fas
Ncl. thalamicus lateralis	lateral thalamic nuclear region	LTh
Ncl. thalamicus mediodorsalis	mediodorsal thalamic nucleus	MD
Ncl. thalamicus mediodorsalis, pars dorsalis	mediodorsal thalamic nucleus, dorsal part	MDD
Ncl. thalamicus mediodorsalis, pars fasciculata	mediodorsal thalamic nucleus, pars fasciculosa	MDFa
Ncl. thalamicus mediodorsalis, pars fibrosa	mediodorsal thalamic nucleus, pars fibrosa	MDFi
Ncl. thalamicus mediodorsalis, pars ventralis	mediodorsal thalamic nucleus, ventral part	MDV
Ncl. thalamicus mediodorsalis, pars magnocellularis	mediodorsal thalamic nucleus, pars magnocellularis	MDMC
Ncl. thalamicus posterolateralis, pars ventralis	ventroposterior lateral thalamic nucleus	VPL
Ncl. thalamicus posteromedialis, pars inferior	ventroposterior inferior thalamic nucleus	VPI
Ncl. thalamicus posteromedialis, pars ventralis	ventroposterior medial thalamic nucleus	VPM
Ncl. thalamicus reticularis	reticular thalamic nucleus	Rt
Ncl. thalamicus ventralis anterior, pars fasciculosus	ventroanterior thalamic nucleus, fasciculosus part *see* fasciculosus nucleus	
Ncl. thalamicus ventralis anterior, pars magnocellularis	ventroanterior thalamic nucleus, magnocellular part	VAMC
Ncl. tractus olfactorius	nucleus of the olfactory tract *see* nucleus of the lateral olfactory tract	
Ncl. tractus opticus	nucleus of the optic tract	OT
Ncl. tractus solitarius	nucleus of the solitary tract	Sol
Ncl. trapezoidalis, *see* Ncl. corpus trapezoideum	trapezoid nucleus	
Ncl. triangularis septi	triangular septal nucleus	TS
Ncl. trigeminalis accessorius	accessory trigeminal nucleus	Acs5
Ncl. trigeminalis mesencephali	mesencephalic trigeminal nucleus	Me5
Ncl. trigeminalis, pars spinalis	dorsomedial spinal trigeminal nucleus	DMSp5
Ncl. trochlearis (nervi trochlearis)	trochlear nucleus	4
Ncl. tuberis lateralis	lateral tuberal nucleus	LTu
Ncl. tuberis medialis	medial tuberal nucleus	MTu
Ncl. tuberomamillaris	tuberomammillary nucleus	TM
Ncl. ventralis anterior thalami	ventral anterior thalamic nucleus	VA
Ncl. ventrolateralis thalami	ventral lateral thalamic nucleus	VL
Ncl. ventromedialis hypothalami, pars centralis	ventromedial hypothalamic nucleus, central part	VMHC
Ncl. ventromedialis thalami, *see* Ncl. thalamicus -	ventromedial thalamic nucleus	
Ncl. vestibularis descendens (spinalis)	spinal vestibular nucleus	SpVe
Ncl. vestibularis lateralis	lateral vestibular nucleus	LVe
Ncl. vestibularis medialis	medial vestibular nucleus	MVe

Ncl. vestibularis superior	superior vestibular nucleus	SuVe
Ncll. accessorii hypothalami	accessory neurosecretory (hypothalamic) nuclei	ANC
Ncll. intermedii hypothalami	intermediate hypothalamic nuclei	IMH
Ncll. intralamellares thalami	intralamellar thalamic nuclei	ILa
Ncll. pontis	pontine nuclei	Pn
Nervus *see* N.	nerve	n
Neurohypophysis	neurohypophysis	NHp
Nn. spinales	spinal nerve	spn
Nodus lymphaticus	lymph node	Ly
Obex obex	Obex	
Oesophagus	esophagus	Eso
Oliva inferior	inferior olive	IO
Oliva inferior *see* Ncl. olivaris -	inferior olive	
Oliva superior	superior olive	SOl
Operculum	operculum	Op
Operculum frontale	frontal operculum	FOp
Operculum parietale	parietal operculum	PaOp
Operculum temporale (facies supratemporalis)	temporal operculum	TOp
Organum (vasculosum) subcommissurale	subcommissural organ	SCO
Organum (vasculosum) subfornicale	subfornical organ	SFO
Organum (vasculosum) laminae terminalis	vascular organ of the lamina terminalis	VOLT
Organum Corti	organ of Corti	Corti
Os ethmoidale	ethmoid bone	Ethm
Os ethmoidale, lam. cribriformis	cribriform plate	CrP
Os ethmoidale, lam. orbitalis	orbital plate	OrbP
Os ethmoidale, lam. perpendicularis	perpendicular plate	PeP
Os frontale	frontal bone	Fro
Os frontale (pars nasalis)	frontal bone, nasal part	FroN
Os frontale (pars orbitalis)	frontal bone, orbital part	FroO
Os frontale (prc. zygomaticus)	frontal bone, zygomatic process	FroZ
Os frontale (squama ossis frontalis)	frontal bone, squamous part	FroS
Os frontale, crista	frontal bone, crest	FroC
Os hyoideum	hyoid bone	Hyoid
Os hyoideum, cornu majus	greater horn of hyoid bone	GHHy
Os hyoideum, cornu minus	lesser horn of hyoid bone	LHHy
Os mandibulae, Mandibula	mandible	Man
Os mandibulare / corpus mandibulae	body of mandible	BMan
Os nasale	nasal bone	Na
Os occipitale	occipital bone	Occ
Os palatinum	palate	Palate
Os parietale	parietal bone	ParB
Os sphenoidale	sphenoid bone	SphB
Os sphenoidale, ala major	sphenoid, greater wing	SphGW
Os sphenoidale, ala minor	sphenoid, lesser wing	SphLW
Os temporale	temporal bone	Temp
Os temporale, pars petrosa	temporal bone, petrosal part	TempP
Os temporale, pars squamosa	squamous part of the temporal bone	Sq
Os zygomaticum	zygomatic bone	Zyg
Ostium pharyngeum tubae auditivae	opening of auditory tube	oaud
Ostium sinus maxillaris	opening of the maxillary sinus	omaxs
Palatum molle	soft palate	SPal
Palpebra	eyelid	Eyelid
Papilla nervi optici	optic papilla	pap
Paraflocculus	paraflocculus	PFl
Parasubiculum	parasubiculum	PaS
Pars tuberalis hypophysealis	tuberal part of hypophysis	TuHp
Pedunclus cerebellaris inferior	inferior cerebellar peduncle (restiform body)	icp
Pedunclus cerebellaris superior	superior cerebellar peduncle (brachium conjunctivum)	scp
Pedunculus (nuclei) lentiformis	peduncle of lenticular nucleus	PedL
Pedunculus cerebellaris medialis	middle cerebellar peduncle	mcp
Pedunculus cerebri, pars basalis	cerebral peduncle	cp
Pedunculus olfactorius *see* Tractus o.	olfactory peduncle *see* olfactory tract	
Pedunculus thalami inferior	inferior thalamic peduncle	ithp
Planum temporale	planum temporale	PTe
Platysma	platysma	Plat
Plexus brachialis	brachial plexus	bplx
Plexus caroticus	carotid plexus	cplx
Plexus caroticus internus	internal carotid plexus	ictpx
Plexus cervicalis	cervical plexus	cerpx
Plexus choroideus	choroid plexus	chp
Plexus choroideus	choroid plexus of 3rd ventricle	chp3V
Plexus choroideus	choroid plexus of 4th ventricle	chp4V
Plexus lumbosacralis	lumbosacral plexus	lsplx
Plexus parotideus	parotid plexus	papx
Plexus sympathicus	sympathetic plexus	splx
Plexus venosus pterygoideus	pterygoid plexus	ptgpx
Plexus venosus pterygoideus internus	internal pterygoid plexus	iptgpx
Plexus venosus retroarticularis	retroarticular plexus	rapx
Plexus venosus retroorbicularis	retroorbicular plexus	ropx
Plexus venosus suboccipitalis	suboccipital venous plexus	socv
Plexus venosus venae vertebralis (int.)	internal vertebral venous plexus	ivvpx
Plica salpingopalatina	salpingopalatinal fold	SPaF
Plica salpingopharyngea	salpingopharyngeal fold	SPhF
Plica sublingualis	sublingual plica	SlPl
Polus frontalis	frontal pole	FrP
Polus occipitalis	occipital pole	OcP
Polus temporalis	temporal pole	TmP
Pons	pons	Pons
Pontes striatales	striatal cell bridges	SB
Praecuneus	precuneus	PCun

Praesubiculum	presubiculum	PrS
Prerubral field (tegmental field)	prerubral field (tegmental field)	PR
Proc. alveolaris maxillae	alveolar process of maxilla	Alv
Proc. clinoideus anterior	anterior clinoid process	AClP
Proc. condylaris mandibulae	condylar process of mandible	Con
Proc. coronoideus mandibulae	coronoid process of the mandible	Cor
Proc. mastoideus	mastoid process of temporal bone	Mst
Proc. palatinus maxillae	maxilla, palatine process	MxPl
Proc. pterygoideus	pterygoid process	Ptg
Proc. pterygoideus, lamina lateralis	lateral lamina of pterygoid process	LLPtg
Proc. spinosus axis	spinous process of axis	SpAx
Proc. styloideus	styloid process	Sty
Proc. transversus	transverse process	TrP
Proc. transversus	transverse process of vertebra	TrPV
Proc. transversus atlantis	transverse process of atlas	TrPAt
Proc. zygomaticus ossis frontalis	zygomatic process of frontal bone	ZyFr
Pulvinar	pulvinar	Pul
Putamen	putamen	Pu
Putamen mediale	putamen, medial part	PuM
Putamen ventrale	putamen, ventral part	Pu
Pyramis	pyramid	Pyr
Radiatio corporis callosi	radiation of corpus callosum	racc
Radiatio olfactoria	olfactory radiation	olfr
Radiatio olfactoria profunda	deep olfactory radiation	dolf
Radiatio optica	optic radiation	or
Radiatio thalamica superior	superior thalamic radiation	str
Radix dorsalis	dorsal root	dr
Radix sensoria nervi trigemini	sensory root of the trigeminal nerve	s5
Radix ventralis	ventral root	vr
Rami glandulares	glandular branches	gld
Rami glandulares	glandular blood vessels	glve
Rami nasales interni	internal nasal (venous) branches	inav
Rami nasales posteriores	posterior nasal branches	pnar
Rami nervi facialis	facial nerve roots	7r
Rami pharyngei	pharyngeal branches	phar
Rami pterygoidei	pterygoid branches of trigeminal nerve	ptg5
Ramus mandibulae	ramus of mandible	Ram
Recessus infundibularis ventriculi tertii	infundibular recess of the 3rd ventricle	IRe
Recessus lateralis ventriculi quarti	lateral recess of the fourth ventricle	LR4V
Recessus mamillaris	mammillary recess of the 3rd ventricle	MaRe
Recessus medianus ventriculi quarti	medial recesses of the fourth ventricle	MR4V
Recessus opticus	optic recess of third ventricle	ORe
Recessus pharyngeus	pharyngeal recess	PhaRe
Recessus pinealis	pineal recess of the third ventricle	PiRe
Recessus piriformis	piriform recess	PirR
Recessus praeopticus	preoptic recess of the third ventricle	P3V
Regio periamygdalaris	periamygdalar region	PAm
Regio retrobulbaris *see* Ncl. olfactorius ant.	retrobulbar region *see* ant. olfactory nucl.	
Regio subparaventricularis	subparaventricular zone	SPZ
Retina	retina	Retina
S. angularis	angular sulcus	angs
S. calcarinus	calcarine sulcus	ccs
S. calcarinus anterior	anterior calcarine sulcus	acs
S. calcarinus inferior	inferior calcarine sulcus	iccs
S. callosomarginalis	callosomarginal sulcus	cms
S. centralis	central sulcus	cs
S. cinguli	cingulate sulcus	cgs
S. circularis insulae	circular insular sulcus	cir
S. collateralis	collateral sulcus	cos
S. corporis callosi	sulcus of corporis callosi *see* callosal sulcus	
S. corporis callosi	callosal sulcus	cas
S. cruciformis	cruciform sulcus	crs
S. dorolateralis	dorolateral sulcus	dls
S. endorhinalis	endorhinal sulcus	ers
S. frontalis inf.	inferior frontal sulcus	ifs
S. frontalis intermedius	intermediate frontal sulcus	imfs
S. frontalis superior	superior frontal sulcus	sfs
S. fronto-marginalis	fronto marginal sulcus	fms
S. fronto-orbitalis	fronto-orbitalis sulcus	fos
S. hippocampi	hippocampal sulcus	his
S. hypothalamicus	hypothalamic sulcus	hs
S. insularis	insular sulcus	is
S. intraparietalis	intraparietal sulcus	ips
S. intrarhinalis	intrarhinal sulcus	irs
S. limitans	sulcus limitans	sl
S. lingualis	lingual sulcus	lgs
S. longitudinalis insulae	longitudinal insular sulcus	lis
S. marginalis insulae	marginal insular sulcus, *see* circular insular s.	
S. medianus	median sulcus	mns
S. occipitalis	occipital sulcus	os
S. occipitalis anterior	anterior occipital sulcus	aos
S. occipitalis transversus	occipittransverse sulcus	otrs
S. occipito-temporalis	occipitotemporal sulcus	ots
S. occipito-temporalis inferior s. collateralis	inferior occipito temporal sulcus	iots
S. olfactorius	olfactory sulcus	olfs
S. orbitalis (sulci orbitales)	orbital sulcus (sulci)	ors
S. orbitalis lateralis	lateral orbital sulcus	los
S. orbitalis medialis	medial orbital sulcus	mos
S. orbitalis posterior	posterior orbital sulcus	pos
S. paracentralis	paracentral sulcus	pacs
S. parahippocampo-lingualis	parahippocampal sulcus, *see* lingual sulcus	

S. parieto-occipitalis	parieto-occipital sulcus	pocs
S. parolfactorius	parolfactory sulcus	pols
S. parolfactorius anterior	anterior parolfactory sulcus	aps
S. parolfactorius posterior	posterior parolfactory sulcus	pps
S. pontinus superior	superior pontine sulcus	sps
S. postcentralis	postcentral sulcus	pocs
S. postcentralis inferior	inferior postcentral sulcus	poci
S. postcentralis superior	superior postcentral sulcus	spocs
S. praecentralis	precentral sulcus	pcs
S. rhinalis	rhinal sulcus	rhs
S. rostralis	rostral sulcus	ros
S. semiannularis	semiannular sulcus	sas
S. subparietalis	subparietal sulcus	sbps
S. temporalis inferior	inferior temporal sulcus	its
S. temporalis medius	middle temporal sulcus	mts
S. temporalis superior	superior temporal sulcus	sts
S. temporalis transversus	transverse temporal sulcus	tts
S. unci	uncal sulcus (diverticulum unci)	us
Sacculus	saccule	Sacc
Saccus endolymphaticus	endolymphatic sac	ELS
Septum	septum	Spt
Septum linguae	lingual septum	LgSpt
Septum nasi (pars ossea)	nasal septum	NSpt
Septum pellucidum	septum pellucidum	SptP
Sinus cavernosus	cavernous sinus	cav
Sinus ethmoidalis (Cellulae ethm.)	ethmoidal sinus (labyrinth and air cells)	eths
Sinus frontalis	frontal sinus	frs
Sinus marginalis	marginalis sinus *see* occipital sinus	
Sinus maxillaris	maxillary sinus	mxs
Sinus occipitalis	occipital sinus	occs
Sinus petrosus inferior	inferior petrosal sinus	ipets
Sinus petrosus superior	superior petrosal sinus	spets
Sinus rectus	straight sinus	ss
Sinus sagittalis inferior	inferior sagittal sinus	iss
Sinus sagittalis superior	superior sagittal sinus	sss
Sinus sigmoideus	sigmoid sinus	sigs
Sinus sphenoidalis	sphenoid sinus	sphs
Sinus sphenoparietalis	sphenoparietal sinus	sphps
Sinus transversus	transverse sinus	trs
Spatium subarachnoidale	subarachnoid space	SArS
Stapes	stapes (ossicle)	Stp
Stapes, caput	head of stapes	HStapes
Sternum	sternum	St
Stratum medullare superficiale	superficial medullary stratum	sms
Stratum sagittale	sagittal stratum	sstr
Stratum sagittale internum	internal sagittal stratum	isst
Stratum subependymale	subependymal stratum	SEpS
Stria longitudinalis	longitudinal stria	lngs
Stria longitudinalis lateralis	lateral longitudinal stria	lls
Stria longitudinalis medialis	medial longitudinal stria	mls
Stria medullaris thalami	stria medullaris of the thalamus	sm
Stria olfactoria lateralis	lateral olfactory stria	lls
Stria olfactoria medialis	medial olfactory stria	mo
Stria sublenticularis	sublenticular stria	sls
Stria terminalis	stria terminalis	st
Striae medullares	striae medullares	smed
Striatum	striatum	Str
Subiculum	subiculum	S
Substantia gelatinosa	substantia gelatinosa	SG
Substantia gliosa subependymalis	substantia gliosa	SGl
Substantia grisea centralis mesencephali (Griseum centrale mesencephali)	central gray, *see* periaqueductal gray	PAG
Substantia grisea centralis spinalis	medullary central gray substance	MCG
Substantia innominata	substantia innominata	SI
Substantia nigra	substantia nigra	SN
Substantia nigra, pars compacta	substantia nigra, pars compacta	SNC
Substantia nigra, pars lateralis	substantia nigra, pars lateralis	SNL
Substantia nigra, pars reticulata	substantia nigra, pars reticulata	SNR
Substantia perforata anterior	anterior perforated substance	APS
Sulci orbitales	orbital sulci	orbs
Sulcus *see* S.		
Sut. lambdoidea	lambdoid suture	lds
Sut. maxillo-zygomatica	maxillo-zygomatic suture	mxzg
Sut. occipito-mastoidea	occipito-mastoid suture	ocm
Sut. parieto-zygomatica	parieto-zygomatic suture	pazg
Sut. sagittalis	sagittal suture	sags
Sut. spheno-frontalis	spheno-frontal suture	sphfs
Sut. spheno-occipitalis	spheno-occipital suture	sphoc
Sut. spheno-petrosa	spheno-petrosal suture	sphpe
Sut. spheno-squamosa	spheno-squamosal suture	sphsq
Sut. spheno-zygomatica	spheno-zygomatic suture	sphzg
Sut. squamosa	squamosal suture	squs
Sut. zygomatico-maxillaris	zygomatico-maxillary suture	zgmx
Sut. zygomatico-parietalis	zygomatico-parietal suture	zgpa
Sut. zygomatico-temporalis	zygomatico-temporal suture	zgte
Taenia choroidea	tenia of choroid plexus	tch
Taenia fimbriae	tenia of fimbria	tfi
Taenia fornicis	tenia of fornix	tfx
Taenia striae terminalis	tenia of stria terminalis	tst
Taenia tecti	tenia tecta	TT
Taenia thalami	tenia thalamus	tt

Tapetum	tapetum	tp
Tbc. articulare	articular tubercle (of TMJ)	ATub
Tbc. cuneatum	cuneate tubercle	CuTu
Tbc. gracilis	gracilis tubercle	GrTu
Tbc. olfactorium	olfactory tubercle	Tu
Tectum	tectum	Tec
Tectum mesencephali	mesencephalic tectum	MTec
Tegmentum	tegmentum	Tg
Tegmentum, pars paracollicularis	paracollicular tegmentum	PCTg
Tela choroidea ventriculi lateralis	tela choroidea of lateral ventricle	tclv
Tela choroidea ventriculi tertii	tela choroidea of third ventricle	tc3v
Telencephalon	telencephalon	Telen
Tentorium cerebelli	tentorium cerebelli	TCb
Thalamus	thalamus	Th
Thalamus, pars posterior	posterior thalamus	PTh
Tonsilla palatina	palatine tonsil	PtT
Tonsilla pharyngea	nasophaaryngeal tonsil	NPhT
Torus levatorius	torus levatorius	TLev
Torus tubarius	torus tubarius	TTub
Tr. amygdalofugalis ventralis	ventral amygdalofugal pathway	vaf
Tr. cerebello-rubro-thalamicus	cerebello-rubro-thalamic fibers	crt
Tr. cerebello-thalamicus	cerebellothalamic tract	cbth
Tr. cortico-hypothalamicus	corticohypothalamic tract	chy
Tr. cortico-hypothalamicus medialis	medial corticohypothalamic tract	mch
Tr. cortico-spinalis (et -nuclearis)	cortico-spinal (and -nuclear) tract	csp
Tr. corticospinalis dorsalis	dorsal corticospinal tract	dcs
Tr. cortico-spinalis lateralis	lateral cortico-spinal tract	lcsp
Tr. cortico-spinalis ventralis	ventral cortico-spinal tract	vcsp
Tr. cuneo-cerebellaris	cuneo-cerebellar tract	cucb
Tr. dentato-thalamicus	dentato-thalamic tract	dt
Tr. dorsolateralis (Klaus)	dorsolateral tract	dlt
Tr. hypothalamo-hypophysealis	hypothalamo-hypophyseal tract	hyh
Tr. mamillo-tegmentalis	mammillo-tegmental tract	mtg
Tr. mamillo-thalamicus	mammillo-thalamic tract	mt
Tr. mesencephalicus nervi trigemini	mesencephalic trigeminal tract	me5
Tr. olfactorius	olfactory tract	olf
Tr. olfactorius im.	intermediate olfactory tract	iolf
Tr. olfactorius lateralis	lateral olfactory tract	lo
Tr. olivo-cerebellaris	olivocerebellar tract	oc
Tr. opticus	optic tract	opt
Tr. pyramidalis	pyramidal tract	py
Tr. reticulo-spinalis	reticulo-spinal tract	rtsp
Tr. rubro-spinalis	rubrospinal tract	rs
Tr. solitarius	solitary tract	sol
Tr. spinalis nervi trigeminal	spinal trigeminal tract	sp5
Tr. spino-cerebellaris dorsalis	dorsal spinocerebellar tract	dsc
Tr. spino-cerebellaris ventralis	ventral spinocerebellar tract	vsc
Tr. spino-olivaris	spino-olivary tract	spo
Tr. spino-thalamicus	spinothalamic tract	spth
Tr. tecto-bulbaris	tectobulbar tract	tb
Tr. tecto-spinalis	tectospinal tract	ts
Tr. tegmenti centralis	central tegmental tract	ctg
Tr. trigemino-thalamicus	trigemino-thalamic tract	tth
Tr. trigemino-thalamicus dorsalis	dorsal trigemino-thalamic tract (*see* Has, FFo)	tth
Tr. tubero-hypophysealis	tubero-hypophyseal tract	thp
Tr. vestibulo-spinalis	vestibulo-spinal tract	vsp
Trachea	trachea	Trachea
Trigonum collaterale	collateral trigone	ctr
Trigonum hypoglossi	hypoglossal trigone	12Tr
Trigonum nervi vagi	vagal trigone	10Tr
Trigonum olfactorium	olfactory trigone	OTr
Truncus brachiocephalicus	brachiocephalic trunk	brctr
Truncus sympathicus	sympathetic trunk	Symp
Tuba auditiva	auditory tube	Aud
Tuber cinereum	tuber cinereum	TuCn
Tuberculum *see* Tbc.		
Uncus hippocampi	uncus hippocampi	Un
Utriculus	utricle	Utr
Uvula	uvula	Uv
V. alveolaris inferior	inferior alveolar vein	ialvv
V. alveolaris posterior	posterior alveolar vein	palv
V. angularis	angular vein	angv
V. auricularis posterior	posterior auricular vein	pauv
V. axillaris	axillary vein	axv
V. azygos	azygos vein	azy
V. basalis (R.)	basal vein	basv
V. brachiocephalica	brachiocephalic vein	brcv
V. cava inferior	inferior vena cava	ivc
V. cava superior	superior vena cava	svc
V. cerebri inferior	inferior cerebral vein	infcv
V. cerebri interna	inferior cerebral vein	icv
V. cerebri magna (G.)	great cerebral vein	gcv
V. cervicalis profunda	deep cervical vein	dpcv
V. cervicalis transversa	transverse cervical vein	trcerv
V. diploica frontalis	diploic vein	dip
V. emissaria canalis hypoglossi	emissary vein, (hypoglossal canal)	emi
V. emissaria mastoidea	emissary vein, (mastoid)	emi
V. facialis	facial vein	facv
V. facialis anterior	anterior facial vein	afv
V. intervertebralis	intervertebral vein	ivert
V. jugularis anterior	anterior jugular vein	ajugv

V. jugularis externa	external jugular vein	ejug
V. jugularis interna	internal jugular vein	ijugv
V. jugularis posterior	posterior jugular vein	pjug
V. lacrimalis	lacrimal vein	lacv
V. lingualis	lingual vein	lgv
V. maxillaris	maxillary vein	mxv
V. occipitalis	occipital vein	occv
V. ophthalmica	ophthalmic vein	ophv
V. ophthalmica inferior	inferior ophthalmic vein	iophv
V. ophthalmica sup.	superior ophthalmic vein	sophv
V. orbicularis posterior	posterior ophthalmic vein	pophv
V. plexus carotidei	vein of carotid plexus	cplxv
V. retromandibularis	retromandibular vein	rmv
V. septi pellucidi	septal vein	sv
V. subclavia	subclavian vein	subclv
V. sublingualis	sublingual vein	sublgv
V. submentalis	submental vein	smv
V. supratrochlearis	supratrochlear vein	sutrv
V. temporalis	temporal vein(s)	tv
V. temporalis superficialis	superficial temporal vein	stempv
V. thalamo-striata	thalamostriate vein	tsv
V. thyroidea superior	superior thyroid vein	sthyv
V. transversa facei	transverse facial vein	tfv
V. vertebralis	vertebral vein	vertv
Vagina carotica	carotid sheath	CtdS
Vas	blood vessel	bv
Velum medullare inferior	inferior medullary velum	IMV
Velum medullare superior	superior medullary velum	SMV
Velum terminale (Aebi)	terminal velum (Aebi)	vt
Vena see V.	vein (unidentified)	v
Ventral pallidum, Pallidum ventrale	ventral pallidum	VP
Ventral striatum	ventral striatum	VStr
Ventriclus tertius	ventral third ventricle	V3V
Ventriculus lateralis	lateral ventricle	LV
Ventriculus lateralis, cornu frontale	frontal horn of lateral ventricle	FLV
Ventriculus lateralis, cornu occipitale	occipital horn of lateral ventricle	OLV
Ventriculus lateralis, cornu temporale	temporal horn of lateral ventricle	TLV
Ventriculus lateralis, pars centralis	central part (body) of lateral ventricle	CVL
Ventriculus lateralis, trigonum collaterale, Atrium	trigone of lateral ventricle	TrLV
Ventriculus quartus	fourth ventricle	4V
Ventriculus sinister	left ventricle	LVent
Ventriculus tertius thyroarytenoid	third ventricle	3V
Vermis cerebelli	vermis of cerebellum	Ver
Vertebra	vertebra	Vert
Vestibulum oris	vestibule of mouth	Vest
Vomer	vomer	Vomer
Zona incerta	zona incerta	ZI
Zona incerta, pars dorsalis	zona incerta, dorsal part	ZID
Zona incerta, pars ventralis	zona incerta, ventral part	ZIV
Zona reticularis, pars intermedia	intermediate reticular zone	IRt

---

[1] anterior limb, genu of -, posterior limb, lenticulothalamic part, retrolenticular part, sublenticular part,

[2] (.br = brevis, .lg = longus)

[3] (.l = lobulus fusiformis)

7 INDEX OF TERMS

A

anteromedial thalamic nucleus		Ncl. anteromedialis thalami, *see* Ncl. thalamicus -	
anteromedial thalamic nucleus	AM	Ncl. thalamicus anteromedialis	182, 184, 186, 287
anteroprincipal thalamic nucleus		Ncl. anteroventralis thalami, *see* Ncl. thalamicus -	
anteroprincipal thalamic nucleus	APr	Ncl. thalamicus anteroprincipalis	182, 184, 186, 188, 190, 192, 194, 196, 198, 287
apical ligament of dens	ald	Lig. apicis dentis	117
aqueduct	Aq		37
arachnoid granulations	argr	Granulationes arachnoidales	84
articular disc of temporo-mandibular joint, *see* also temporomandibular disc	Disc	Discus articularis mandibulae	42, 43, 109
articular tubercle (of TMJ)	ATub	Tbc. articulare	109
aryepiglotticus muscle	AryE	M. aryepiglotticus	68
ascending palatine artery	apal	A. palatina ascendens	45, 47, 48, 49, 50
ascending pharyngeal artery	aph	A. pharyngea ascendens	48, 49, 50, 72
atlanto axial membrane	AtAx		117
atlanto occipital joint	AtOcJ	Artic. atlanto occipitalis	80, 115
atlanto occipital membrane	AtOcM	Membrana atlanto-occipitalis	45, 117
atlas (C1 vertebra)	Atlas	Atlas	45, 46, 47, 76, 80, 84, 117, 118
auditory tube	Aud	Tuba auditiva	68, 112, 113, 115
auditory tube cartilage	AudC	Cartilago tubae auditivae	113
auriculotemporal nerve	aute	N. auriculotemporalis	42, 43
axis (C2 vertebra)	Axis	Axis	49, 76, 80, 84, 117, 118

B

band of Giacomini	bG	Bandeletta Giacomini	190, 192, 194, 196, 280, 281
basal nucleus of Meynert	B	Ncl. basalis (Meynert)	284
basal nucleus, compact part	BC	Ncl. basalis, pars compacta	172, 176, 178, 182, 184, 188, 284
basal nucleus, diffuse part	BD	Ncl. basalis, pars diffusa	284
basal operculum	Bop		143, 145, 279
basilar artery	bas	A. basilaris	38, 39, 40, 41, 76
basilar cistern	BasCi	Cisterna basilaris	41
basolateral amygdaloid nucleus	BL	Ncl. amygdaloideus basolateralis	172, 176, 180, 188, 190, 282
basolateral amygdaloid nucleus, dorsal part	BLD	Ncl. amygdaloideus basolateralis, p.dorsalis	182, 184, 186, 282
basolateral amygdaloid nucleus, ventrolateral part	BLVL	Ncl. amygdaloideus basolateralis, pars ventrolateralis	178, 184, 186, 282
basolateral amygdaloid nucleus, ventromedial part	BLI	Ncl. amygdaloideus basolateralis, pars intermedius	182, 184, 186, 282
basolateral amygdaloid nucleus, ventromedial part	BLPL	Ncl. amygdaloideus basolateralis, pars paralaminaris	178, 182, 184, 186, 282
basolateral amygdaloid nucleus, ventromedial part	BLVM	Ncl. amygdaloideus basolateralis, pars ventromedialis	170, 172, 176, 178, 180, 182, 186, 282
basomedial amygdaloid nucleus	BM	Ncl. amygdaloideus basomedialis	168, 170, 172, 176, 178, 180, 184, 188, 190, 282
basomedial amygdaloid nucleus, centromedial part	BMCM		186, 282
basomedial amygdaloid nucleus, dorsolateral part	BMDL		186, 282
basomedial amygdaloid nucleus, dorsomedial part	BMDM		186, 282
basomedial amygdaloid nucleus, ventromedial part	BMVM		186, 282
bed nucleus of the anterior commissure	BAC	Ncl. commissurae ant., Ncl. interstitialis commissurae anterior	284
bed nucleus of the stria terminalis	BST	Ncl. interstitialis striae terminalis	116
bed nucleus of the stria terminalis, central division	BSTC	Ncl. interstitialis striae terminalis, pars interamygdaloidia	162, 164, 166, 168, 170, 172, 284, 285
bed nucleus of the stria terminalis, lateral division	BSTL	Ncl. interstitialis striae terminalis, pars lateralis	162, 166, 168, 170, 284
bed nucleus of the stria terminalis, lateral division, juxtacapsular part	BSTLJ	Ncl. interstitialis striae terminalis, pars juxtacapsularis	164, 172, 284
bed nucleus of the stria terminalis, medial division	BSTM	Ncl. interstitialis striae terminalis, pars anterior	164, 166, 168, 170, 284
bed nucleus of the stria terminalis, posterior part	BSTP	Ncl. interstitialis striae terminalis, pars posterior	172, 178, 284
bed nucleus of the stria terminalis, ventral division	BSTV	Ncl. interstitialis striae terminalis, pars ventralis	170, 172
body of caudate nucleus	BCd	Corpus nuclei caudati	82
body of corpus callosum	bcc	Corpus callosum, corpus	70, 73, 74, 77, 82, 116, 154, 156, 158, 160, 162, 164, 166, 168, 172, 176, 180, 184, 188, 190, 192, 194, 196, 198, 200, 202, 204, 206, 208, 210, 212, 214, 216
body of fornix	bfx	Corpus fornicis	77, 78, 82, 184, 186, 188, 190, 192, 194, 196, 198, 200, 202, 204, 206, 208, 210, 212, 214
body of fornix	bfx	Fornix, corpus	77, 78, 82, 184, 186, 188, 190, 192, 194, 196, 198, 200, 202, 204, 206, 208, 210, 212, 214
body of hyoid bone	BHy	Corpus ossis hyoidei	52
body of mandible	BMan	Os mandibulare / corpus mandibulae	60
brachium of the inferior colliculus	bic	Brachium colliculi inferioris	216, 220, 223, 225
brachium of the superior colliculus	bsc	Brachium colliculi superioris	220
buccal fat pad	BFat	Corpus adiposum buccae	56, 64
buccal nerve	bucn	N. buccalis	42, 43, 45, 46, 47, 48, 49, 50
buccinator muscle	BucM	M. buccinator	46, 47, 48, 49, 50, 51, 52, 56, 60, 111, 113

C

CA1 field of the hippocampus	CA1	Hippocampus (Cornu Ammonis)	184, 186, 188, 190, 192, 194, 196, 198, 200, 202, 204, 206, 208, 210, 212, 214, 216, 218, 220, 223, 225, 227, 229, 231
CA2 field of the hippocampus	CA2	Hippocampus	192, 194, 196, 198, 200, 202, 204, 206, 208, 210, 212, 214, 216, 218, 220, 223, 225, 227, 229, 231
CA3 field of the hippocampus	CA3	Hippocampus	194, 196, 198, 200, 202, 204, 206, 208, 210, 212, 214, 216, 218, 220, 223, 225
calcar avis	cal	Calcar avis	237
calcarine sulcus	ccs	S. calcarinus	232, 241, 243, 247, 249, 251, 253, 255, 257, 259, 261, 281
callosal sulcus	cas	S. corporis callosi	143, 145, 149, 150, 152, 154, 281
callosal vein	calv		145
callosomarginal sulcus	cms	S. callosomarginalis	281
capsule of red nucleus	cr	Ncl. ruber, capsula	196, 198, 200, 202
carotid plexus	cplx	Plexus caroticus	51
cartilage of the auditory tube	CAT		45
caudate fundus	FCd	Fundus caudati	149, 151, 153, 155, 162, 285
caudate nucleus	Cd	Ncl. caudatus	114, 145, 184 ,186, 188, 190, 192, 194, 196, 198, 200, 202, 204, 206, 208, 210, 212, 214, 216, 218, 220, 223, 268, 285
caudate putamen *see* striatum	CPu	Caudato-Putamen	
cavernous sinus	cav	Sinus cavernosus	39, 40, 68, 72
central amygdaloid nucleus	Ce	Ncl. amygdaloideus centralis	176, 178, 180, 192, 282
central amygdaloid nucleus, lateral part	CeL		184, 186, 188, 190, 282
central amygdaloid nucleus, medial part	CeM		184, 186, 188, 190, 282
central artery of retina	cret	A. centralis retinae	60
central gray, *see* periaqueductal gray	PAG	Substantia grisea centralis mesencephali (Griseum centrale mesencephali)	215
central nucleus	cen	Ncl. centralis	287
central part (body) of lateral ventricle	CVL	Ventriculus lateralis, pars centralis	74, 78
central sulcus	cs	S. centralis	77, 263, 265
central tegmental tract	ctg	Tr. tegmenti centralis	212, 214, 216
centromedial thalamic nucleus		Ncl. medialis centralis thalami, *see* Ncl. thalamicus -	78
centromedian thalamic nucleus	CM	Centrum medianum *see* Ncl. centromedianus	78, 200, 202, 204, 206, 287
centromedian thalamic nucleus	CM	Ncl. thalamicus centralis medialis	78, 196, 198, 208, 210, 212
centromedian thalamic nucleus, magnocellular part	CMMC	Ncl. thalamicus centralis medialis, pars magnocellularis	204, 210, 287
centromedian thalamic nucleus, parvocellular part	CMPC	Ncl. thalamicus centralis medialis, pars parvocellularis	287
centromedian thalamic nucleus, ventral part	CMV	Ncl. thalamicus centralis medialis, pars ventralis	287
cerebellar hemisphere	CH	Haemisphaerium cerebelli	82, 85, 86
cerebello-rubro-thalamic fibers	crt	Tr. cerebello-rubro-thalamicus	196, 198, 200, 202, 204
cerebellum	Cb	Cerebellum	37, 112, 113, 114
cerebral aqueduct (Sylvius)	Aq	Aqueductus (Sylvii)	212, 214, 216, 218, 220, 223
cerebral cortex	Cx	Cx. cerebri	266
cerebral peduncle	cp	Pedunculus cerebri, pars basalis	37, 77, 78, 114, 186, 188, 190, 192, 194, 196, 198, 200, 202, 204, 206, 208, 210, 212
cervical interspinal muscle	CISM	M. interspinalis cervicis	88
cervical nerve	cem	N. cervicalis	47, 51, 52, 76, 80, 115
cervical plexus	cerpx	Plexus cervicalis	76
chorda tympani nerve	cty	Chorda tympani	43, 45
choroid artery	cha	A. choroidea	34, 36, 38
choroid plexus	chp	Plexus choroideus	33, 35, 37, 86
ciliary muscle	CilM	M. ciliaris	41
cingulate gyrus	CG	Gyrus cinguli	28, 29, 30, 31, 32, 33, 34, 35, 36, 65, 66, 69, 70, 73, 74, 77, 78, 82, 85, 86, 89, 90, 93, 114, 116, 118, 135, 137, 139, 141, 143, 145, 149, 150, 153, 154, 156, 158, 160, 162, 164, 166, 168, 170, 172, 176, 184, 192, 196, 200, 202, 204, 206, 208, 210, 212, 214, 216, 218, 220, 223, 225, 227, 229, 231, 233, 235, 237, 239, 241, 243, 280
cingulate sulcus	cgs	S. cinguli	133, 135, 137, 139, 141, 143, 145, 149, 150, 156, 243, 281
cingulum	cg	Cingulum	220
circular insular sulcus	cir	S. circularis insulae	154, 156, 158, 160, 162, 164, 166, 168, 172, 176, 180, 182, 281
cistern	Ci	Cisterna	39
claustrum	Cl	Claustrum	35, 37, 70, 73, 74, 77, 78, 112, 147, 150, 153, 200, 202, 204, 206
collateral sulcus	cos	S. collateralis	196, 198, 204, 206, 210, 214, 216, 218, 220, 223, 225, 227, 229, 231, 235, 237, 239, 241, 247, 249, 251, 253, 255, 257, 259, 261, 281
column of fornix *see* anterior column		Columna fornicis, *see* fornix	
comb system	comb	Fibrae perforantes pedunculi	186, 188, 190, 192, 194, 196, 198
commissural nucleus of the thalamus	Com	Ncl. commissuralis thalami	287
commissure of the inferior colliculi	cic	Commissura colliculi inferioris	225
commissure of the superior colliculi	csc	Commissura colliculi superioris	216, 218, 221
common anular tendon	CAnT	Anulus tendineus	41
common carotid artery	cctd	A. carotis communis	51, 52, 72, 76

extreme capsule	ex	Capsula extrema	35, 73, 149, 150, 153, 154, 156, 159, 160, 162, 164, 166, 168, 172, 176, 180, 190, 192, 194, 196, 198, 200, 202, 204, 206
eye	eye	Bulbus oculi	41, 56

F

facial artery	fac	A. facialis	46, 47, 48, 49, 51, 52, 56, 60, 64, 68, 72, 109, 111, 113
facial artery, glandular branches	fagl	A. facialis (rr. glandulares)	50
facial canal *see* facial nerve canal		Canalis	
facial canal *see* facial nerve canal		Canalis facialis	
facial nerve canal	7C	Canalis nervi facialis	43
facial nerve or its root	7n	N. facialis	40, 41, 42, 45, 76, 80, 107
facial vein	facv	V. facialis	45, 46, 47, 48, 49, 52, 56, 60, 64, 68, 72, 109, 111, 113
falx cerebelli	FxCb	Falx cerebelli	56
falx cerebri	FxC	Falx cerebri	64
fascia dentata *see* dentate gyrus	FD	Fascia dentata	196, 198, 200, 202, 204
fasciculosus nucleus	Fa		184, 186, 188, 190, 287
fasciculosus thalamic nucleus	Fas	Ncl. thalamicus fasciculosus	287
fasciculus retroflexus	fr	Fc. retroflexus	200, 202, 204, 206, 208, 210, 212
fasciola cinerea	FC	Fasciola cinerea	280, 281
fasciolar gyrus	FG	Gyrus fasciolaris	86, 114, 227, 229, 231, 280, 281
fimbria of the hippocampus	fi	Fimbria hippocampi	35, 37, 112, 198, 200, 202, 204, 206, 208, 210, 212, 214, 216, 218, 221
forceps major of the corpus callosum	fmj	Corpus callosum, forceps major	33
forceps minor of the corpus callosum	fmi	Corpus callosum, forceps minor	33, 141, 143, 155
fornix	fx	Fornix	33, 35, 85, 118, 168, 170, 172, 176, 178, 180, 182
fourth ventricle	4V	Ventriculus quartus	38, 39, 41, 82
frontal bone	Fro	Os frontale	37
frontal bone, crest	FroC	Os frontale, crista	56, 109
frontal bone, nasal part	FroN	Os frontale (pars nasalis)	38, 39
frontal bone, orbital part	FroO	Os frontale (pars orbitalis)	38, 39, 56
frontal bone, squamous part	FroS	Os frontale (squama ossis frontalis)	60
frontal horn of lateral ventricle	FLV	Ventriculus lateralis, cornu frontale	33, 35, 68, 70, 73, 145, 149, 151, 153, 155, 159, 164, 166, 168, 170
frontal limbic area	FLA	Area limbica frontalis (intermedio-limbica)	65, 66, 69, 70, 73, 74, 77, 78
frontal lobe	FL	Lobus frontalis	60
frontal nerve of V	5 fr	N. frontalis	38, 39, 60
frontal operculum	FOp	Operculum frontale	32, 33, 110, 112, 143, 145, 147, 149, 151, 153, 155, 159, 160, 162, 164, 166, 168, 170, 172, 176, 178, 279
frontal pole	FrP	Polus frontalis	57, 58, 61, 279
frontal sinus	frs	Sinus frontalis	37, 40, 56, 60
fronto marginal sulcus	fms	S. fronto-marginalis	129, 131, 133, 281
frontomarginal gyrus	FMG	Gyrus frontomarginalis	129, 131, 133
fronto-orbitalis sulcus	fos	S. fronto-orbitalis	281
fronto-polar area	FPA	Area frontopolaris	279
fundus striati	FStr	Fundus striati	37, 116, 285
fusiform gyrus	FuG	Gyrus fusiformis (occipito-temp.lat. =T4)	35, 65, 66, 69, 70, 73, 74, 77, 78, 82, 85, 86, 89, 90, 93, 94, 108, 110, 112, 114, 204, 206, 208, 210, 212, 214, 216, 218, 221, 223, 225, 227, 229, 231, 233, 235, 237, 239, 241, 243, 247, 249, 251, 253, 280

G

galea aponeurotica	gapo	Galea aponeurotica	37
genioglossus muscle	GGM	M. genioglossus	50, 51, 52, 56, 60, 117, 118
geniohyoid muscle	GeHy	M. genohyoideus	52, 56, 60, 117, 118
genu of the corpus callosum	gcc	Corpus callosum, genu	33, 35, 143, 145, 147, 149, 151, 153
genu of the internal capsule	gic	Capsula interna, genu	186, 188
genu of the internal capsule	gic	Genu capsulae internae	186
glandular branches	gld	Rami glandulares	51, 52
globus pallidus	GP	Globus pallidus	35, 78, 112, 114, 116, 162, 268, 286
glossopharyngeal nerve	9n	N. glossopharyngeus	42, 43, 45, 46, 47, 48, 49, 50, 64, 68, 72, 76, 80, 111, 113
great cistern	GrCi	Cisterna magna (cerebello-medullaris)	84
great magna terminal island	GTI	Insula terminalis magna	160, 162, 164, 166, 168, 170, 285
greater horn of hyoid bone	GHHy	Cornu majus ossis hyoidei	50, 51, 52
greater horn of hyoid bone	GHHy	Os hyoideum, cornu majus	50
greater nasal cartilage	GNaC	Cartilago nasi	45
greater occipital nerve	gocn	N. occipitalis major	41, 42, 43, 44, 45, 46, 47, 48, 113, 115
greater palatine artery	gpa	A. palatina major	44, 46, 47
greater palatine foramen	GPalF	For. palatinum majus	56, 60
greater palatine nerve	gpaln	N. palatinus major	44, 56
greater petrosal nerve	7gp	N. petrosus (superficialis) major	41, 76
greater zygomatic muscle	GZgM	M. zygomaticus major	44, 45, 46, 47, 48, 49, 50, 56, 107, 109
gyrus fornicatus *see* isthmus of cingulate gyrus		Gyrus fornicatus	280
gyrus rectus	GRe	Gyrus rectus	38, 58, 61, 65, 66, 69, 70, 116, 118, 131, 133, 135, 137, 139, 141, 143, 145, 147, 149, 151, 153, 155, 157, 279

H

habenula	Hb	Habenula	35, 212

M

medial dorsal thalamic nucleus, pars fasciculosa	MDFa	Ncl. thalamicus mediodorsalis, pars fasciculata	192, 194, 196, 198, 202, 206, 208, 210 212, 287
medial dorsal thalamic nucleus, pars fibrosa	MDFi	Ncl. thalamicus mediodorsalis, pars fibrosa	192, 194, 196, 198, 202, 206, 208, 210, 212, 215, 287
medial dorsal thalamic nucleus, pars magnocellularis	MDMC	Ncl. thalamicus mediodorsalis, pars magnocellularis	203, 206, 208, 210, 287
medial dorsal thalamic nucleus, ventral part	MDV	Ncl. thalamicus mediodorsalis, pars ventralis	192, 194, 196, 198, 203, 206, 208, 211, 212, 287
medial forebrain bundle	mfb	Fc. longitudinalis telencephali medialis	162, 169, 171, 173, 174, 177, 179, 181, 183, 185, 188
medial geniculate nucleus	MG	Corpus geniculatum mediale	114, 211, 288
medial geniculate nucleus, dorsoanterior (magnocellular) part	MGDA		212, 215, 288
medial geniculate nucleus, dorsoposterior part	MGDP		213, 215, 216, 288
medial geniculate nucleus, fibrosus part	MGFi		
medial geniculate nucleus, limitans part	MGLi		215, 216, 288
medial geniculate nucleus, parvocellular part	MGPC		213, 288
medial habenular nucleus	MHb	Ncl. habenule medialis	215, 288
medial lemniscus	ml	Lemniscus medialis	213, 215, 217, 219, 221
medial longitudinal fasciculus	mlf	Fc. longitudinalis medialis	217, 219, 221
medial longitudinal stria	mls	Stria longitudinalis medialis	151, 157, 162, 173, 174, 177, 179, 192, 196
medial mammillary nucleus	MM	Ncl. mamillaris medialis	190, 290
medial mammillary nucleus, magnocellular part	MMC	Ncl. mamillaris medialis, pars magnocellularis	185, 187, 188, 290
medial mammillary nucleus, parvocellular part	MPC	Ncl. mamillaris medialis, pars parvocellularis	185, 187, 189, 290
medial medullary lamina of the globus pallidus	mml	Lamina (lamella) pallidi interna	169, 171, 173, 174, 177, 179, 185, 189, 190, 192, 194, 196
medial occipito-temporal gyrus *see* lingual g.	MOTG	Gyrus occipito-temporalis medialis	280
medial orbital gyrus	MOrG	Gyrus orbitalis medius	133, 135, 137, 139, 141, 143, 145, 147, 149, 151, 279
medial orbital sulcus	mos	S. orbitalis medialis	281
medial preoptic nucleus	MPO	Ncl. praeopticus medialis	169, 289
medial pterygoid muscle	Mptg	M. pterygoideus medialis	44, 45, 46, 47, 48, 49, 50, 64, 68, 111, 113, 115
medial pulvinar nucleus	Mpul	Ncl. pulvinaris medialis	217, 219, 221, 223, 225, 288
medial rectus muscle	MRec	M. rectus medialis	40, 41, 56, 60, 64, 115
medial scalenus muscle	MScal	M. scalenus medius	47, 48
medial septal nucleus	MS	Ncl. septi medialis	173, 174, 177, 179, 181, 286
medial transverse frontopolar gyrus	TFPGM	Gyrus frontoplaris transversus med.	129, 131, 133, 279
medial tuberal nucleus	MTu	Ncl. tuberis medialis	179, 290
median preoptic nucleus	MnPO	Ncl. praeopticus medianus	169
medulla oblongata	Md	Medulla oblongata	43
medullary substance of frontal lobe	ms		143, 145, 147
mentalis muscle	MentM	M. mentalis	52
mesencephalic tectum	MTec	Tectum mesencephali	116
mesencephalon, midbrain	Mes	Mesencephalon	266
middle cerebellar peduncle	mcp	Pedunculus cerebellaris medialis	78, 114
middle cerebral artery	mcer	A. cerebri media	26, 28, 30, 32, 34, 36, 37, 38, 72, 76, 80, 110
middle constrictor of the pharynx	MCM		49, 50, 51
middle ear	MidE	Auris media	113
middle (medial) frontal gyrus	MFG	Gyrus frontalis medius	29, 30, 31, 32, 33, 34, 34, 36, 57, 58, 61, 65, 66, 69, 70, 73, 74, 77, 78, 82, 85, 86, 110, 112, 114, 129, 131, 133, 135, 137, 139, 141, 143, 279
middle meatus of nasal cavity	MidM	Meatus nasi med.	56
middle meningeal art., frontal branch	mmf	A. meningea media (r. frontalis)	39, 68
middle meningeal art., parietal branch	mmp	A. meningea media (r. parietalis)	76, 84
middle meningeal artery	mm	A. meningea media	40, 41, 72, 76, 113
middle nasal concha	MNaC	Concha nasalis media	56, 60, 64
middle (medial) temporal gyrus	MTG	Gyrus temporalis medius	31, 32, 34, 35, 36, 37, 38, 39, 65, 66, 69, 70, 73, 74, 77, 78, 82, 85, 86, 89, 90, 93, 94, 107, 108, 110, 112, 233, 235, 237, 239, 241, 243, 247, 249, 251, 253, 255, 257, 259, 279
middle (medial) temporal sulcus	mts	S. temporalis medius	281
minor posterior rectus capitis muscle	MiPRe		43
minor zygomaticus muscle	MiZyM	M. zygomaticus minor	44, 45, 46, 47
motor branch of trigeminal nerve	m5	N. trigeminus, radix motoria	42, 43
multifidus muscle	Mult	M. multifidus	48, 49, 50, 51, 52, 84, 115
mylohyoid muscle	MyHy	M. mylohyoideus	49, 50, 51, 52, 56, 60, 113, 115, 117, 118
mylohyoid nerve	myhy	N. mylohyoideus	51, 64, 68

N

nasal bone	Na	Os nasale	41, 43
nasal septum	NSpt	Septum nasi (pars ossea)	43, 56, 60
nasalis muscle	NaM	M. nasalis	42, 43, 44, 45, 46, 47
nasociliar nerve	5nc	N. nasociliaris	115
nasolacrimal duct	nlac	Ductus nasolacrimalis	43
nasopalatine artery	npal	A. nasopalatina	47
nasopalatine nerve	npal	N. nasopalatinus	118
nasopharyngeal tonsil	NPhT	Tonsilla pharyngea	117
nuchal fascia	nuf	Fascia nuchae	39, 41, 43, 45, 49
nuchal ligament	nl	Lig. nuchae	42, 45, 47

parafascicular thalamic nucleus	PF		197, 200, 203, 205, 206, 209, 211, 287
parafornical nucleus	PaF	Ncl. parafornicalis	181, 183, 185, 289
parahippocampal gyrus	PHG	Gyrus parahippocampalis	34, 36, 112, 114, 206, 209, 211, 213, 215, 217, 219, 221, 223, 225, 227, 229, 231, 233, 280
parahippocampal sulcus, *see* lingual sulcus		S. parahippocampo-lingualis	281
paraoptic nucleus	Pa2	Ncl. paraopticus	179, 290
parasubiculum	PaS	Parasubiculum	191, 192, 197, 199, 200, 203, 204, 206, 209, 211
paratenial thalamic nucleus	PT	Ncl. parataenialis thalami	181, 185, 187, 189, 191, 193, 194, 197, 203, 207, 287
paraterminal gyrus	PTG	Gyrus paraterminalis (*see* G. subcallosus)	70, 73, 157, 159, 161, 183, 279, 280
paraventricular hypothalamic nucleus	Pa	Ncl. paraventricularis hypothalami	171, 173, 174, 177, 179, 289
paraventricular hypothalamic nucleus, anterior parvocellular part	PaAP	Ncl. paraventricularis hypothalami, pars parvocellularis	169, 179
paraventricular hypothalamic nucleus, fornical part	PaFo	Ncl. paraventricularis hypothalami	174, 289
paraventricular hypothalamic nucleus, magnocellular part	PaMc	Ncl. paraventricularis hypothalami, pars magnocellularis	171, 179, 289
paraventricular hypothalamic nucleus, posterior part	PaPo	Ncl. paraventricularis hypothalami, pars posterior	181, 183, 289
paraventricular thalamic nucleus	PV	Ncl. paraventricularis thalami	185, 189, 191, 193, 195, 197, 199, 201, 203, 205, 207, 209, 287
parietal bone	ParB	Os parietale	37, 38
parietal operculum	PaOp	Operculum parietale	32; 86, 89, 108, 110, 279
parieto-occipital sulcus	pocs	S. parieto-occipitalis	281
parieto-occipital transition area	POTZ		253, 255, 257, 259, 261, 279
parotid duct	ptdd	Ductus parotideus	47, 48, 60, 64, 68, 107, 109, 111
parotid gland	Par	Gdl. parotidea	43, 44, 45, 47, 48, 49, 50, 72, 76, 107, 109, 111, 113
parotid plexus	papx	Plexus parotideus	43, 49
peduncle of lenticular nucleus	PedL	Pedunculus (nuclei) lentiformis	185, 187, 189, 191, 285
periamygdalar area	PAA	Area periamygdaloidea (Hassler)	171
periamygdaloid cortex	PAC	Cx. periamygdaloideus	114
periaqueductal gray	PAG	Substantia grisea centralis mesencephali (Griseum centrale mesencephali)	215, 217, 219, 221, 223, 225
perifornical nucleus	PeF	Ncl. perifornicalis	289
peripeduncular area	PPA	Area peripeduncularis	209, 211
peripeduncular nucleus	PP	Ncl. peripeduncularis	213, 215
perirhinal cortex	PRC	Cx. perirhinalis	205
periventricular hypothalamic nucleus	Pe	Ncl. periventricularis hypothalami	289
perpendicular plate	PeP	Os ethmoidale, lam. perpendicularis	56
pharyngeal branches	phar	Rami pharyngei	68, 72
pharyngeal recess	PhaRe	Recessus pharyngeus	72
pineal gland	Pi	Corpus pineale	35, 82, 85, 217, 219, 221, 223
piriform cortex	Pir	Cx. piriformis	70, 73, 114, 281
piriform recess	PirR	Recessus piriformis	68
pituitary gland *see* hypophysis	Pit	Hypophysis cerebri	33, 39, 72
planum polare	PPo		77, 78, 147, 279
planum temporale	PTe	Planum temporale	32, 34, 35, 36, 37, 66, 69, 70, 73, 74, 77, 78, 82, 85, 86, 89, 107, 108, 110, 280
platysma	Plat	Platysma	49, 50, 51, 52, 56, 60, 64, 107, 109, 111, 113, 115, 117
pons	Pons	Pons	39, 77, 78, 116, 118, 193, 194, 197, 199, 201, 203, 205, 207, 209, 211
pontine cistern	PoCi	Cisterna pontis	76
postcentral gyrus	PoG	Gyrus postcentralis	23, 24, 25, 26, 27, 28, 29, 30, 31, 32, 33, 34, 35, 77, 78, 82, 85, 86, 89, 90, 93, 94, 97, 98, 107, 108, 110, 112, 114, 116, 118, 233, 279
postcentral sulcus	pocs	S. postcentralis	281
posterior arch of atlas	PAT	Arcus osterior atlantis	117
posterior auricular artery	pau	A. auricularis posterior	46, 47, 72, 76, 80
posterior auricular vein	pauv	V. auricularis posterior	38, 39, 40, 41, 46, 47, 80, 84
posterior cerebral artery	pcer	A. cerebri osterior	30, 32, 34, 36, 38, 76, 80, 84
posterior commissure	opc	Commissura, posterior	213, 215, 217
posterior communicating artery	pcoma	A. communicans posterior	38
posterior cortical amygdaloid nucleus	PCo	Ncl. amygdaloideus corticalis posterior	181, 183, 185, 187, 189, 282
posterior crus of fornix	pfx	Fornix, crus posterius	217, 219, 221, 223, 225, 227
posterior forceps *see* forceps major		Forceps major	
posterior hypothalamic area	PHA	Area hypothalamica posterior	181, 189, 191, 282, 283, 290
posterior inferior cerebellar artery	pica	A. cerebelli posterior inferior	38, 80, 88
posterior limb of the internal capsule	pic	Capsula interna, pars posterior	35, 191, 193, 194, 197, 199, 201, 203, 205, 206, 209, 211, 213, 217, 219
posterior limitans thalamic nucleus	Pli		221
posterior major rectus capitis muscle	PMjRe	M. rectus capitis posterior major	44, 45, 46, 47, 88, 92, 111, 113, 115
posterior minor rectus capitis muscle	PMiRe	M. rectus capitis posterior minor	42, 44, 45, 88, 92, 111, 115
posterior nasal artery	pna	A. nasalis posterior	64
posterior orbicular muscle	POrbM	M. orbicularis posterior	40
posterior orbital gyrus	POrG		139, 141, 143, 145, 147, 279
posterior orbital sulcus	pos	S. orbitalis posterior	251, 253, 255, 257, 259, 261
posterior parolfactory sulcus	PPS	S. parolfactorius posterior	155, 157, 159, 281
posterior septal nucleus	PS	Ncl. septi posterior	284
posterior superior alveolar artery	psa	A. alveolaris superior posterior	45, 56, 60
posterior superior alveolar nerve	psan	N. alveolaris superior postenor	45
preamygdalar claustrum	PACl	Claustrum temporale, subregio praeamygdaleum	163, 165, 169, 173, 174, 177, 179, 283

preamygdaloid cortex	PrAC	Cx. praeamygdaloideus	281
precentral gyrus	PrG	Gyrus praecentralis	23, 24, 25, 26, 27, 28, 29, 30, 31, 32, 33, 34, 35, 74, 77, 78, 82, 85, 86, 89, 90, 93, 94, 107, 108, 110, 112, 114, 116, 118, 279
precentral sulcus	pcs	S. praecentralis	281
precommissural archicortex	PCA	Archicortex praecommissuralis	159, 161
precommissural fornix	pcfx	Fornix praecommissuralis (longus)	161, 162, 165
precuneus	PCun	Praecuneus	28, 32, 33, 35, 90, 93, 94, 97, 98, 101, 102, 114, 116, 118, 233, 235, 237, 239, 241, 243, 247, 249, 251, 253, 255, 257, 261, 279
pregeniculate nucleus	PGn	Ncl. praegeniculatus	288
preoptic area	POA	Area praeoptica	289
preoptic nucleus	PO	Ncl. praeopticus	289
preoptic recess of the third ventricle	P3V	Recessus praeopticus	118, 161, 163, 165
prepiriform claustrum	PPCl	Claustrum temporale, subregio praepiriformis	153, 155, 157, 159, 161, 163, 165, 169
presubiculurn	PrS	Praesubiculum	187, 191, 193, 197, 199, 201, 203, 205, 207, 209, 211, 213, 215
pretectal area	PTc	Area praetectalis	213, 215, 217, 219
prevertebral fascia	pvf	Fascia praevertebralis	45
principal mammillary fasciculus	pm	Fc. mamillaris	185
pterygoid canal	PtgC	Canalis pterygoideus	68
pterygoid hamulus *see* hamulus of the pterygoid bone		Hamulus pterygoideus	
pterygoid plexus	ptgpx	Plexus venosus pterygoideus	43, 68, 109, 111, 113
pterygoid process	Ptg	Proc. pterygoideus	44, 45
pterygopalatine artery	ptgpal	A. pterygopalatina	
pterygopalatine fossa	PtPf	Fossa pterygopalatina	64, 115
pterygopalatine ganglion, *see* spheno-palatine ganglion		Ggl. pterygopalatinurn	43
pulvinar	Pul	Pulvinar	35, 82, 85, 116, 288
pulvinar nucleus	Pul	Ncl. pulvinaris	114
putamen	Pu	Putamen	35, 70, 73, 74, 77, 78, 112, 114, 147, 163, 165, 169, 171, 173, 175, 177, 181, 185, 187, 191, 193, 195, 197, 199, 201, 203, 205, 207, 209, 211, 213, 215, 217, 219, 221, 268, 285
putamen, medial part	PuM	Putamen mediale	285
putamen, ventral part	PuV	Putarnen ventrale	185, 187, 189, 191, 193, 195, 197, 199, 201, 203, 285
putaminal fundus	FPu	Fundus putaminis	149, 151, 153, 155, 162, 164, 166, 168, 170, 172, 285
pyramidal tract	py	Tr. pyramidalis	118

Q

quadrigeminal plate (*see* Carpenter)	QuPl	Lamina quadrigemina	84, 85

R

radiation of corpus callosum	racc	Radiatio corporis callosi	139, 141, 143, 145, 147, 149, 151, 153, 155, 157, 233, 235, 237
rectus gyrus *see* gyrus rectus		Gyrus rectus	39
red nucleus	R	Ncl. ruber	36, 78, 116, 118, 199, 266, 268
red nucleus, parvocellular part	RPC	Ncl. ruber, pars parvocellularis	201, 203, 205, 207, 209, 211
reticular thalamic nucleus	Rt	Ncl. thalamicus reticularis	78, 82, 85, 175, 177, 179, 181, 183, 185, 187, 189, 191, 193, 195, 197, 199, 201, 203, 205, 207, 209, 211, 213, 215, 217, 219, 221, 223, 225, 288
retroarticular plexus	rapx	Plexus venosus retroarticularis	42, 43
retrobulbar region	RBR	Area retrobulbaris	147, 151
retrobulbar region *see* ant. olfactory nucl.		Regio retrobulbaris *see* Ncl. olfactorius ant.	
retromandibular vein	rmv	V. retromandibularis	46, 47, 48, 50, 68, 72, 107, 109, 111, 113
retrosplenial agranular cortex	RSA	Cx. retrosplenialis agranularis	280
retrosplenial granular cortex	RSG	Cx. retrosplenialis granularis	280
reuniens thalamic nucleus	Re	Ncl. reuniens thalami	187, 189, 191, 193, 195, 197, 199, 201, 203, 205, 207, 287
rhinal sulcus	rhs	S. rhinalis	281
risorius muscle	Ris	M. risorius	50, 51
rostral sulcus	ros	S. rostralis	135, 137, 139, 141, 143, 145, 147, 281
rostfum of the corpus callosum	rcc	Corpus callosum, rostrum	69

S

sagittal stratum	sstr	Stratum sagittale	247, 249, 251, 253, 255, 257, 259
salpingopalatinal fold	SPaF	Plica salpingopalatina	117
salpingopharyngeal fold	SPhF	Plica salpingopharyngea	117
salpingopharyngeus muscle	SalPh	M. salpingopharyngeus	45
scalenus muscle	ScalM	M. scalenus	48, 49, 50, 51, 52, 76, 80, 84, 111
semiannular sulcus	sas	S. semiannularis	175, 177, 181, 183, 185, 187, 281
semicircular canals	SCC	Canalis semicircularis	80
semicircular ducts	SCD		111
semilunar gyrus	SLG	Gyrus semilunaris	70, 73, 163, 165, 169, 173, 185, 187, 189, 281
semispinal capitis muscle	SSpCa	M. semispinalis capitis	39, 41, 42, 43, 44, 45, 46, 48, 49, 50, 51, 52, 84, 88, 92, 96, 111, 113, 115
semispinal cervicis muscle	SSpCe	M. semispinalis cervicis	49, 50, 51, 52, 88

semispinalis muscle	SSpM	M. semispinalis	38, 40, 47, 49
septal (nasal) cartilage	SeC	Cartilago septi nasi	45, 47
septal area	SA	Area septi	266, 281
septal vein	sv	V. septi pellucidi	143, 153, 155, 157, 159, 161, 164, 169, 171, 173, 175, 177
septofimbrial nucleus	Sfi	Ncl. septofimbrialis	163, 165, 169, 284
septohippocampal nucleus	SHi	Ncl. septohippocampalis	284
septum nasi cartilage	SNaC		46
septum pellucidum	SptP	Septum pellucidum	73, 157, 284
sexual dimorphic ncl.	SxD	Ncl. intermedius hypothalami	171, 289
short insular gyri	SIG	Gyri breves insulae	279
sigmoid sinus	sigs	Sinus sigmoideus	38, 39, 40, 41, 42, 43, 80, 84, 88, 109, 113
soft palate	SPal	Palatum molle	68, 117, 118
sphenoid bone	SphB	Os sphenoidale	38, 39, 41, 43
sphenoid sinus	sphs	Sinus sphenoidalis	40, 41, 64, 68, 72, 118
sphenoid, greater wing	SphGW	Os sphenoidale, ala major	109, 111
sphenomandibular ligament	sphmI	Lig. sphenomandibulare	68
sphenopalatine (pterygopalatine) art.	spa	A. sphenopalatina	42, 43, 64
sphenopalatine ganglion	SphP	Ggl. sphenopalatinum	42, 64
sphenoparietal sinus	sphps	Sinus sphenoparietalis	38, 39, 40, 41
spheno-petrosal suture	sphpe	Sut. spheno-petrosa	41
spheno-zygomatic suture	sphzg	Sut. spheno-zygomatica	39
spinal accessory nerve	lln	N. accessorius, pars spinalis	42, 43, 45, 46, 47, 48, 49, 50, 51, 76, 80, 111, 113
spinal cord	Spinal	Medulla spinalis	47
spinalis muscle	SpM	M. spinalis	50, 51, 52
spinothalamic tract	spth	Tr. spino-thalamicus	217
spinous process of axis	SpAx	Proc. spinosus axis	47, 48, 88
splenium of the corpus callosum	scc	Corpus callosum, splenium	33, 85, 86, 219, 221, 223, 225, 227, 229, 231, 233, 235, 237
splenius capitis muscle	SpCa	M. splenius capitis	40, 41, 42, 43, 44, 45, 46, 47, 48, 49, 50, 51, 52, 84, 88, 92, 96, 107, 109, 111, 113, 115
splenius cervicis muscle	SpCe	M. splenius cervicis	48, 49, 50, 51, 52, 111, 113, 115
sternohyoid muscle	StHy	M. sternohyoideus	60, 64, 115
sternomastoid muscle	StM	M. sternocleidomastoideus	43, 44, 45, 46, 47, 49, 50, 51, 52, 72, 76, 80, 84, 88, 92, 107, 109
sternomastoid muscle, tendon	StT	M. sternocleidomastoideus, tendo	42, 109
straight sinus	ss	Sinus rectus	88, 92
stria medullaris of the thalamus	sm	Stria medullaris thalami	177, 179, 181, 183, 185, 187, 189, 191, 193, 195, 197, 199, 201, 203, 205, 207, 209, 211, 213
stria terminalis	st	Stria terminalis	33, 35, 78, 85, 112, 114, 116, 179, 187, 189, 191, 193, 195, 197, 199, 201, 203, 205, 207, 209, 211, 213, 215, 217, 219, 221, 223, 225
striae medullares	smed	Striae medullares	35
striatal cell bridges	SB	Pontes striatales	74, 77, 82, 114, 149, 151, 153, 154, 183, 187, 193, 195, 201, 205
striate cortex	17	Area striata	29, 30, 31, 33, 34, 35, 36, 98, 101, 102, 241, 243, 247, 249, 251, 253, 255, 257, 259, 261, 263, 265, 266, 267, 280
styloglossus muscle	StyGl	M. styloglossus	46, 47, 48, 49, 50, 64, 68, 72, 111, 113
stylohyoid ligament	shl	Lig. stylohyoideum	64, 68
stylohyoid muscle	StyHy	M. stylohyoideus	46, 47, 48, 49, 50, 51, 52, 68, 72, 111, 113
styloid process	Sty	Proc. styloideus	42, 43, 44, 45, 46, 72
stylopharyngeus muscle	StyPh	M. stylopharyngeus	45, 46, 47, 48, 49, 50, 72, 111, 113
subarachnoid space	SArS	Spatium subarachnoidale	47
subcallosal area	SCA	Area subcallosa	70, 118, 149, 151, 153, 155, 157, 159, 161, 280
subcallosal bundle (sup. fronto-occipital bundle)	scal	Fc. subcallosus	149, 151, 153, 155, 165, 169, 171, 173 177, 179, 181, 217, 219, 221, 223
subcallosal gyrus	SuCG	Gyrus subcallosus (PNA)	145, 147
subcallosal stratum	SCS		139, 141, 145, 147, 189, 191, 193, 197, 201, 203, 205, 207, 209, 211, 213, 219, 233
subcaudate terminal island	SCT1	Insula terminalis subcaudata	163, 285
subependymal layer	SEL	Lamina subependymalis	177, 179
subependymal stratum	SEpS	Stratum subependymale	243
subfornical organ	SFO	Organum (vasculosum) subfornicale	175, 177
subhabenular nucleus	SubH	Ncl. subhabenularis	213, 215, 217, 287
subiculum	S	Subiculum	37, 74, 77, 78, 85, 185, 187, 189, 191, 193, 195, 197, 199, 201, 203, 205, 207, 209, 211, 213, 215, 217, 219, 221, 223, 225, 227, 229, 233
sublenticular part of the internal capsule	slic	Capsula interna, pars sublenticularis	215, 217, 219
sublenticular stria	sls	Stria sublenticularis	175
sublingual artery and vein	slg	A., V. sublingualis	56
sublingual duct	sld	Ductus sublingualis	56
sublingual gland	SLGl	Gdl. sublingualis	51, 52, 56, 60, 115
sublingual plica	SlPl	Plica sublingualis	56
sublingual vein	sublgv	V. sublingualis	56
submandibular duct	smd	Ductus submandibularis	51, 52, 56, 60, 64, 117
submandibular gland	SMGl	Gdl. submandibularis	49, 50, 51, 52, 64, 68, 109, 111, 113
submental artery	sma	A. submentalis	56, 60
submental vein	smv	V. submentalis	68, 72
suboccipital venous plexus	socv	Plexus venosus suboccipitalis	113
subparafascicular thalamic, nucleus	SPF	Ncl. subparafascicularis thalami	179, 205, 207
subparaventricular zone	SPZ	Regio subparaventricularis	289
subparietal sulcus	sbps	S. subparietalis	235, 237, 239, 241, 243, 247, 249, 251, 253, 255, 257, 281

uncinate fasciculus	unc	Fc. uncinatus	157, 159, 161, 163, 165, 169, 171, 173, 175, 177, 179, 181, 183, 185, 289
uncinate gyrus	UG	Gyrus uncinatus	280, 281
uncus hippocampi	Un	Uncus hippocampi	73, 74, 161, 163, 165, 169, 171, 173, 175, 177, 179, 181,183, 187, 189, 191, 193, 195, 197, 199, 201, 203, 280, 281
uvula	Uv	Uvula	45, 47, 48, 49, 64, 68

V

vagus nerve	10n	N. vagus	42, 43, 45, 46, 47, 48, 49, 50, 51, 52, 76, 80, 111, 113
vein (unidentified)	v	Vena *see* V.	49, 50, 51
ventral amygdalofugal pathway	vaf	Tr. amygdalofugalis ventralis	175, 177
ventral anterior thalamic nucleus	VA	Ncl. ventralis anterior thalami	179, 183, 287
ventral caudate nucleus	VCd	Ncl. caudatus, pars ventralis	162, 164, 166, 168, 170, 172, 285
ventral claustrum	VCl	Claustrum ventrale	159, 161, 163, 165, 169, 171, 173, 175, 177, 179, 181, 183, 187, 189, 191, 193, 195, 197, 199, 283
ventral lateral thalamic nucleus	VL	Ncl. ventrolateralis thalami	78, 189, 191, 287
ventral pallidum	VP	Ventral pallidum, Pallidum ventrale	193, 195, 197, 199, 286
ventral periventricular hypothalamic nucleus	VPe	Ncl. periventricularis hypothalami, pars ventralis	289
ventral posterolateral thalamic nucleus, anterior part	VPLA		197, 199
ventral posterolateral thalamic nucleus, inferior part	VPI		
ventral preoptic nucleus	VPO	Ncl. praeopticus ventralis	289
ventral root	vr	Radix ventralis	80
ventral septal nucleus	VS	Ncl. septi ventralis	284
ventral tegmental area (Tsai)	VTA	Area tegmentalis ventralis (Tsai)	193, 195, 203, 205, 207, 209
ventral third ventricle	V3V	Ventriclus tertius	77
ventroanterior thalamic nucleus	VA		185, 187, 189, 191, 193, 195
ventroanterior thalamic nucleus, fasciculosus part *see* fasciculosus nucleus		Ncl. thalamicus ventralis anterior, pars fasciculosus	
ventroantenor thalamic nucleus, magnocellular part	VAMC	Ncl. thalamicus ventralis anterior, pars magnocellularis	189, 191, 193
ventrointermedius nucleus	VIM		195, 287
ventrointermedius nucleus, external part	VIME		203, 205, 207
ventrointermedius nucleus, internal part	VIMI		203, 205, 207, 209
ventrolateral anterior thalamic nucleus, external part	VLAE		193, 195, 197, 199, 287
ventrolateral posterior thalamic nucleus	VLP		195, 197, 199, 203, 287
ventrolateral posterior thalamic nucleus, external part	VLPE		201
ventrolateral posterior thalamic nucleus, internal part	VLPI		201
ventrolateral anterior thalamic nucleus, internal part	VLAI		193, 195, 197, 199
ventromedial hypothalamic nucleus	VMH	Ncl. hypothalamicus ventromedialis	175, 177, 181, 183, 289
ventromedial, hypothalamic nucleus, central part	VMHC	Ncl. ventromedialis hypothalami, pars centralis	289
ventromedial thalamic nucleus		Ncl. ventromedialis thalami, *see* Ncl. thalamicus -	185
ventroposterior inferior thalamic nucleus inferior	VPI	Ncl. thalamicus posteromedialis, pars.	209, 211
ventroposterior internus nucleus, parvocellular part	VPIPC		205, 207
ventroposterior lateral thalamic nucleus	VPL ventralis.	Ncl. thalamicus posterolateralis, pars	209, 211, 213, 215, 217
ventroposterior medial thalamic nucleus	VPM	Ncl. thalamicus posteromedialis, pars ventralis	201, 203, 205, 207, 209, 211
vermis of cerebellum	Ver	Vermis cerebelli	35, 82, 86
vertebra	Vert	Vertebra	48, 49, 50, 51, 52, 76, 80, 84, 88
vertebral artery	vert	A. vertebralis	42, 43, 44, 45, 46, 47, 48, 49, 50, 51, 52, 80, 84, 113, 115
vertical limb of the diagonal band	VDB	Ncl. diagonalis, pars verticalis	163, 165, 284
vestibulocochlear nerve	8n	N. vestibulocochlearis	40, 41, 80
vocal ligament	vl	Lig. vocale	64
vocalis muscle	Voc	M. vocalis	64, 68
vomer	Vomcr	Vomer	43, 45, 46, 56, 60, 64

Z

zona incerta	ZI	Zona incerta	179, 181, 183, 185, 187, 189, 191, 193, 195, 199, 201, 203, 205, 207, 209, 211, 288
zona incerta, dorsal part	ZID	Zona incerta, pars dorsalis	197, 288
zona incerta, ventral part	ZIV	Zona incerta, pars ventralis	197, 288
zygomatic arch	ZygA	Arcus zygomaticus	60, 64, 68, 107
zygomatic bone	Zyg	Os zygomaticum	41, 43, 45, 56, 109
zygomatic muscle	ZgM		111

---

[1] (.br = brevis, .lg = longus)

[2] anterior limb, genu of –, posterior limb, lenticulothalamic part, retrolenticular part, sublenticular part.

[3] (.l = lobulus fusiformis)